Pharmacological Potential of Marine Natural Products

Pharmacological Potential of Marine Natural Products

Guest Editor
Chang-Lun Shao

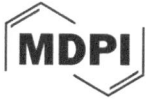

Basel • Beijing • Wuhan • Barcelona • Belgrade • Novi Sad • Cluj • Manchester

Guest Editor
Chang-Lun Shao
Ocean University of China
Qingdao
China

Editorial Office
MDPI AG
Grosspeteranlage 5
4052 Basel, Switzerland

This is a reprint of the Special Issue, published open access by the journal *Marine Drugs* (ISSN 1660-3397), freely accessible at: https://www.mdpi.com/journal/marinedrugs/special_issues/60ZLT2TC09.

For citation purposes, cite each article independently as indicated on the article page online and as indicated below:

Lastname, A.A.; Lastname, B.B. Article Title. *Journal Name* **Year**, *Volume Number*, Page Range.

ISBN 978-3-7258-2795-4 (Hbk)
ISBN 978-3-7258-2796-1 (PDF)
https://doi.org/10.3390/books978-3-7258-2796-1

© 2024 by the authors. Articles in this book are Open Access and distributed under the Creative Commons Attribution (CC BY) license. The book as a whole is distributed by MDPI under the terms and conditions of the Creative Commons Attribution-NonCommercial-NoDerivs (CC BY-NC-ND) license (https://creativecommons.org/licenses/by-nc-nd/4.0/).

Contents

Preface vii

Jialin Li, Tao Chen, Jianchen Yu, Hao Jia, Chen Chen and Yuhua Long
New Sorbicillinoids from the Mangrove Endophytic Fungus *Trichoderma reesei* SCNU-F0042
Reprinted from: *Marine Drugs* **2023**, *21*, 442, https://doi.org/10.3390/md21080442 1

Ge Zou, Taobo Li, Wencong Yang, Bing Sun, Yan Chen, Bo Wang, et al.
Antioxidative Indenone and Benzophenone Derivatives from the Mangrove-Derived Fungus *Cytospora heveae* NSHSJ-2
Reprinted from: *Marine Drugs* **2023**, *21*, 181, https://doi.org/10.3390/md21030181 11

Nicola Franchi, Loriano Ballarin and Francesca Cima
Botryllin, a Novel Antimicrobial Peptide from the Colonial Ascidian *Botryllus schlosseri*
Reprinted from: *Marine Drugs* **2023**, *21*, 74, https://doi.org/10.3390/md21020074 21

Zhuling Shao, Yingying Tian, Shan Liu, Xiao Chu and Wenjun Mao
Anti-Diabetic Activity of a Novel Exopolysaccharide Produced by the Mangrove Endophytic Fungus *Penicillium janthinellum* N29
Reprinted from: *Marine Drugs* **2023**, *21*, 270, https://doi.org/10.3390/md21050270 40

Mireguli Maimaitiming, Ling Lv, Xuetao Zhang, Shuli Xia, Xin Li, Pingyuan Wang, et al.
Semi-Synthesis and Biological Evaluation of 25(*R*)-26-Acetoxy-3β,5α-Dihydroxycholest-6-One
Reprinted from: *Marine Drugs* **2023**, *21*, 191, https://doi.org/10.3390/md21030191 62

Qian-Qian Jing, Jun-Na Yin, Ya-Jie Cheng, Qun Zhang, Xi-Zhen Cao, Wei-Feng Xu, et al.
Study on the Anti-*Mycobacterium marinum* Activity of a Series of Marine-Derived 14-Membered Resorcylic Acid Lactone Derivatives
Reprinted from: *Marine Drugs* **2024**, *22*, 135, https://doi.org/10.3390/md22030135 75

Chang Xu, Guangping Cao, Hong Zhang, Meng Bai, Xiangxi Yi and Xinjian Qu
Avellanin A Has an Antiproliferative Effect on TP-Induced RWPE-1 Cells via the PI3K-Akt Signalling Pathway
Reprinted from: *Marine Drugs* **2024**, *22*, 275, https://doi.org/10.3390/md22060275 90

Xi-Zhen Cao, Bo-Qi Zhang, Cui-Fang Wang, Jun-Na Yin, Waqas Haider, Gulab Said, et al.
A Terphenyllin Derivative CHNQD-00824 from the Marine Compound Library Induced DNA Damage as a Potential Anticancer Agent
Reprinted from: *Marine Drugs* **2023**, *21*, 512, https://doi.org/10.3390/md21100512 103

Islam Ahmed Abdelmawgood, Noha Ahmed Mahana, Abeer Mahmoud Badr, Ayman Saber Mohamed, Abdeljalil Mohamed Al Shawoush, Tarek Atia, et al.
Echinochrome Ameliorates Physiological, Immunological, and Histopathological Alterations Induced by Ovalbumin in Asthmatic Mice by Modulating the Keap1/Nrf2 Signaling Pathway
Reprinted from: *Marine Drugs* **2023**, *21*, 455, https://doi.org/10.3390/md21080455 119

Yao-Sheng Liu, Wen-Liang Chen, Yu-Wei Zeng, Zhi-Hong Li, Hao-Lin Zheng, Ni Pan, et al.
Isaridin E Protects against Sepsis by Inhibiting Von Willebrand Factor-Induced Endothelial Hyperpermeability and Platelet–Endothelium Interaction
Reprinted from: *Marine Drugs* **2024**, *22*, 283, https://doi.org/10.3390/md22060283 140

Nannan Song, Yanfei Tang, Yangui Wang, Xian Guan, Wengong Yu, Tao Jiang, et al.
A SIRT6 Inhibitor, Marine-Derived Pyrrole-Pyridinimidazole Derivative 8a, Suppresses Angiogenesis
Reprinted from: *Marine Drugs* **2023**, *21*, 517, https://doi.org/10.3390/md21100517 156

Chieh-Chen Huang, Yuan-Hsin Lo, Yu-Jou Hsu, Yuan-Bin Cheng, Chia-Chi Kung, Cher-Wei Liang, et al.
Anti-Atopic Dermatitis Activity of *Epi*-Oxyzoanthamine Isolated from Zoanthid
Reprinted from: *Marine Drugs* **2023**, *21*, 447, https://doi.org/10.3390/md21080447 . . . . **170**

Malia Lasalo, Thierry Jauffrais, Philippe Georgel and Mariko Matsui
Marine Microorganism Molecules as Potential Anti-Inflammatory Therapeutics
Reprinted from: *Marine Drugs* **2024**, *22*, 405, https://doi.org/10.3390/md22090405 . . . . **185**

Preface

Approximately 70% of the Earth's surface is covered by ocean, which is a defining feature of the Earth's geography. The marine environment has unique characteristics, including high pressure, high salinity, low temperature, anaerobic conditions, and low nutrient levels. The special ecological environment in the ocean endows marine organisms (such as corals, sponges, sea squirts, bryozoans, mollusks, etc.) with unique survival strategies, metabolic mechanisms, and genetic diversity. During the processes of survival and evolution, marine organisms have developed functional metabolites—marine natural products (MNPs). More than 40,000 MNPs have been isolated and identified, exhibiting a wide range of biological activities, including anticancer, antibacterial, anti-inflammatory, antiviral, and hypolipidemic activities. These natural molecules have sparked great interest in exploring their pharmacological potential and elucidating their efficacy in drug development.

In recent decades, MNPs have become a vital resource for innovative drug development. To date, 17 marine-derived drugs have been approved for market use. Furthermore, there are 33 drugs in different stages of clinical trials, including 6 in phase III, 17 in phase II, and 10 in phase I. These drugs are primarily being developed for use as cancer treatment, as well as for managing pain and treating viral infections.

This Special Issue comprises 12 articles and a review, which describe the discovery and biological activity studies of different classes of bioactive MNPs. It addresses the potential for research into these natural products' antitumor, antibacterial, anti-inflammatory, antiviral, and type 2 diabetes mellitus (T2DM) treatment properties. Further potential applications of MNPs have been identified through in vivo and in vitro activity studies and mechanistic exploration. Therefore, it is evident that MNPs are a key source for developing new drugs. The development of additional activity evaluation models and novel product discovery will undoubtedly facilitate the creation of a more expansive and diverse foundation for the advancement of new, safe, and efficacious drugs.

This Special Issue is aimed at a wide range of MNP researchers, with a view to providing more possibilities for the development of novel drugs while providing more insights for experimentalists. In light of the growing medical burden and the toxic side effects and adverse reactions associated with existing pharmaceuticals, there is a pressing need to develop new, effective, and safe drugs. MNPs will continue to provide enormous potential for the development of new drugs.

Chang-Lun Shao
Guest Editor

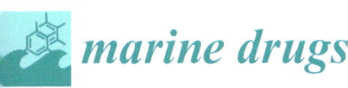

Article

New Sorbicillinoids from the Mangrove Endophytic Fungus *Trichoderma reesei* SCNU-F0042

Jialin Li [1], Tao Chen [1], Jianchen Yu [2], Hao Jia [1], Chen Chen [1] and Yuhua Long [1,*]

1. GDMPA Key Laboratory for Process Control and Quality Evaluation of Chiral Pharmaceuticals, School of Chemistry, South China Normal University, Guangzhou 510006, China; jialinli@m.scnu.edu.cn (J.L.); chent296@mail2.sysu.edu.cn (T.C.); haojia@m.scnu.edu.cn (H.J.); chenchen2021@m.scnu.edu.cn (C.C.)
2. Key Laboratory of Tropical Disease Control, Ministry of Education, Department of Biochemistry, Zhongshan School of Medicine, Sun Yat-Sen University, Guangzhou 510080, China; yujch3@mail.sysu.edu.cn
* Correspondence: longyh@scnu.edu.cn

Abstract: Three new dimeric sorbicillinoids (**1–3**) and one new 3,4,6-trisubstituted α-pyrone (**5**), along with seven analogues (**4** and **6–11**), were isolated from the mangrove endophytic fungus *Trichoderma reesei* SCNU-F0042 under the guidance of molecular networking approach. Their chemical structures were established by 1D and 2D NMR HR-ESI-MS and ECD analysis. In a bioassay, compound **2** exhibited moderate SARS-CoV-2 inhibitory activity with an EC_{50} value of 29.0 μM.

Keywords: mangrove endophytic fungus; *Trichoderma reesei*; sorbicillinoids; SARS-CoV-2 inhibitory activity; molecular networking

1. Introduction

Trichoderma sp. is a widespread filamentous fungus of ascomycetes in various types of soils [1]. Among them, the mangrove-derived fungal genus *Trichoderma* produces a diverse array of secondary metabolites including alkaloids, polyketides, terpenoids, phenols, lactones, and various hybrids of the aforementioned classes [2–6]. Sorbicillinoids, a marker secondary metabolite of *Trichoderma reesei* (*T. reesei*), have a characteristic sorbyl side chain and a cyclic hexaketide nucleus in the structures [7,8]. Since sorbicillin was first discovered from *Penicillium notatum* in 1948, more than 100 analogs of sorbicillinoids have been reported and they can be classified into monomeric-, bi-, tri-, and hybrid sorbicillinoids by the number of sorbicillinoid construction units [9,10]. Many of them exhibited a wide range of biological activities, such as cytotoxic [11], antibacterial [12], antifungal [13], anti-inflammatory [14], phytotoxic [15], and α-glucosidase inhibitory activity [16].

Molecular networking, a strategy that organizes and analyses MS/MS data based on chemical similarity, can be used for dereplication in natural products discovery [17]. After extraction and concentration, the EtOAc extract was subjected to LC-MS/MS analysis, then the data were uploaded to the Global Natural Product Social Molecular Networking (GNPS; www.gnps.ucsd.edu) platform, followed by MN analysis using the online workflow. A comprehensive examination of the MS^2 spectra libraries allowed the annotation of the node at m/z 497.217 ($C_{28}H_{33}O_8$, $[M + H]^+$) as the bislongiquinolide (**4**) based on its fragmentation pattern [18]. By the guidance of bislongiquinolide node, more new bioactive sorbicillinoids remain to be discovered in the metabolites from the fungus *Trichoderma reesei* SCNU-F0042 (Figure 1 and Figure S28). Eventually, under the guidance of molecular networking, three new dimeric sorbicillinoids (**1–3**) and one new 3,4,6-trisubstituted α-pyrone (**5**), as well as seven analogues (**4** and **6–11**) were isolated from the mangrove-derived fungus *Trichoderma reesei* SCNU-F0042 (Figure 2). Details of the isolation, structure elucidation, and bioactivities of these compounds are reported herein.

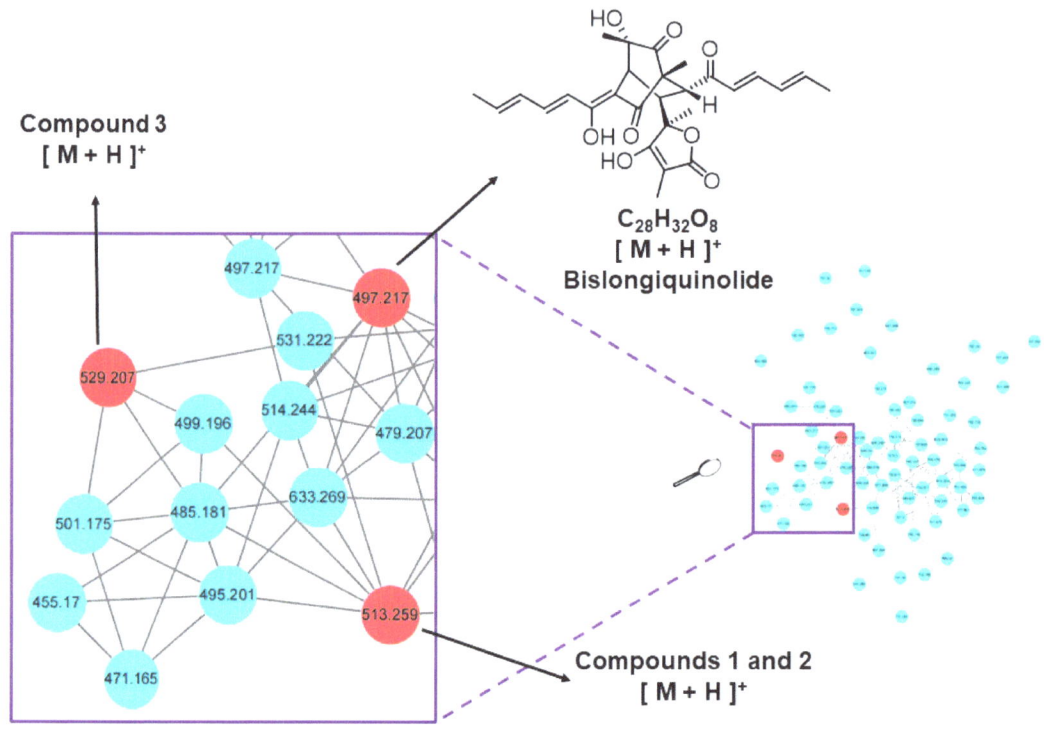

Figure 1. Cluster of nodes from *T. reesei* with compounds 1–4.

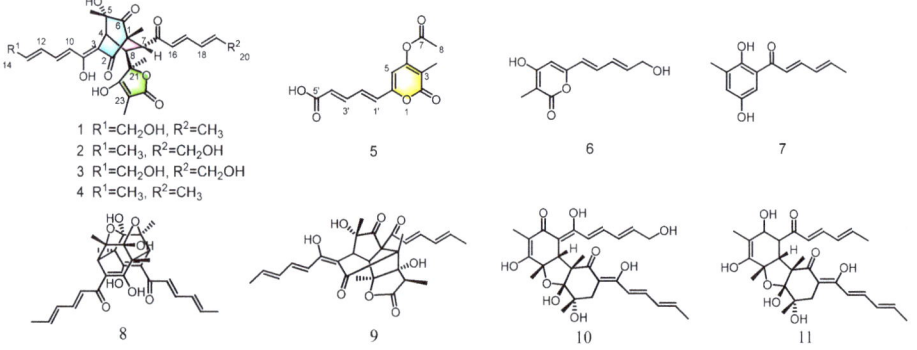

Figure 2. Structure of compounds 1–11.

2. Results

14-hydroxybislongiquinolide (**1**) was yellowish amorphous powder. Its molecular formula was determined as $C_{28}H_{32}O_9$ by ^{13}C NMR and negative-ion HRESIMS data (m/z 511.1975, [M-H]$^-$, calcd for $C_{28}H_{31}O_9$, 511.1974), indicating 13 indices of hydrogen deficiency. The ^1H NMR data (Table 1, Figure S1) of **1** showed resonances of five methyls [δ_H 1.89 (3H, d, J = 6.1 Hz), 1.45(3H, s), 1.38(3H, s), 1.18(3H, s), and 0.99(3H, s)], one oxygenated methylene [δ_H 4.22(2H, d, J = 4.4 Hz), three methines [δ_H 3.36(H, d, J = 5.6 Hz), 3.34(H, s), and 3.22(H, d, J = 5.6 Hz)], and eight olefinic protons [δ_H 7.35(H, dd, J = 14.5, 11.2 Hz), 7.20(H, dd, J = 15.3, 10.7 Hz), 6.55–6.59(H, m), 6.43–6.49(H, m), 6.38–6.42(H, m), 6.31–6.35(H, m), 6.25–6.29(H, m), and 6.18(H, d, J = 15.3 Hz)]. The ^{13}C NMR data (Table 1, Figure S2) revealed 28 carbon resonances corresponding to four carbonyls (δ_C 210.3, 203.1, 198.3, and 179.1), five methyls (δ_C 24.1, 23.3, 19.1, 11.4, and 6.4), one oxygenated methylene (δ_C 63.0), three methines (δ_C 52.2, 43.9, and 43.6), twelve olefinic C-atoms (δ_C 185.5, 168.6, 147.9, 144.9, 143.0, 142.5, 131.7, 129.9, 128.8, 121.6, 111.7, and 94.7), and three quaternary (δ_C 84.8, 75.9, and 63.7). These NMR data were similar to those of bislongiquinolide (**4**), which was previously isolated from the fungi *Trichoderma longibrachiatum* Rifai aggr., indicating that they had the same core skeleton structure [18]. The major difference was the replacement of the C-14 methyl group of the alkene in the side chain in bislongiquinolide by an hydroxymethyl ($\delta_{C/H}$ 63.0/4.22) in **1**, which was further supported by the key ^{1}H−^{1}H COSY correlations (Figures 3 and S3) of H-10/H-11/H-12/H-13/H$_2$-14 and HMBC correlations (Figure S5) from H$_2$-14(δ_H 4.22) to C-12(δ_C 129.9), C-13(δ_C 143.0) and from H-16(δ_H 6.18), H-17(δ_H 7.20) to C-15(δ_C 203.1). To determine relative and absolute configurations of compound **1**, the method of nuclear overhauser effect spectroscopy (NOESY) correlations (Figure 4), coupling constants (Table 1), circular dichroism (CD) spectra (Figure 5), and biogenetic considerations were used. The *E* geometries of double bonds about Δ^{10}, Δ^{12}, Δ^{16}, and Δ^{18} were deduced based on the coupling constants of H-11 (*J* = 14.5, 11.2 Hz) and H-17 (*J* = 15.3, 10.7 Hz). In addition, the NOE correlations (s 4 and S6) of 5-CH$_3$(δ_H 1.18)/H-10(δ_H 6.43–6.49) and H-4(δ_H 3.34)/H-10(δ_H 6.43–6.49) suggest Δ^3 was the Z-type and 5-CH$_3$ and H-4 were located on the side chain from C-9 through C-14. The NOESY correlations of H-10(δ_H 6.43–6.49) (δ_H 1.38) and H-4(δ_H 3.34)/21-CH$_3$ (δ_H 1.38) were oriented H-4 and 21-CH$_3$ to the side chain from C-9 to C-14, which is the same as 5-CH$_3$. The NOESY correlations of 1-CH$_3$ (δ_H 0.99)/H-17 (δ_H 7.20) and H-17(δ_H 7.20)/23-CH$_3$ (δ_H 1.45) indicated that the same orientation of 1-CH$_3$ and 23-CH$_3$ with another side chain from C-7 through C-20. The 7R*, 8S* relative configuration was suggested by the coupling constant (*J*$_{7,8}$ = 5.6 Hz) [18]. Thus, the relative configuration of compound **1** should be 1R*, 4S*, 5S*, 7R*, 8S*, 21S*, which adopted the same configuration of the bicyclo [2.2.2] octanedione core as bislongiquinolide (**4**) [18]. The absolute configurations of compound **1** proposed to the absolute configurations were 1R, 4S, 5S, 7R, 8S, 21S, which were the same as bislongiquinolide (**4**) comparisons of the information between them, including the similar optical rotation values, the biosynthetic pathway, the trend in CD curves (Figure 5), and the chemical shifts [19]. Hence, compound **1** was identified as the 14-hydroxylated analogue of bislongiquinolide (**4**), and named as 14-hydroxybislongiquinolide.

20-hydroxybislongiquinolide (**2**) was isolated as a yellowish amorphous powder. The molecular formula of **2**, the same as **1**, was determined as C$_{28}$H$_{32}$O$_9$ by HRESIMS in observing a protonated molecular ion at *m/z* 511.1975 [M-H]$^-$ (calcd for C$_{28}$H$_{31}$O$_9$, 511.1974). In addition, the hydrogen protons and carbons of **1** and **2** were also of the same type by comparison of the NMR data. However, the position of the hydroxymethyl group was changed from C-14 to C-20, which was confirmed by the key ^{1}H−^{1}H COSY correlations (Figure 3 and Figure S10) of H-16/H-17/H-19/H-19/H$_2$-20, as well as HMBC correlations (Figure S12) from H$_2$-20(δ_H 4.22) to C-18(δ_C 128.5), C-19(δ_C 147.6) and from H-17(δ_H 7.25), H-16(δ_H 6.32) to C-15(δ_C 202.5). The relative configuration of **2** was the same as **1** based on their similar NOESY correlations (Figure 4). Together, they shared the same ECD Cotton effect at 226, 280 and 320 nm of **2** in the experimental ECD spectrum, which was identical to that of **1** (Figure 5). Thus, the absolute configuration of **2** was identified as 1R, 4S, 5S, 7R, 8S, 21S. The structure of **2** was established and named as 20-hydroxybislongiquinolide.

14, 20-dihydroxybislongiquinolide (**3**) was obtained as a yellowish amorphous powder and it was analyzed by HRESIMS (*m/z* 527.1925 [M−H]$^-$, calcd. 527.1923) for the molecular formula C$_{28}$H$_{32}$O$_{10}$, which had an extra oxygen atom than **1**. Its ^{1}H and ^{13}C NMR data (Table 1, Figures S15 and S16) were very similar to those of **1**, with the exception that the methyl signals (C-20, $\delta_{C/H}$ 19.1/1.89) in **1** were replaced by hydroxymethyl signals (C-20, $\delta_{C/H}$ 63.0/4.22). This deduction was also confirmed by the key ^{1}H−^{1}H COSY correlations (Figures 3 and S17) of H-10/H-11/H-12/H-13/H$_2$-14 and H-16/H-17/H-18/H-19/H$_2$-20. The relative configuration of **3** was also the same as **1** deduced from the NOESY correlations (Figure 4). At the same time, the experimental ECD of **3** also has a negative Cotton effect at

226 and 320 nm, as well as positive Cotton effect at 280 nm, just like that of **1** (Figure 5). Therefore, the absolute configuration of **3** was identified as 1R, 4S, 5S, 7R, 8S, 21S and **3** was determined as 14, 20-dihydroxybislongiquinolide.

Table 1. ^{1}H and ^{13}C NMR data for compounds **1**–**3** (methanol-d_4).

NO	1		2		3	
	δ_H (J in Hz)	δ_C, Type	δ_H (J in Hz)	δ_C, Type	δ_H (J in Hz)	δ_C, Type
1	-	63.7, C	-	63.5, C	-	63.6, C
2	-	198.3, C	-	197.5, C	-	197.8, C
3	-	111.7, C	-	110.2, C	-	110.5, C
4	3.34, s	43.6, CH	3.33, s	43.5, CH	3.35, s	43.6, CH
5	-	75.9, C	-	75.8, C	-	75.8, C
6	-	210.3, C	-	210.2, C	-	210.2, C
7	3.36, d (5.6)	52.2, CH	3.31 [a]	52.8, CH	3.33 [a]	52.6, CH
8	3.22, d (5.6)	43.9, CH	3.28 [a]	43.9, CH	3.26 [a]	43.9, CH
9	-	168.6, C	-	169.5, C	-	169.4, C
10	6.43–6.49 [a]	121.6, CH	6.28–6.33	119.6, CH	6.43–6.46	121.5, CH
11	7.35, dd (14.5, 11.2)	142.5, CH	7.30, dd (14.7, 11.2)	143.7, CH	7.37, dd (13.4, 11.5)	142.7, CH
12	6.55–6.59 [a]	129.9, CH	6.39–6.43 [a]	132.4, CH	6.52–6.60 [a]	129.8, CH
13	6.25–6.29 [a]	143.0, CH	6.19–6.25 [a]	140.6, CH	6.26–6.32 [a]	143.3, CH
14	4.22, d (4.4)	63.0, CH$_2$	1.90, d (6.4)	18.9, CH$_3$	4.23, d (4.1)	62.8, CH$_2$
15	-	203.1, C	-	202.5, C	-	202.1, C
16	6.18, d (15.3)	128.8, CH	6.30–6.36 [a]	130.0, CH	6.31–6.40 [a]	130.1, CH
17	7.20, dd (15.3, 10.7)	147.9, CH	7.25, dd (15.4, 10.4)	146.8, CH	7.27, dd (15.2, 10.3)	146.6, CH
18	6.31–6.35 [a]	131.7, CH	6.48–6.53 [a]	128.5, CH	6.49–6.52 [a]	128.6, CH
19	6.38–6.42 [a]	144.9, CH	6.45–6.48 [a]	147.6, CH	6.48–6.51 [a]	147.5, CH
20	1.89, d (6.1)	19.1, CH$_3$	4.22, d (4.0)	62.7, CH$_2$	4.23, d (4.1)	63.0, CH$_2$
21	-	84.8, C	-	84.6, C	-	84.6, C
22	-	185.5, C	-	182.0, C	-	182.9, C
23	-	94.7, C	-	96.2, C	-	96.1, C
24	-	179.1, C	-	178.2, C	-	178.2, C
1-CH$_3$	0.99, s	11.4, CH$_3$	0.99, s	11.3, CH$_3$	0.99, s	11.3, CH$_3$
5-CH$_3$	1.18, s	24.1, CH$_3$	1.18, s	24.2, CH$_3$	1.19, s	24.2, CH$_3$
21-CH$_3$	1.38, s	23.3, CH$_3$	1.40, s	23.4, CH$_3$	1.33, s	23.3, CH$_3$
23-CH$_3$	1.45, s	6.4, CH$_3$	1.48, s	6.5, CH$_3$	1.47, s	6.4, CH$_3$

[a] Overlapped by other signals.

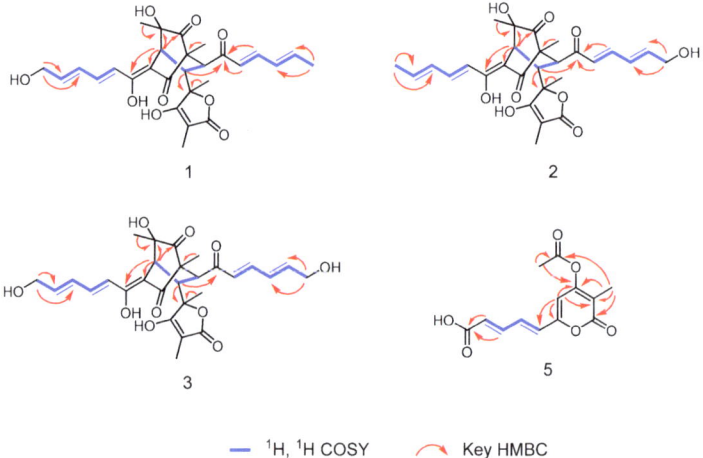

Figure 3. ^{1}H, ^{1}H COSY, and key HMBC correlations of compounds **1**–**3** and **5**.

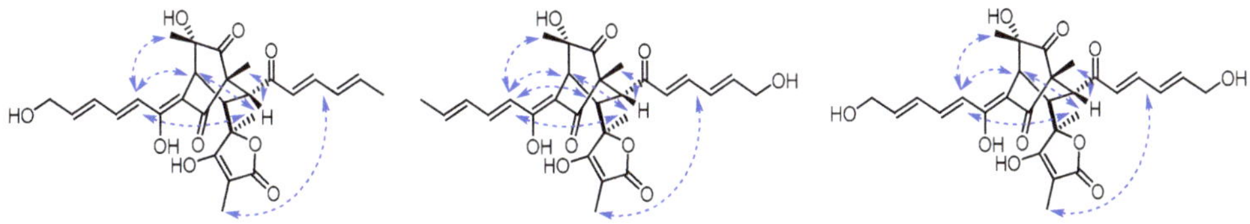

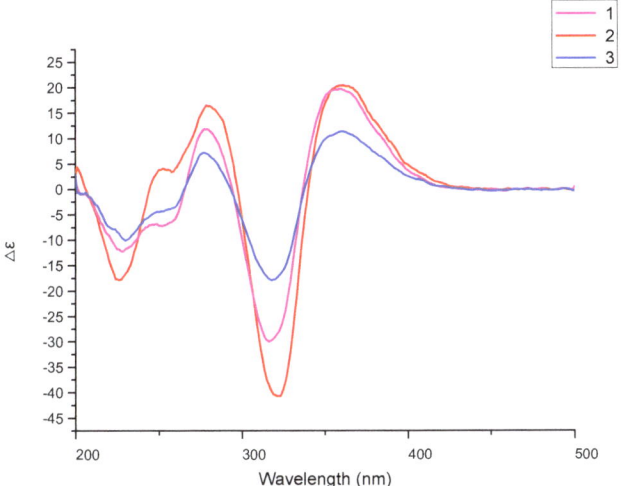

Figure 4. Key NOESY correlations of compounds **1–3**.

Figure 5. Circular dichroism (CD) spectra of compounds **1–3**.

Acetylchrysopyrone B (**5**), a yellowish amorphous powder, has a molecular formula of $C_{13}H_{12}O_6$ determined by HREIMS data (m/z 263.0560 [M-H]$^-$; calcd for $C_{13}H_{11}O_6$, 263.0561), with 8 degrees of unsaturation. The ^{1}H NMR spectral data (Table 2, Figure S22), along with the HSQC data, informed the presence of two methyls [δ_H 2.34(3H, s) and 1.91(3H, s)] and five olefinic protons [δ_H 7.37(1H, dd, J = 15.2, 11.5 Hz), 7.15(1H, dd, J = 15.2, 11.5 Hz), 6.70 (1H, d, J = 15.2 Hz), 6.28 (1H, d, J = 15.2 Hz), and 6.47(1H, s)]. The ^{13}C NMR and HSQC spectra (Figures S23 and S25) displayed 13 carbon resonances, including two carbonyls (δ_C 167.9 and 163.6), one carboxyl (δ_C 167.4), eight olefinic C-atoms (δ_C 158.9, 155.6, 143.4, 132.2, 130.2, 126.6, 115.5, and 106.6) and two methyls (δ_C 20.8 and 10.3). The above spectroscopic features suggested that **5** had a close structural relationship to chrysopyrone B [20], and the only difference was the appearance of the acetyl group connected to 4−OH, which was confirmed by the HMBC correlations from H$_3$-8 to C-4 and C-7, and from H$_3$-3 to C-4 and C-7 (Figure 3 and Figure S26). The geometry of double bonds $\Delta^{1'}$ and $\Delta^{3'}$ were deduced based on the coupling constants of H-2' and H-3' (J = 15.2, 11.5 Hz), suggesting the *E*-type of D1' and D3' double bonds. Therefore, the structure of **5** was proposed and named acetylchrysopyrone B.

The structures of the known compounds, bislongiquinolide (**4**) [18], saturnispol H (**6**) [21], sorbicillin (**7**) [22], trichodimerol (**8**) [23], bisorbicillinolide (**9**) [24], saturnispol B (**10**) [21], and bisvertinolone (**11**) [25], were recognized by comparing with their spectroscopic data reported in the literature. In terms of biological activity, the known compounds **4** and **6–11** have been evaluated for antibacterial [18,21,26], anti-inflammatory [14], radical scavenging activity [24], and PPARγ agonist [27], etc.

Table 2. ^{1}H and ^{13}C NMR data for compound 5 (acetone-d_6).

NO	δ_H (J in Hz)	δ_C, Type
2	-	163.6, C
3	-	115.5, C
4	-	158.9, C
5	6.47, s	106.6, CH
6	-	155.6, C
7	-	167.9, C
8	2.34, s	20.8, CH$_3$
1'	6.70, d (15.2)	130.2, CH
2'	7.15, dd (15.2, 11.5)	132.2, CH
3'	7.37, dd (15.2, 11.5)	143.4, CH
4'	6.28, d (15.2)	126.6, CH
5'	-	167.4, C
3-CH$_3$	1.91, s	10.3, CH$_3$

Biological activities of all new compounds were evaluated in virus bioassays. The results showed that compound **2** displayed moderate antiviral activity against SARS-CoV-2 the causative agent of COVID-19 infection, as assessed in 293T cells, exhibiting an EC$_{50}$ value of 29.0 µM, while compounds **1**, **3**, and **5** displayed no activity at 80 µM. All the tested compounds showed no cytotoxicity at 80 µM. Remdesivir (IC$_{50}$ = 1.2 µM) was used as a positive control (Table 3).

Table 3. Results of anti-SARS-CoV-2 activity and cytotoxicity for 293T cell.

Compound	Inhibition of SARS-CoV-2 Viruses (EC$_{50}$/µM) [b]	Cytotoxicity for 293T Cell (IC$_{50}$/µM) [b]
1	NS [c]	>80
2	29.0	>80
3	NS	>80
5	NS	>80
Remdesivir [a]	1.2	>80

[a] Positive control; [b] Data are shown as mean from three parallel experiments; [c] NS means not sensitive at 80 µM.

3. Experimental Section

3.1. General Experimental Procedures

Optical rotations were recorded on an Anton Paar (MCP 500) polarimeter at 25 °C (Graz, Austria), and ECD spectra were acquired on an Applied Photophysics Chirascan spectropolarimeter (Surrey, UK). HRESIMS spectra were obtained on a ThermoFisher LTQ–Orbitrap–LCMS spectrometer (Palo Alto, CA, USA). A Bruker AVANCE NEO 600 MHz spectrometer (Bruker BioSpin, Rheinstetten, Germany) was used to record the 1D and 2D NMR using TMS as an internal reference at room temperature. Column chromatography (CC) was performed on silica gel (100–200 and 200–300 mesh; Qingdao Marine Chemical Factory, Qingdao, China) and Sephadex LH-20 (25–100 µm; GE Healthcare BioSciences AB, Stockholm, Sweden). HPLC analysis uses a Waters 2695 system (Waters, Milford, MA, USA) with an ACE Excel 5 C18-AR column (250 × 4.6 mm, 5 µm; Hichrom Limited, Leicestershire, UK).

3.2. Fungal Material

The fungal strain *Trichoderma reesei* SCNU-F0042 was isolated from the fresh bark of the mangrove plant *Bruguiera gymnorhiza* collected from Qi'ao Island Mangrove Nature Reserve, Zhuhai City, Guangdong Province, China. The fungus was obtained using the standard protocol for isolation. The sequence data of the fungal strain have been deposited at Gen Bank with accession no. OP978317. A BLAST search result showed that the sequence was the most similar (99%) to the sequence of *Trichoderma reesei* (compared to OK445677.1)

A voucher strain was deposited in School of Chemistry, South China Normal University, Guangzhou, China, with the access code *Trichoderma reesei* SCNU-F0042.

3.3. General Experimental Procedures

Spores of the fungal strain were inoculated into solid autoclaved rice medium in 400 1L Erlenmeyer flasks, each of which contained 50 g rice and 50 mL 0.3% sea salt, culturing in room temperature under static condition for 30 days. The mycelia and solid rice medium were soaked with MeOH and extracted with EtOAc three times. The organic solvents were evaporated under 48 °C with reduced pressure and obtained 158.6 g of organic crude extract. The extract was isolated by column chromatography over silica gel eluting with a gradient of PE/EA (1:0–0:1) to yield 5 fractions (Frs. 1–5). Fr. 3 (2.87 g) was subjected to Sephadex LH−20 (DCM/MeOH v/v, 1:1) to afford four sub-fractions (SFrs. 3.1–3.4). SFr. 3.2 (674.2 mg) was applied to silica gel CC (DCM/MeOH v/v, 60:1.5) to give compound **4** (28.1 mg) and compound **5** (8.2 mg). Fr. 4 (3.62 g) was subjected to Sephadex LH−20 (DCM/MeOH v/v, 1:1) to afford four sub-fractions (SFrs. 4.1–4.3). SFr. 4.2 (641.3 mg) was applied to silica gel CC (DCM/MeOH v/v, 60:2) to give compound **7** (5.1 mg), compound **9** (4.4 mg) and compound **11** (7.6 mg). Fr. 5 (1.82 g) was subjected to Sephadex LH−20 (DCM/MeOH v/v, 1:1) to afford three sub-fractions (SFrs. 5.1–5.3). SFr. 5.2 (582.1 mg) was applied to silica gel CC (DCM/MeOH v/v, 60:4) to afford two sub-fractions (SFrs. 5.2.1 and SFrs. 5.2.4). SFrs. 5.2.1 (85.3 mg) was further purified by Sephadex LH-20 CC eluted with MeOH to give compound **1** (8.2 mg). SFrs. 5.2.2 (68.1 mg) was further purified by silica gel CC (DCM/MeOH v/v, 60:3) to give compound **2** (4.3 mg). SFrs. 5.2.3 (56.5 mg) was further purified by silica gel CC (DCM/MeOH v/v, 60:3.5) to give compound **6** (4.6 mg) and compound **8** (4.2 mg). Fr. 6 (1.43 g) was subjected to Sephadex LH−20 (DCM/MeOH v/v, 1:1) to afford four sub-fractions (SFrs. 6.1–6.4). SFr. 6.2 (321.7 mg) was applied to silica gel CC (DCM/MeOH v/v, 60:4.5) to afford three sub-fractions (SFrs. 6.2.1—SFrs. 6.2.3). SFrs. 6.2.2 (32.5 mg) was further purified by Sephadex LH-20 CC eluted with MeOH to give compound **3** (3.1 mg). SFrs. 6.2.3 (46.0 mg) was further purified by silica gel CC (DCM/MeOH v/v, 60:4) eluted with MeOH to give compound **10** (6.1 mg)

3.4. Spectral and Physical Data of Compounds **1**–**3** *and* **5**

14-hydroxybislongiquinolide (**1**): Yellowish amorphous powder; $[\alpha]_{25}^{D}$ + 143 (c = 0.1, MeOH); UV (MeOH) λ_{max} (log ε) 294(4.36), 366(4.28) nm; IR (neat) v_{max} 3380, 2965, 1735, 1661, 1452, 1442, 1381, 1258, 1200, 1152, 852, 802, 758 cm^{-1}; ^{1}H and ^{13}C NMR data; see Table 1. HRESIMS: m/z 511.1975 [M-H]$^-$ (calcd for C$_{28}$H$_{31}$O$_9$, 511.1974).

20-hydroxybislongiquinolide (**2**): Yellowish amorphous powder; $[\alpha]_{25}^{D}$ + 175 (c = 0.1, MeOH); UV (MeOH) λ_{max} (log ε) 291(4.44), 369(4.36) nm; IR (neat) v_{max} 3325, 2985, 1741, 1670, 1465, 1453, 1379, 1243, 1202, 1148, 856, 805, 747 cm^{-1}; ^{1}H and ^{13}C NMR data; see Table 1. HRESIMS: m/z 511.1975 [M-H]$^-$ (calcd for C$_{28}$H$_{31}$O$_9$, 511.1974).

14, 20-dihydroxybislongiquinolide (**3**): Yellowish amorphous powder; $[\alpha]_{25}^{D}$ + 150 (c = 0.1, MeOH); UV (MeOH) λ_{max} (log ε) 287(4.21), 369(4.06) nm; IR (neat) v_{max} 3451, 2975, 1733, 1656, 1470, 1445, 1383, 1255, 1198, 1146, 870, 802, 751 cm^{-1}; ^{1}H and ^{13}C NMR data; see Table 1. HRESIMS: m/z 527.1925 [M-H]$^-$ (calcd for C$_{28}$H$_{31}$O$_{10}$, 527.1923).

Acetylchrysopyrone B (**5**): Yellowish amorphous powder; $[\alpha]_{25}^{D}$ + 174 (c = 0.10, McOH); UV (MeOH) λ_{max} (log ε) 260(4.12), 355(4.07) nm; IR (neat) v_{max} 3185, 1735, 1651, 1562, 1423, 1367, 1260, 1145, 1019, 995 cm^{-1}; ^{1}H and ^{13}C NMR data; see Table 2. HRESIMS: m/z 263.0560 [M-H]$^-$ (calcd for C$_{13}$H$_{11}$O$_6$, 263.0561).

3.5. LC-MS/MS and Molecular Networking Analysis

The EtOAc extract of *Trichoderma reesei* SCNU-F0042 was analyzed by LC−MS/MS. In positive-ionization conditions (m/z 200−800), the mobile phase consisted of 1‰ HCOOH formic acid in H$_2$O and CH$_3$CN. The elution gradient conditions for the LC mobile phase were as follows, based on times (t): t = 0−1 min, hold at 90% H$_2$O/CH$_3$CN; t = 1−10 min, increased linearly to 40% H$_2$O/CH$_3$CN; t = 10−13 min, increased linearly to 10% H$_2$O/

CH$_3$CN; t = 13–16 min, hold at 10% H$_2$O/CH$_3$CN; t = 16–16.2 min, increased linearly to 90% H$_2$O/CH$_3$CN; t = 16.2–20 min, hold at 90% H$_2$O/CH$_3$CN with the flow rate of 0.3 mL/min. A total of 1 µL of the sample (c 1 mg/mL, CH$_3$CN) was injected. The MS/MS data of EtOAc extract was first saved as .mzML format files through MSConvert software. The molecular networking was performed using the GNPS data analysis workflow and the spectral clustering algorithm. Parameters for molecular network generation were set as follows: precursor mass tolerance m/z 2.0 Da, fragment ion tolerance m/z 0.5 Da, cosine score above 0.7, minimum matched fragment ions 6, minimum cluster size 2, network TopK10. Data were visualized using Cytoscape 3.8.2 software.

3.6. SARS-CoV-2 Inhibition Assay

3.6.1. Cell Lines and Virus

HEK 293T-hACE2 (ATCC CRL-3216 derived) was described previously [28]. African green monkey kidney epithelial cell line Vero were obtained from The Cell Bank of the Chinese Academy of Sciences, CBCAS, Shanghai, China. HEK 293T-hACE2 and Vero were maintained in Dulbecco's modified Eagle's medium (Invitrogen, Carlsbad, CA, USA), containing 10% fetal bovine serum (FBS, GIBCO, Carlsbad, CAe), 2 mM L-glutamine 100 µg/mL streptomycin and 100 units/mL penicillin (Invitrogen) at 37 °C under 5% CO$_2$ BA.2 (GDPCC 2.00299) was obtained from Guangdong Center for Human Pathogen Culture Collection (GDPCC), Guangdong Provincial Center for Disease Control and Prevention BA.2 were amplified in Vero cells.

3.6.2. Plasmids

ACE2 packaging construct (GeneCopoeia, EX-U1285-Lv105) uses a cytomegalovirus (CMV) promoter to express ACE2 and bears a puromycin selection marker in the integrating cassette.

3.6.3. RT-qPCR Analysis

HEK 293T-hACE2 cells were seeded in 12-well flat-bottom plate at a density of 1.2 × 10^4 cells/well. After 24 h, cells were incubated in media consisting of BA.2 (MOI of 0.01) and different concentrations of each compound for 1 h at 37 °C. After the incubation, cells were washed with sterile phosphate-buffered saline (PBS) once and incubated with media mixed with different concentrations of each compound, respectively, for further 48 h. Total RNA of each well was extracted from the cell culture supernatant using LogPure Viral DNA/RNA Kit (Magen, Guangzhou, China). Reverse transcription and qPCR were performed with Detection Kit for Novel Coronavirus (2019-nCoV) RNA (DA0932, DAAN GENE, Guangzhou, China). Samples were read on the QuantStudio7 Flex real-time PCR detection system (Thermo Fisher Scientific, Shanghai, China). The qPCR was performed in duplicates for each sample, and results were calculated using $2^{-\Delta CT}$, where CT is threshold cycle [29].

3.7. Cell Viability Assay

The test compounds at a serial final concentration of 50 to 1 µM were evaluated against HEK 293T-hACE2 using the MTT method. Tested cell lines were cultured in Dulbecco's modified Eagle's medium (DMEM) (Invitrogen, Carlsbad, CA, USA) supplemented with 5% fetal bovine serum (Hyclone, Logan, UT, USA), 2 mM L-glutamine, 100 mg/mL streptomycin, and 100 units/mL penicillin (Invitrogen). The cultures were maintained at 37 °C in a humidified atmosphere of 5% CO$_2$.

4. Conclusions

In summary, three new dimeric sorbicillinoids (**1**–**3**) and one new 3,4,6-trisubstituted α-pyrone (**5**), together with seven analogues (**4** and **6**–**11**), were isolated from the cultures of the mangrove endophytic fungus *Trichoderma reesei* SCNU-F0042 under the guidance of MS/MS based on molecular networking. Compound **2** exhibited moderate inhibitory effects on anti-SARS-CoV-2 activity with an EC$_{50}$ value of 29.0 µM without cytotoxicity observed. Our study enriched the structural and biological activity diversity of sorbicillinoids.

Supplementary Materials: The following supporting information can be downloaded at: https://www.mdpi.com/article/10.3390/md21080442/s1, Figure S1: ^{1}H NMR spectrum of compound **1**; Figure S2. ^{13}C NMR spectrum of compound **1**; Figure S3. ^{1}H, ^{1}H- COSY spectrum of compound **1**; Figure S4. HSQC spectrum of compound **1**; Figure S5. HMBC spectrum of compound **1**; Figure S6. NOESY spectrum of compound **1**; Figure S7. HR-ESI-MS spectrum of compound **1**; Figure S8. ^{1}H NMR spectrum of compound **2**; Figure S9.^{13}C NMR spectrum of compound **2**; Figure S10. ^{1}H, ^{1}H-COSY spectrum of compound **2**; Figure S11. HSQC spectrum of compound **2**; Figure S12. HMBC spectrum of compound **2**; Figure S13. NOESY spectrum of compound **2**; Figure S14. HR-ESI-MS spectrum of compound **2**. Figure S15. ^{1}H NMR spectrum of compound **3**; Figure S16.^{13}C NMR spectrum of compound **3**; Figure S17. ^{1}H, ^{1}H-COSY spectrum of compound **3**; Figure S18. HSQC spectrum of compound **3**; Figure S19. HMBC spectrum of compound **3**; Figure S20. NOESY spectrum of compound **3**; Figure S21. HR-ESI-MS spectrum of compound **3**. Figure S22. ^{1}H NMR spectrum of compound **5**; Figure S23.^{13}C NMR spectrum of compound **5**; Figure S24. ^{1}H, ^{1}H-COSY spectrum of compound **5**; Figure S25. HSQC spectrum of compound **5**; Figure S26. HMBC spectrum of compound **5**; Figure S27. HR-ESI-MS spectrum of compound **5**; Figure S28. Molecular networking of the EtOAc extract from strain *Trichoderma reesei* SCNU-F0042.

Author Contributions: Conceptualization, Y.L.; methodology, J.L. and Y.L.; software, J.L. and T.C.; formal analysis, Y.L.; investigation, J.L., T.C., J.Y., H.J. and C.C.; resources, Y.L.; data curation, Y.L.; writing—original draft preparation, J.L.; writing—review and editing, J.L. and Y.L.; validation, J.L.; visualization, J.L., T.C., J.Y., H.J., C.C. and Y.L.; supervision, Y.L.; project administration, Y.L.; funding acquisition, Y.L. All authors have read and agreed to the published version of the manuscript.

Funding: This research was funded by the Guangdong Marine Economy Development Special Project (No. GDNRC [2023]39 and GDNRC [2022]35) and National Natural Science Foundation of China (No. 41876153).

Conflicts of Interest: The authors declare no conflict of interest.

References

1. Reino, J.L.; Guerrero, R.F.; Hernández-Galán, R.; Collado, I.G. Secondary Metabolites from Species of the Biocontrol Agent *Trichoderma*. *Phytochem. Rev.* **2008**, *7*, 89–123. [CrossRef]
2. Chen, S.; Cai, R.; Liu, Z.; Cui, H.; She, Z. Secondary Metabolites from Mangrove-associated fungi: Source, Chemistry and Bioactivities. *Nat. Prod. Rep.* **2022**, *39*, 560–595. [CrossRef]
3. Zhang, L.; Niaz, S.I.; Khan, D.; Wang, Z.; Zhu, Y.; Zhou, H.; Lin, Y.; Li, J.; Liu, L. Induction of Diverse Bioactive Secondary Metabolites from the Mangrove Endophytic Fungus *Trichoderma* sp. (Strain 307) by Co-Cultivation with *Acinetobacter johnsonii* (Strain B2). *Mar. Drugs* **2017**, *15*, 35. [CrossRef] [PubMed]
4. Zhao, D.-L.; Zhang, X.-F.; Huang, R.-H.; Wang, D.; Wang, X.-Q.; Li, Y.-Q.; Zheng, C.-J.; Zhang, P.; Zhang, C.-S. Antifungal Nafuredin and Epithiodiketopiperazine Derivatives from the Mangrove-Derived Fungus *Trichoderma harzianum* D13. *Front. Microbiol.* **2020**, *11*, 1495. [CrossRef]
5. Zhang, M.; Zhao, J.-L.; Liu, J.-M.; Chen, R.-D.; Xie, K.-B.; Chen, D.-W.; Feng, K.-P.; Zhang, D.; Dai, J.-G. Neural Anti-Inflammatory Sesquiterpenoids from the Endophytic Fungus *Trichoderma* sp. Xy24. *J. Asian Nat. Prod. Res.* **2017**, *19*, 651–658. [CrossRef]
6. Shiono, Y.; Miyazaki, N.; Murayama, T.; Koseki, T.; Harizon; Katja, D.G.; Supratman, U.; Nakata, J.; Kakihara, Y.; Saeki, M.; et al. GSK-3β Inhibitory Activities of Novel Dichroloresorcinol Derivatives from *Cosmospora vilior* Isolated from a Mangrove Plant. *Phytochem. Lett.* **2016**, *18*, 122–127. [CrossRef]
7. Harned, A.M.; Volp, K.A. The Sorbicillinoid Family of Natural Products: Isolation, Biosynthesis, and Synthetic Studies. *Nat. Prod. Rep.* **2011**, *28*, 1790–1810. [CrossRef] [PubMed]
8. Cao, Y.; Yang, R.; Zheng, F.; Meng, X.; Zhang, W.; Liu, W. Dual Regulatory Role of Chromatin Remodeler ISW1 in Coordinating Cellulase and Secondary Metabolite Biosynthesis in *Trichoderma reesei*. *Mbio* **2022**, *13*, 03456. [CrossRef]
9. Cram, D.J.; Tishler, M. Mold Metabolites; Isolation of Several Compounds from Clinical Penicillin. *J. Am. Chem. Soc.* **1948**, *70*, 4238. [CrossRef]
10. Meng, J.; Wang, X.; Xu, D.; Fu, X.; Zhang, X.; Lai, D.; Zhou, L.; Zhang, G. Sorbicillinoids from Fungi and Their Bioactivities. *Molecules* **2016**, *21*, 715. [CrossRef]
11. Rehman, S.; Yang, L.-J.; Zhang, Y.-H.; Wu, J.-S.; Shi, T.; Haider, W.; Shao, C.-L.; Wang, C.-Y. Sorbicillinoid Derivatives from Sponge-Derived Fungus *Trichoderma reesei* (HN-2016-018). *Front. Microbiol.* **2020**, *11*, 1334. [CrossRef] [PubMed]

12. Meng, J.; Wang, B.; Cheng, W. Study on the Secondary Metabolites of *Thichoderma sturnisporum*. *Chin. J. Mar. Drugs* **2017**, *36*, 27–31.
13. Ngo, M.T.; Nguyen, M.V.; Han, J.W.; Park, M.S.; Kim, H.; Choi, G.J. In Vitro and In Vivo Antifungal Activity of Sorbicillinoids Produced by *Trichoderma longibrachiatum*. *J. Fungi* **2021**, *7*, 428. [CrossRef] [PubMed]
14. Zhang, P.; Deng, Y.; Lin, X.; Chen, B.; Li, J.; Liu, H.; Chen, S.; Liu, L. Anti-inflammatory Mono- and Dimeric Sorbicillinoids from the Marine-Derived Fungus *Trichoderma reesei* 4670. *J. Nat. Prod.* **2019**, *82*, 947–957. [CrossRef]
15. Meng, J.; Gu, G.; Dang, P.; Zhang, X.; Wang, W.; Dai, J.; Liu, Y.; Lai, D.; Zhou, L. Sorbicillinoids from the Fungus *Ustilaginoidea virens* and Their Phytotoxic, Cytotoxic, and Antimicrobial Activities. *Front. Chem.* **2019**, *7*, 435. [CrossRef]
16. Pang, X.; Zhou, X.; Lin, X.; Yang, B.; Tian, X.; Wang, J.; Xu, S.; Liu, Y. Structurally Various Sorbicillinoids from the Deep-Sea Sediment Derived Fungus *Penicillium* sp. SCSIO06871. *Bioorg. Chem.* **2021**, *107*, 104600. [CrossRef]
17. Yang, J.Y.; Sanchez, L.M.; Rath, C.M.; Liu, X.; Boudreau, P.D.; Bruns, N.; Glukhov, E.; Wodtke, A.; Felicio, R.; Fenner, A.; et al. Molecular Networking as a Dereplication Strategy. *J. Nat. Prod.* **2013**, *76*, 1686–1699. [CrossRef]
18. Andrade, R.; Ayer, W.A.; Trifonov, L.S. The Metabolites of *Trichoderma longibrachiatum*. III. Two New Tetronic Acids: 5 Hydroxyvertinolide and Bislongiquinolide. *Aust. J. Chem.* **1997**, *50*, 255–257. [CrossRef]
19. Yu, J.; Han, H.; Zhang, X.; Ma, C.; Sun, C.; Che, Q.; Gu, Q.; Zhu, T.; Zhang, G.; Li, D. Discovery of Two New Sorbicillinoids by Overexpression of the Global Regulator LaeA in a Marine-Derived Fungus *Penicillium dipodomyis* YJ-11. *Mar. Drugs* **2019**, *17*, 446. [CrossRef]
20. Han, W.; Cai, J.; Zhong, W.; Xu, G.; Wang, F.; Tian, X.; Zhou, X.; Liu, Q.; Liu, Y.; Wang, J. Protein Tyrosine Phosphatase 1B (PTP1B) Inhibitorsfrom the Deep-Sea Fungus *Penicillium chrysogenum* SCSIO 07007. *Bioorg. Chem.* **2020**, *96*, 103646. [CrossRef]
21. Meng, J.; Cheng, W.; Heydari, H.; Wang, B.; Zhu, K.; Konuklugil, B.; Lin, W. Sorbicillinoid-Based Metabolites from a Sponge Derived Fungus *Trichoderma saturnisporum*. *Mar. Drugs* **2018**, *16*, 226. [CrossRef]
22. Zhao, P.-J.; Li, G.-H.; Shen, Y.-M. New Chemical Constituents from the Endophyte *Streptomyces* Species LR4612 Cultivated on *Maytenus hookeri*. *Chem. Biodivers.* **2006**, *3*, 337–342. [CrossRef] [PubMed]
23. Andrade, R.; Ayer, W.A.; Trifonov, L.S. The Metabolites of *Trichoderma longibrachiatum*. Part II The Structures of Trichodermolide and Sorbiquinol. *Can. J. Chem.* **1996**, *74*, 371–379. [CrossRef]
24. Abe, N.; Murata, T.; Hirota, A. Novel Oxidized Sorbicillin Dimers with 1,1-Diphenyl-2-Picrylhydrazyl-Radical Scavenging Activity from a Fungus. *Biosci. Biotechnol. Biochem.* **1998**, *62*, 2120–2126. [CrossRef] [PubMed]
25. Trifonov, L.S.; Hilpert, H.; Floersheim, P.; Dreiding, A.S.; Rast, D.M.; Skrivanova, R.; Hoesch, L. Bisvertinols: A New Group of Aimeric Vertinoids from *Verticillium intertextum*. *Tetrahedron* **1986**, *42*, 3157. [CrossRef]
26. Kontani, M.; Sakagami, Y.; Marumo, S. First β-1,6-glucan biosynthesis inhibitor, bisvertinolone isolated from fungus, *Acremonium strictum* and its absolute stereochemistry. *Tetrahedron Lett.* **1994**, *35*, 2577. [CrossRef]
27. Liu, J.; Gao, S.; Zhou, W.; Chen, Y.; Wang, Z.; Zeng, Z.; Zhou, H.; Lin, T. Dihydrotrichodimerol Purified from the Marine Fungus *Acremonium citrinum* Prevents NAFLD by Targeting PPARα. *J. Nat. Prod.* **2023**, *86*, 1189–1201. [CrossRef]
28. Oguntuyo, K.Y.; Stevens, C.S.; Hung, C.; Ikegame, S.; Acklin, J.A.; Kowdle, S.S.; Carmichael, J.C.; Chiu, H.P.; Azarm, K.D.; Haas G.D.; et al. Quantifying Absolute Neutralization Titers against SARS-CoV-2 by a Standardized Virus Neutralization Assay Allows for Cross-Cohort Comparisons of COVID-19 Sera. *Mbio* **2021**, *12*, 02492. [CrossRef]
29. Tóth, G.; Horváti, K.; Kraszni, M.; Ausbüttel, T.; Pályi, B.; Kis, Z.; Mucsi, Z.; Kovács, G.M.; Bősze, S.; Boldizsár, I. Arylnaphthalene Lignans with Anti-SARS-CoV-2 and Antiproliferative Activities from the Underground Organs of *Linum austriacum* and *Linum perenne*. *J. Nat. Prod.* **2023**, *86*, 672–682. [CrossRef]

Disclaimer/Publisher's Note: The statements, opinions and data contained in all publications are solely those of the individual author(s) and contributor(s) and not of MDPI and/or the editor(s). MDPI and/or the editor(s) disclaim responsibility for any injury to people or property resulting from any ideas, methods, instructions or products referred to in the content.

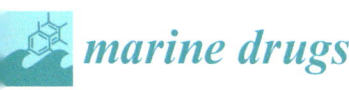

Article

Antioxidative Indenone and Benzophenone Derivatives from the Mangrove-Derived Fungus *Cytospora heveae* NSHSJ-2

Ge Zou [1], Taobo Li [1], Wencong Yang [1], Bing Sun [1], Yan Chen [1], Bo Wang [1], Yanghui Ou [2], Huijuan Yu [2,*] and Zhigang She [1,*]

[1] School of Chemistry, Sun Yat-Sen University, Guangzhou 510275, China
[2] Guangdong Key Laboratory of Animal Conservation and Resource Utilization, Guangdong Public Laboratory of Wild Animal Conservation and Utilization, Institute of Zoology, Guangdong Academy of Sciences, Guangzhou 510260, China
* Correspondence: yuhj@giz.gd.cn (H.Y.); cesshzhg@mail.sysu.edu.cn (Z.S.)

Abstract: Seven new polyketides, including four indenone derivatives, cytoindenones A–C (**1**, **3**–**4**), 3′-methoxycytoindenone A (**2**), a benzophenone derivative, cytorhizophin J (**6**), and a pair of tetralone enantiomers, (±)-4,6-dihydroxy-5-methoxy-α-tetralone (**7**), together with a known compound (**5**) were obtained from the endophytic fungus *Cytospora heveae* NSHSJ-2 isolated from the fresh stem of the mangrove plant *Sonneratia caseolaris*. Compound **3** represented the first natural indenone monomer substituted by two benzene moieties at C-2 and C-3. Their structures were determined by the analysis of 1D and 2D NMR, as well as mass spectroscopic data, and the absolute configurations of (±)-**7** were determined on the basis of the observed specific rotation value compared with those of the tetralone derivatives previously reported. In bioactivity assays, compounds **1**, **4**–**6** showed potent DPPH· scavenging activities, with EC_{50} values ranging from 9.5 to 16.6 µM, better than the positive control ascorbic acid (21.9 µM); compounds **2**–**3** also exhibited DPPH· scavenging activities comparable to ascorbic acid.

Keywords: mangrove endophytic fungus; *Cytospora heveae*; indenone; benzophenone; DPPH·scavenging activity

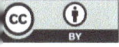

1. Introduction

Indenones are characterized by a cyclopentenone ring fused with an aromatic benzene ring, providing a rigid bicyclic ring framework which enables the extensive evaluation of structure–activity relationship analysis of target therapeutic molecules [1], and indenone derivatives have been synthesized extensively for drug discovery [2–5]. The indenone moiety usually exists in natural products as a structural fragment or a small independent molecule [6–11], and 2,3-diaryl indenone analogues are rarely reported [12–14]. These compounds were considered to be dimers of benzophenone, xanthone, diphenyl ether moieties and indanone moieties, and there was no natural 2,3-diphenyl indenone monomer reported previously. Indenones have multiple bioactivities, including cytotoxicity, DPPH· scavenging activity, anti-inflammatory activity, anti-osteoporosis activity, human DNA dealkylation repair enzyme AlkBH3 inhibitory activity, and PPAR γ agonistic activity [2–5,8,13–15].

Mangrove-associated fungi are known to be an essential source of natural products for the discovery of new drug leads [16,17]. In our continuing search for structurally diverse and biologically active metabolites from mangrove endophytic fungi [18–22], a chemical investigation for new secondary metabolites from mangrove endophytic fungus *Cytospora heveae* NSHSJ-2, which was isolated from the fresh stem of the mangrove plant *Sonneratia caseolaris*, led to the isolation and characterization of seven new polyketides (Figure 1), including four new indenone derivatives, cytoindenones A–C (**1**, **3**–**4**), 3′-methoxycytoindenone A (**2**), a new benzophenone derivative, cytorhizophin J (**6**), and a pair of undescribed tetralone enantiomers, (±)-4,6-dihydroxy-5-methoxy-α-tetralone (**7**), together with a known compound, cytosporaphenones E (**5**) [23]. Among them, compound **3** represented the first natural indenone monomer substituted by two benzene moieties at C-2 and C-3. Herein, the isolation, structure elucidation, and DPPH· radical scavenging activities of these compounds are described.

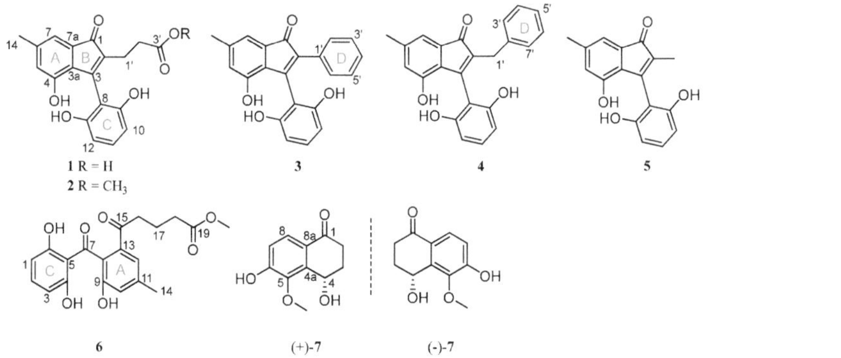

Figure 1. Structure of compounds **1–7**.

2. Results

2.1. Structure Elucidation

Compound **1** was obtained as brown oil. Its molecular formula was assigned as $C_{19}H_{16}O_6$ on the basis of HRESIMS analysis at m/z 363.08383 [M + Na]$^+$ (calcd. For $C_{19}H_{16}O_6Na$, 363.08391), which was determined to possess 12 degrees of unsaturation. In the ^{1}H NMR spectrum (Table 1), the signals for five olefinic protons (δ_H 7.06, 6.79, 6.65, 6.50 and 6.50), two methylenes (δ_H 2.49 and 2.42) and one methyl (δ_H 2.24) were observed. The ^{13}C NMR data (Table 2) exhibited 19 carbon resonances, including two carbonyls (δ_C 198.2 and 174.3), two aromatic rings (A and C) (δ_C 156.2, 156.2, 151.7, 140.7, 134.3, 130.7, 127.1, 124.5, 116.4, 110.6, 108.0, 108.0), two olefinic carbons for one double bond (δ_C 152.1, 134.4), two methylenes (δ_C 32.4 and 20.4) and one methyl (δ_C 21.0).

Table 1. ^{1}H NMR data of **1–4** (J in Hz).

No.	**1** [a]	**2** [b]	**3** [c]	**4** [c]
5	6.65, s	6.54, s	6.63, s	6.58, s
7	6.79, s	6.82, s	6.87, s	6.75, s
10	6.50, d (8.1)	6.57, d (8.3)	6.33, d (8.1)	6.40, d (8.2)
11	7.06, t, (8.1)	7.15, t (8.3)	6.99, t (8.1)	7.02, t (8.2)
12	6.50, d (8.1)	6.57, d (8.3)	6.33, d (8.1)	6.40, d (8.2)
14	2.24, s	2.17, s	2.27, s	2.22, s
1'	2.42, m	2.42, t (7.1)		3.41, s
2'	2.49, m	2.66, t (7.1)	7.30, m	
3'			7.15, m	7.09, m
4'		3.58, s	7.13, m	7.07, m
5'			7.15, m	7.02, t (8.2)
6'			7.30, m	7.07, m
7'				7.09, m

[a] Data were recorded in Actone-d_6 at 400 MHz for ^{1}H NMR. [b] Data were recorded in CDCl$_3$ at 400 MHz for ^{1}H NMR. [c] Data were recorded in CD$_3$OD at 600 MHz for ^{1}H NMR.

Table 2. ^{13}C NMR data of **1–4**.

No.	**1** [a]	**2** [b]	**3** [c]	**4** [c]
1	198.2, C	197.5, C	199.1, C	200.2, C
2	134.4, C	135.2, C	133.6, C	134.8, C
3	152.1, C	148.3, C	154.0, C	154.8, C
3a	127.1, C	123.7, C	127.1, C	127.4, C
4	151.7, C	150.0, C	153.1, C	152.3, C
5	124.5, CH	124.7, CH	125.1, CH	125.0, CH
6	140.7, C	141.5, C	141.9, C	141.1, C
7	116.4, CH	118.2, CH	116.9, CH	116.6, CH
7a	134.3, C	132.5, C	134.4, C	134.6, C
8	110.6, C	108.4, C	112.1, C	111.4, C
9	156.2, C	153.6, C	156.5, C	156.6, C
10	108.0, CH	109.4, CH	107.9, CH	107.8, CH
11	130.7, CH	131.9, CH	130.7, CH	130.8, CH
12	108.0, CH	109.4, CH	107.9, CH	107.8, CH
13	156.2, C	153.6, C	156.5, C	156.6, C
14	21.0, CH$_3$	21.3, CH$_3$	21.2, CH$_3$	21.1, CH$_3$
1′	20.4, CH$_2$	19.6, CH$_2$	133.7, C	30.5, CH$_2$
2′	32.4, CH$_2$	31.0, CH$_2$	129.9, CH	140.9, C
3′	174.3, C	175.1, C	128.5, CH	129.7, CH
4′		52.2, CH$_3$	127.9, CH	128.9, CH
5′			128.5, CH	126.5, CH
6′			129.9, CH	128.9, CH
7′				129.7, CH

[a] Data were recorded in Actone-d_6 at 100 MHz for ^{13}C NMR. [b] Data were recorded in CDCl$_3$ at 100 MHz for ^{13}C NMR. [c] Data were recorded in CD$_3$OD at 150 MHz for ^{13}C NMR.

The HMBC correlations from H-1′, to C-1, C-2, C-3, from H-14 to C-5, C-6, C-7, from H-5 to C-3a, C-4, and from H-7 to C-1, C-3a suggested the presence of an indenone fragment (rings A and B) (Figure 2). Additionally, the ^{1}H-^{1}H COSY correlations of H-10/H-11/H-12, together with the HMBC correlations from H-12 to C-3, C-8 and C-13, and from H-11 to C-13, completed the 2,6-dihydroxybenzoyl fragment (ring C), which connected to the indenone ring at C-3. The structures of ring A, B and C were further confirmed by comparison of ^{1}H and ^{13}C NMR spectra between **1** and **5** [23]. Furthermore, the ^{1}H-^{1}H COSY correlation of H-1′/H-2′ and the HMBC correlations from H-1′, H-2′ to C-3′, from H-1′ to C-1, C-2, C-3, and from H-2′, to C-2 indicated the presence of the 2-carboxyethyl group, which was assigned to be connected to the indenone ring at C-2. Thus, the structure of **1** was deduced, named cytoindenone A.

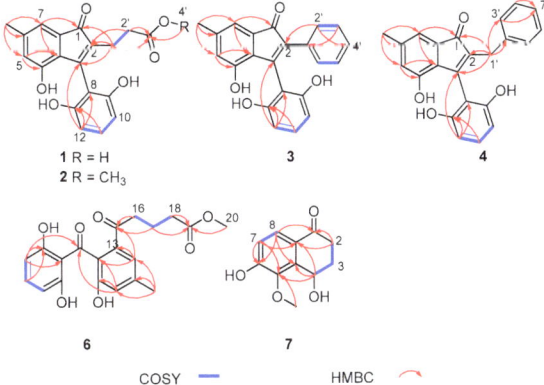

Figure 2. Key COSY and HMBC correlations of **1–4** and **6–7**.

Compound **2** was isolated as brown oil. Its molecular formula was determined as $C_{20}H_{18}O_6$ (12 degrees of unsaturation) in terms of HREIMS analysis at m/z 377.09985 $[M + Na]^+$ (calcd. for $C_{20}H_{18}O_6Na$, 377.09956). Analysis of the ^1H and ^{13}C NMR spectroscopic data of **2** (Tables 1 and 2) revealed mostly similarities with that of **1**, except that the hydroxyl group was substituted with the methoxy group (δ_H 3.58, δ_C 52.2) at C-3′. Combined with the HMBC from H-4′ to C-3′ (Figure 2), the structure of compound **2** was clearly confirmed, named 3′-methoxycytoindenone A.

Compound **3** was acquired as brown oil and had a molecular formula of $C_{22}H_{16}O_4$, determined by HRESIMS data m/z 367.09424 $[M + Na]^+$ (calcd. 367.09408) with 15 degrees of unsaturation. The ^1H NMR spectrum of **3** displayed the signal for ten olefinic protons (δ_H 7.30, 7.30, 7.15, 7.15, 7.13, 6.99, 6.87, 6.63, 6.33 and 6.33) and one methyl (δ_H 2.27). The ^{13}C NMR data exhibited one carbonyl (δ_C 199.1), three aromatic rings (δ_C 156.5, 156.5, 153.1, 141.9, 134.4, 133.7, 130.7, 129.9, 129.9, 128.5, 128.5, 127.9, 127.1, 125.1, 116.9, 112.1, 107.9 and 107.9), two olefinic carbons for one double bond (δ_C 154.0, 133.6) and one methyl (δ_C 21.2) (Tables 1 and 2). According to 1D NMR and 2D NMR data, the rings A, B and C of **2** were similar to that of **1**. The obvious difference was the absence of the 2-carboxyethyl group at the C-2 position of compound **1** and the presence of a phenyl group (ring D) at the C-2 position of compound **3**. Meanwhile, the ^1H-^1H COSY correlations of H-3′/H-4′/H-5′ failed to be identified because the chemical shifts of H-3′, H-4′ and H-5′ were overlapped, the ^1H-^1H COSY correlations of H-2′/H-3′, the HMBC from H-2′ to C-2, C-5′, and from H-3′ to C-1′ also indicated that ring D was formed and connected to the indenone ring at C-2, and the structure of compound **3** was determined, named cytoindenone B.

Compound **4** was obtained as brown oil. The molecular formula was determined as $C_{23}H_{18}O_4$ on the basis of HRESIMS data at m/z 381.10980 $[M + Na]^+$ (calcd. for $C_{23}H_{18}O_4Na$, 381.10973), which was thus determined to possess 15 degrees of unsaturation. The ^1H and ^{13}C NMR spectroscopic data were listed in Tables 1 and 2, which suggested that the structure of compound **4** was similar to compound **3**, except the presence of methylenes (δ_H 3.41, δ_C 30.5). Similarly, the ^1H-^1H COSY correlations of H-3′/H-4′/H-5′/H-6′/H-7′ failed to be identified because of the overlapping chemical shifts. Combined with the HMBC from H-1′ to C-1, C-2, C-3, C-2′, C-3′, and from H-3′, H-4′ to C-5′ (Figure 2), ring D was formed and C-1′ was connected to the indenone ring and ring D at C-2 and C-2′, and the structure of compound **5** was clearly confirmed, named cytoindenone C.

Compound **6** was isolated as white powder and assigned an HRESIMS ion peak at m/z 395.11005 ($[M + Na]^+$, calcd. for $C_{20}H_{20}O_7Na$, 395.11012), which perfectly matched the molecular formula of $C_{20}H_{20}O_7$ with 11 degrees of unsaturation. The ^1H NMR spectrum of **6** displayed the signal for five olefinic protons (δ_H 7.25, 7.18, 6.87, 6.27 and 6.27), one methoxyl (δ_H 3.63), three methylenes (δ_H 2.96, 2.32 and 1.85) and one methyl (δ_H 2.36). The ^{13}C NMR data revealed 20 carbon resonances, involving two carbonyls (δ_C 204.1 and 202.2), one ester carbonyl (d_C 175.5), two aromatic rings (δ_C 163.2, 163.2, 155.0, 140.8, 137.8, 137.0, 130.0, 121.6, 121.6, 112.7, 108.1, 108.1), one methoxyl (δ_C 52.0), three methylenes (δ_C 38.9, 33.7 and 20.6) and one methyl (δ_C 21.3) (Table 3). According to 1D NMR and 2D NMR data, the benzophenone moiety of **6** was similar to cytorhizophin C [24]. The only difference between them were that the popionyl group at the C-13 position of cytorhizophin C was replaced by the 5-methoxy-5-oxopentanoyl group of compound **6**. The ^1H-^1H COSY correlations of H-16/H-17/H-18, together with the HMBC correlations from H-16 to C-13 and C-15, from H-17 to C-15, and from H-18, H-20 to C-19 indicated that the 5-methoxy-5-oxopentanoyl group was located at C-13. Therefore, the structure of **6** was deduced and named cytorhizophin J.

Table 3. ^{1}H and ^{13}C NMR data for **6**.

No.	δ_C, Type	δ_H Mult (J in Hz)
	6 ^{a}	
1	108.1, CH	6.27, d (8.2)
2	137.0, CH	7.18, t (8.2)
3	108.1, CH	6.27, d (8.2)
4	163.2, C	
5	112.7, C	
6	163.2, C	
7	204.1, C	
8	130.0, C	
9	155.0, C	
10	121.6, CH	6.87, s
11	140.8, C	
12	121.6, CH	7.25, s
13	137.8, C	
14	21.3, CH$_3$	2.36, s
15	202.2, C	
16	38.9, CH$_2$	2.96, t (7.5)
17	20.6, CH$_2$	1.85, m
18	33.7, CH$_2$	2.32, t (7.3)
19	175.5, C	
20	52.0, CH$_3$	3.63, s

^{a} Data were recorded in CD$_3$OD at 400 MHz for ^{1}H NMR and 100 MHz for ^{13}C NMR.

Compound **7** was acquired as colorless oil. Its molecular formula C$_{11}$H$_{12}$O$_4$ (six degrees of unsaturation) was established on the basis of HREIMS analysis at m/z 209.08093 [M + H]$^+$ (calcd. For C$_{11}$H$_{13}$O$_4$, 209.08084). Analysis of the ^{1}H and ^{13}C NMR spectroscopic data of **7** (Table 4) revealed mostly similarities to 3,4-dihydro-4β,6-dihydroxy-5-methoxy-2α-methyl-1(2H)-naphthalenone [25]. The main difference between them were the absence of one methine at δ_H 2.98 (1H, m, H-2β) and one methyl at δ_H 1.11 (3H, d, J = 6.8 Hz, 2-Me) in 3,4-dihydro-4β,6-dihydroxy-5-methoxy-2α-methyl-1(2H)-naphthalenone and the presence of one methylene at δ_H 2.99 (1H, m, H$_a$-2) and 2.43 (1H, dt, J = 17.2, 3.6, H$_b$-2) in **7**, which was confirmed by the ^{1}H-^{1}H COSY correlations of H$_{a,b}$-2/H$_{a,b}$-3/H-4, and the HMBC correlations (Figure 2) from H$_{a,b}$-2 to C-1, C-8a. Thus, compound **7** was assigned as shown in Figure 1, and named 4,6-dihydroxy-5-methoxy-α-tetralone. However, chiral HPLC analysis of **7** showed two peaks (t_R 21.3 min and 24.6 min), and subsequent chiral HPLC purification of (±)-**7** led to the separation of the two enantiomers (+)-**7** and (−)-**7**. The absolute configurations of (+)-**7** and (−)-**7** were determined as 4S and 4R by the comparison of the observed specific rotation value [(+)-**7**: $[\alpha]_D^{25}$ + 31.3, (+)-**7**: $[\alpha]_D^{25}$ − 31.5)] of compounds (±)-**7** with those for (4S)-4,8-dihydroxy-α-tetralone ($[\alpha]_D^{27}$ + 24.5), (4S)-5-hydroxy-4-methoxy-α-tetralone ($[\alpha]_D^{27}$ + 50.0), (4R)-4,8-dihydroxy-α-tetralone ($[\alpha]_D^{27}$ − 26.0) and (4R)-5-hydroxy-4-methoxy-α-tetralone ($[\alpha]_D^{27}$ − 50.0) (Figure S39) [26].

Table 4. ^{1}H and ^{13}C NMR data for **7**.

No.	δ_C, Type	δ_H Mult (J in Hz)
		7 [a]
1	199.6, C	
2	33.0, CH$_2$	2.99, m
		2.43, dt (17.2, 3.6)
3	31.6, CH$_2$	2.26, m
		2.17, m
4	61.7, CH	5.26, t (3.1)
4a	139.9, C	
5	146.2, C	
6	157.5, C	
7	117.8, C	6.92, d (8.6)
8	125.4, CH	7.67, d (8.6)
8a	125.6, C	
9	61.9, CH$_3$	

[a] Data were recorded in CD$_3$OD at 400 MHz for ^{1}H NMR and 100 MHz for ^{13}C NMR.

2.2. Biological Evaluation

Compounds **1–7** were tested for their DPPH· scavenging activity. As seen in Table 5, the results indicated that compounds **1, 4–6** showed significant DPPH· scavenging activities with EC$_{50}$ values ranging from 9.5 to 16.6 μM, better than the positive control ascorbic acid (21.9 μM) [27,28]; compounds **2–3** also exhibited DPPH· scavenging activities comparable to ascorbic acid.

Table 5. DPPH· scavenging activities of compounds **1–9**.

Compound	% Inhibition (100 μM)	EC$_{50}$ (μM)
1	90.8	11.5 ± 0.1
2	72.5	21.5 ± 1.0
3	69.0	19.7 ± 1.8
4	78.2	16.6 ± 0.4
5	81.0	12.4 ± 0.5
6	87.3	9.5 ± 0.1
(+)-7	12.0	–
(−)-7	4.2	–
ascorbic acid [a]	91.4	21.9 ± 0.3

[a] positive control.

The antioxidant activities of phenolic compounds were widely investigated and the phenolic content and the side chain functional groups had significant influences on DPPH· scavenging activities [29,30]. Comparing the activities of compounds **1–2**, when the carboxyl group at C-3′ was esterified by the methyl group, the antioxidant activity of **2** decreases significantly. Comparing the activities of compounds **2–5**, the higher activity of compound **5** was due to the accessibility of the phenolic OH group by DPPH·. The activities of compounds **2–4** were due to the presence of bulky groups at C-2 obstructing DPPH· access to the phenolic OH group. Compound **6** could be regarded as a precursor of compound **2**, which formed ring B through C7–C16 aldol-type cyclization. Compound **6** exhibited the strongest antioxidant activity due to the disconnection of ring B and the smallest steric hindrance of phenolic ring C. Compounds (+)-**7** and (−)-**7** showed no antioxidant activities due to the reduction of the phenolic content.

3. Experimental Section

3.1. General Experimental Procedures

Optical rotations were performed on an MCP300 (Anton Paar, Shanghai, China) UV data were measured on a Shimadzu UV-2600 spectrophotometer (Shimadzu, Kyoto,

Japan). The ECD experiment data were conducted with a J-810 spectropolarimeter (JASCO, Tokyo, Japan). IR spectra were measured on an IR Affinity-1 spectrometer (Shimadzu, Kyoto, Japan). Melting points were recorded on a Fisher-Johns hot-stage apparatus. The NMR spectra were tested on a Bruker Avance spectrometer (Bruker, Beijing, China) (Compounds **3**–**4**: 600 MHz for ^{1}H and 150 MHz for ^{13}C; compounds **1**–**2** and **5**–**7**: 400 MHz for ^{1}H and 100 MHz for ^{13}C, respectively). HRESIMS data were conducted on a ThermoFisher LTQ-Orbitrap-LC-MS spectrometer (Palo Alto, CA, USA). Column chromatography (CC) was performed on silica gel (200–300 mesh, Marine Chemical Factory, Qingdao, China) and Sephadex LH-20 (Amersham Pharmacia, Piscataway, NJ, USA). Semi-preparative HPLC (Ultimate 3000 BioRS, Thermo Scientific, Germany) were conducted using the Chiral INA column (5 μm, 4.6 × 250 mm, Phenomenex, Piscataway, NJ, USA), and the Chiralcel ODH column (5 μm, 4.6 × 250 mm, Daicel, Tokyo, Japan) for chiral separation.

3.2. Fungal Material

The fungal strain NSHSJ-2 used in this study was isolated from the fresh stem of mangrove plant *Sonneratia caseolaris*, which was collected in June 2020 from the Nansha Mangrove National Nature Reserve in Guangdong Province, China. The strain was identified as *Cytospora heveae* (compared to no. OQ423127) upon the analysis of ITS sequence data of the rDNA gene. The ITS sequence data obtained from the fungal strain has been submitted to GenBank with accession no. OL780505.1. A voucher strain was deposited in our laboratory.

3.3. Fermentation, Extraction and Isolation

The fungus *Cytospora heveae* NSHSJ-2 was fermented on solid cultured medium (sixty 1000 mL Erlenmeyer flasks, each containing 50 g of rice and 50 mL of distilled water with 3% sea salt) for 30 days at 25 °C. The cultures were extracted three times with MeOH to yield 22.9 g of residue. Then, the crude extract was eluted by using a gradient elution with petroleum ether/EtOAc from 9:1 to 0:10 (*v/v*) on silica gel CC to get six fractions (Fr. A–F). Fr. D (297 mg) was subjected to silica gel CC (CH$_2$Cl$_2$/MeOH, *v/v*, 800:1 to 200:1) to obtain three subfractions (Fr. D$_1$–D$_3$). Fr. D$_2$ (9.4 mg) was separated by normal phase HPLC on a chiral column (INA), using hexane/isopropanol (80:20, *v/v*, flow rate: 1.0 mL/min) as the solvent system, to yield compounds **3** (1.6 mg, t_R 14.0 min) and **4** (4.3 mg, t_R 21.2 min). Fr. D$_3$ (83.4 mg) was applied to Sephadex LH-20 CC (CH$_2$Cl$_2$/MeOH, *v/v*, 1:1) to yield compound **5** (26 mg). Fr. E (749 mg) was subjected to silica gel CC (CH$_2$Cl$_2$/MeOH, *v/v*, 100:1 to 20:1) to afford four fractions (Fr. E$_1$–E$_4$). Fr. E$_2$ (204 mg) was subjected to silica gel CC (petroleum ether/EtOAc, *v/v*, 7:3) to yield compounds **2** (46.5 mg). Fr. E$_3$ (56.4 mg) was subjected to silica gel CC (petroleum ether/EtOAc, *v/v*, 6:4) to yield compounds **6** (15.4 mg) and (±)-**7** (9.4 mg). The chiral HPLC separation of (±)-**7** was accomplished over a chiral column (ODH) (column size: 4.6 × 250 mm, 5 μm; flow rate: 1.0 mL/min; solvent: n-hexane-isopropanol = 90:10) to yield (+)-**7** (1.4 mg, t_R 21.3 min) and (−)-**7** (7.3 mg, t_R 24.6 min). Fr. E$_4$ (103 mg) was purified by Sephadex LH-20 CC and eluted with MeOH to obtain compound **1** (27.9 mg).

Cytoindenone A (**1**): brown oil; UV (MeOH) λ_{max} (log ε): 205 (1.24), 247 (0.53) nm; IR v_{max} 3282, 2949, 2835, 1695, 1435, 1276, 1010, 781 cm^{-1}; HRESIMS *m/z* 363.08383 [M + Na]$^+$ (calcd. for C$_{19}$H$_{16}$O$_6$Na, 363.08391); ^{1}H NMR (400 MHz, Actone-*d$_6$*) data and ^{13}C NMR (100 MHz, Actone-*d$_6$*) data (see Tables 1 and 2).

3′-methoxycytoindenone A (**2**): brown oil; UV (MeOH) λ_{max} (log ε): 204 (0.90), 248 (0.42) nm; IR v_{max} 3360, 2954, 2920, 1697, 1622, 1462, 1278, 1012, 783 cm^{-1}; HRESIMS *m/z* 377.09985 [M + Na]$^+$ (calcd. for C$_{20}$H$_{18}$O$_6$Na, 377.09956); ^{1}H NMR (400 MHz, CDCl$_3$) data and ^{13}C NMR (100 MHz, CDCl$_3$) data (see Tables 1 and 2).

Cytoindenone B (**3**): brown oil; UV (MeOH) λ_{max} (log ε): 203 (0.32), 272 (0.15) nm; IR v_{max} 3365, 2949, 2850, 1689, 1618, 1462, 1280, 1014, 792 cm^{-1}; HRESIMS *m/z* 367.09424 [M + Na]$^+$ (calcd. for C$_{22}$H$_{16}$O$_4$Na, 367.09408); ^{1}H NMR (600 MHz, CD$_3$OD) data and ^{13}C NMR (150 MHz, CD$_3$OD) data (see Tables 1 and 2).

Cytoindenone C (**4**): brown oil; UV (MeOH) λ_{max} (log ε): 205 (0.80), 249 (0.35) nm IR ν_{max} 3358, 2922, 2852, 1683, 1618, 1462, 1276, 1012, 700 cm^{-1}; HRESIMS m/z 381.10980 [M + Na]$^+$ (calcd. for C$_{23}$H$_{18}$O$_4$Na, 381.10973); ^{1}H NMR (600 MHz, CD$_3$OD) data and ^{13}C NMR (150 MHz, CD$_3$OD) data (see Tables 1 and 2).

Cytorhizophin J (**6**): white powder, mp 190.2–191.6 °C; UV (MeOH) λ_{max} (log ε) 216 (1.43), 270 (0.67) nm; IR ν_{max} 3342, 2924, 1716, 1627, 1456, 1338, 1226, 1031, 925, cm^{-1} HRESIMS m/z 395.11005 [M + Na]$^+$ (calcd. for C$_{20}$H$_{20}$O$_7$Na, 395.11012); ^{1}H NMR (400 MHz CD$_3$OD) and ^{13}C NMR (100 MHz, CD$_3$OD) data (see Table 3).

($\pm$)-4,6-dihydroxy-5-methoxy-α-tetralone (**7**): colorless oil; UV (MeOH) λ_{max} (log ε) 205 (1.63), 230 (1.29), 282 (1.01) nm; IR ν_{max} 3261, 2943, 2839, 1660, 1578, 1305, 1290, 1190 1012 cm^{-1}; ^{1}H NMR (400 MHz, CD$_3$OD) data and ^{13}C NMR (100 MHz, CD$_3$OD) data (see Table 4); HRESIMS m/z 209.08093 [M + H]$^+$ (calcd for C$_{11}$H$_{13}$O$_4$, 209.08084). (+)-**7** $[\alpha]_D^{25}$ + 31.3 (c 0.1 MeOH); ECD (c = 0.18 mg/mL, MeOH) λ_{max} ($\Delta\varepsilon$) 205 (+13.5), 230 (+8.4) 284 (+7.0), 327 ($-$6.0). ($-$)-**7**, $[\alpha]_D^{25}$ $-$ 31.5 (c 0.1 MeOH); ECD (c = 0.17 mg/mL, MeOH) λ_{max} ($\Delta\varepsilon$) 205 ($-$14.9), 225 ($-$6.1), 277 ($-$5.4), 320 (+5.8).

3.4. Biological Assays

The DPPH·radical scavenging activities of compounds **1**–**7** were determined according to the reported method [14,28]. The DPPH· radical scavenging test was performed in 96-well microplates. Testing materials (compounds **1**–**7**) were added to 100 µL (0.16 mmol/L) DPPH solution in MeOH at a range of 100 µL solutions of different concentrations (6.25–100 µM). Ascorbic acid was prepared as positive control at the same concentrations (Table 5). Absorbance was recorded at λ = 517 nm after 45 min of incubation in the dark. The DPPH·radical scavenging activity was calculated using the formula:

$$\text{DPPH radical scavenging activity (\%)} = [(\text{Abs}_{control} - \text{Abs}_{sample})/\text{Abs}_{control}] \times 100$$

4. Conclusions

In summary, seven new polyketides including four indenone derivatives, cytoindenones A–C (**1**, **3**–**4**), 3'-methoxycytoindenone A (**2**), a new benzophenone derivative cytorhizophin J (**6**) and a pair of undescribed tetralone enantiomers, ($\pm$)-4,6-dihydroxy-5-methoxy-1-tetralone (**7**), together with a known compound (**5**), were isolated from the endophytic fungus *Cytospora heveae* NSHSJ-2. Compound 3 represented the first natural indenone monomer substituted by two benzene moieties at C-2 and C-3. Their structures were confirmed by the analysis of NMR, HR-MS and ECD spectra. All of the compounds were tested for their antioxidative activities. Compounds **1**, **4**–**6** showed potent DPPH· scavenging activities with EC$_{50}$ values ranging from 9.5 to 16.6 µM, better than the positive control ascorbic acid (21.9 µM); compounds **2**–**3** also exhibited DPPH· scavenging activities comparable to ascorbic acid.

Supplementary Materials: The following are available online at https://www.mdpi.com/article/10 .3390/md21030181/s1, Figure S1: HRESIMS spectrum of compound **1**; Figure S2: ^{1}H NMR spectrum of compound **1** (400 MHz, Actone-d_6); Figure S3: ^{13}C NMR spectrum of compound **1** (100 MHz, Actone-d_6); Figure S4: ^{1}H-^{1}H COSY spectrum of compound **1**; Figure S5: HSQC spectrum of compound **1**; Figure S6: HMBC spectrum of compound **1**; Figure S7: HRESIMS spectrum of compound **2**; Figure S8: ^{1}H NMR spectrum of compound **2** (400 MHz, CDCl$_3$); Figure S9: ^{13}C NMR spectrum of compound **2** (100 MHz, CDCl$_3$); Figure S10: ^{1}H-^{1}H COSY spectrum of compound **2**; Figure S11: HSQC spectrum of compound **2**; Figure S12: HMBC spectrum of compound **2**; Figure S13: HRESIMS spectrum of compound **3**; Figure S14: ^{1}H NMR spectrum of compound **3** (600 MHz, CD$_3$OD); Figure S15: ^{13}C NMR spectrum of compound **3** (150 MHz, CD$_3$OD); Figure S16: ^{1}H-^{1}H COSY spectrum of compound **3**; Figure S17: HSQC spectrum of compound **3**; Figure S18: HMBC spectrum of compound **3**; Figure S19: HRESIMS spectrum of compound **4**; Figure S20: ^{1}H NMR spectrum of compound **4** (600 MHz, CD$_3$OD); Figure S21: ^{13}C NMR spectrum of compound **4** (150 MHz, CD$_3$OD); Figure S22: ^{1}H-^{1}H COSY spectrum of compound **4**; Figure S23: HSQC spectrum of compound **4**; Figure S24: HMBC spectrum of compound **4**; Figure S25: HRESIMS spectrum of compound **6**; Figure S26: ^{1}H

NMR spectrum of compound **6** (400 MHz, CD$_3$OD); Figure S27: ^{13}C NMR spectrum of compound **6** (100 MHz, CD$_3$OD); Figure S28: ^{1}H-^{1}H COSY spectrum of compound **6**; Figure S29: HSQC spectrum of compound **6**; Figure S30: HMBC spectrum of compound **6**; Figure S31: HRESIMS spectrum of compound **7**; Figure S32: ^{1}H NMR spectrum of compound **7** (400 MHz, CD$_3$OD); Figure S33: ^{13}C NMR spectrum of compound **7** (100 MHz, CD$_3$OD); Figure S34: ^{1}H-^{1}H COSY spectrum of compound **7**; Figure S35: HSQC spectrum of compound **7**; Figure S36: HMBC spectrum of compound **7**; Figure S37: ECD spectrum of compound (+)-7; Figure S38: ECD spectrum of compound (−)-7; Figure S39: Structure of compounds 3,4-dihydro-4β,6-dihydroxy-5-methoxy-2α-methyl-1(2H)-naphthalenone, (4S)-4,8-dihydroxy-α-tetralone, (4R)-4,8-dihydroxy-α-tetralone, (4S)-5-hydroxy-4-methoxy-α-tetralone and (4R)- 5-hydroxy-4-methoxy-α-tetralone.

Author Contributions: G.Z. performed the experiments and wrote the paper; T.L., W.Y. and B.S. participated in the experiments; Y.C., B.W. and Y.O. analyzed the data and discussed the results; H.Y. and Z.S. reviewed the manuscript; Z.S. designed and supervised the experiments. All authors have read and agreed to the published version of the manuscript.

Funding: We thank the National Natural Science Foundation of China (U20A2001, 42276114, 82104228), the Key-Area Research and Development Program of Guangdong Province (2020B1111030005), and the GDAS Special Project of Science and Technology Development (Grant No. 2021GDASYL–20210103057) for the generous support.

Data Availability Statement: Data are contained within the article and Supplementary Material.

Conflicts of Interest: The authors declare no conflict of interest.

References

1. Prasher, P.; Sharma, M. Medicinal chemistry of indane and its analogues: A mini review. *ChemistrySelect* **2021**, *6*, 2658–2677. [CrossRef]
2. Nigam, R.; Babu, K.R.; Ghosh, T.; Kumari, B.; Akula, D.; Rath, S.N.; Das, P.; Anindya, R.; Khan, F.A. Indenone derivatives as inhibitor of human DNA dealkylation repair enzyme AlkBH3. *Bioorgan. Med. Chem.* **2018**, *26*, 4100–4112. [CrossRef] [PubMed]
3. Hao, X.D.; Chang, J.; Qin, B.Y.; Zhong, C.; Chu, Z.B.; Huang, J.; Zhou, W.J.; Sun, X. Synthesis, estrogenic activity, and anti-osteoporosis effects in ovariectomized rats of resveratrol oligomer derivatives. *Eur. J. Med. Chem.* **2015**, *102*, 26–38. [CrossRef] [PubMed]
4. Ahn, J.H.; Shin, M.S.; Jung, S.H.; Kang, S.K.; Kim, K.R.; Rhee, S.D.; Jung, W.H.; Yang, S.D.; Kim, S.J.; Woo, J.R.; et al. Indenone Derivatives: A Novel Template for Peroxisome Proliferator-Activated Receptor γ (PPARγ) Agonists. *J. Med. Chem.* **2006**, *49*, 4781–4784. [CrossRef]
5. Liu, J.; Liu, L.; Zheng, L.; Feng, K.W.; Wang, H.T.; Xu, J.P.; Zhou, Z.Z. Discovery of novel 2,3-dihydro-1H-inden-1-ones as dual PDE4/AChE inhibitors with more potency against neuroinflammation for the treatment of Alzheimer's disease. *Eur. J. Med. Chem.* **2022**, *238*, 114503. [CrossRef] [PubMed]
6. Ernst-Russell, M.A.; Chai, C.L.L.; Wardlaw, J.H.; Elix, J.A. Euplectin and Coneuplectin, New Naphthopyrones from the Lichen *Flavoparmelia euplecta*. *J. Nat. Prod.* **2000**, *63*, 129–131. [CrossRef] [PubMed]
7. Li, X.L.; Ru, T.; Navarro-Vázquez, A.; Lindemann, P.; Nazaré, M.; Li, X.W.; Guo, Y.W.; Sun, H. Weizhouochrones: Gorgonian-Derived Symmetric Dimers and Their Structure Elucidation Using Anisotropic NMR Combined with DP4+ Probability and CASE-3D. *J. Nat. Prod.* **2022**, *85*, 1730–1737. [CrossRef]
8. Du, Y.E.; Byun, W.S.; Lee, S.B.; Hwang, S.; Shin, Y.H.; Shin, B.; Jang, Y.J.; Hong, S.; Shin, J.; Lee, S.K.; et al. Formicins, N-Acetylcysteamine-Bearing Indenone Thioesters from a Wood Ant-Associated Bacterium. *Org. Lett.* **2020**, *22*, 5337–5341. [CrossRef]
9. Luo, H.F.; Zhang, L.P.; Hu, C.Q. Five novel oligostilbenes from the roots of *Caragana sinica*. *Tetrahedron* **2001**, *57*, 4849–4854. [CrossRef]
10. Sema, D.K.; Lannang, A.M.; Tatsimo, S.J.N.; Rehman, M.; Yousuf, S.; Zoufou, D.; Iqbal, U.; Wansi, J.D.; Sewald, N.; Choudhary, M.I. New indane and naphthalene derivatives from the rhizomes of *Kniphofia reflexa* Hutchinson ex Codd. *Phytochem. Lett.* **2018**, *26*, 78–82. [CrossRef]
11. Jaki, B.; Heilmann, J.; Sticher, O. New Antibacterial Metabolites from the Cyanobacterium *Nostoc commune* (EAWAG 122b). *J. Nat. Prod.* **2000**, *63*, 1283–1285. [CrossRef]
12. Kim, H.; Yang, I.; Ryu, S.Y.; Won, D.H.; Giri, A.G.; Wang, W.H.; Choi, H.; Chin, J.; Hahn, D.; Kim, E.; et al. Acredinones A and B, Voltage-Dependent Potassium Channel Inhibitors from the Sponge-Derived Fungus *Acremonium* sp. F9A015. *J. Nat. Prod.* **2015**, *78*, 363–367. [CrossRef]
13. Liu, Z.M.; Qiu, P.; Li, J.; Chen, G.Y.; Chen, Y.; Liu, H.J.; She, Z.G. Anti-inflammatory polyketides from the mangrove-derived fungus *Ascomycota* sp. SK2YWS-L. *Tetrahedron* **2018**, *74*, 746–751. [CrossRef]

14. Tan, C.B.; Liu, Z.M.; Chen, S.H.; Huang, X.S.; Cui, H.; Long, Y.H.; Lu, Y.J.; She, Z.G. Antioxidative Polyketones from the Mangrove-Derived Fungus *Ascomycota* sp. SK2YWS-L. *Sci. Rep.* **2016**, *6*, 36609. [CrossRef] [PubMed]
15. Zhong, C.; Liu, X.H.; Chang, J.; Yu, J.M.; Sun, X. Inhibitory effect of resveratrol dimerized derivatives on nitric oxide production in lipopolysaccharide-induced RAW 264.7 cells. *Bioorg. Med. Chem. Lett.* **2013**, *23*, 4413–4418. [CrossRef] [PubMed]
16. Chen, S.H.; Cai, R.L.; Liu, Z.M.; Cui, H.; She, Z.G. Secondary metabolites from mangrove-associated fungi: Source, chemistry and bioactivities. *Nat. Prod. Rep.* **2022**, *39*, 560–595. [CrossRef] [PubMed]
17. Xu, J. Bioactive natural products derived from mangrove-associated microbes. *RSC Adv.* **2015**, *5*, 841–892. [CrossRef]
18. Tan, Q.; Yang, W.C.; Zhu, G.; Chen, T.; Wu, J.; Zhu, Y.J.; Wang, B.; Yuan, J.; She, Z.G. A Pair of Chromone Epimers and an Acetophenone Glucoside from the Mangrove Endophytic Fungus *Mycosphaerella* sp. L3A1. *Chem. Biodivers.* **2022**, *19*, e202200998. [CrossRef]
19. Chen, T.; Yang, W.C.; Li, T.B.; Yin, Y.H.; Liu, Y.F.; Wang, B.; She, Z.G. Hemiacetalmeroterpenoids A–C and Astellolide Q with Antimicrobial Activity from the Marine-Derived Fungus *Penicillium* sp. N-5. *Mar. Drugs* **2022**, *20*, 514. [CrossRef]
20. Chen, Y.; Yang, W.C.; Zou, G.; Wang, G.S.; Kang, W.Y.; Yuan, J.; She, Z.G. Cytotoxic Bromine- and Iodine-Containing Cytochalasins Produced by the Mangrove Endophytic Fungus *Phomopsis* sp. QYM-13 Using the OSMAC Approach. *J. Nat. Prod.* **2022**, *85*, 1229–1238. [CrossRef]
21. Zang, Z.M.; Yang, W.C.; Cui, H.; Cai, R.L.; Li, C.Y.; Zou, G.; Wang, B.; She, Z.G. Two Antimicrobial Heterodimeric Tetrahydroxanthones with a 7,7′-Linkage from Mangrove Endophytic Fungus *Aspergillus flavus* QQYZ. *Molecules* **2022**, *27*, 2691. [CrossRef] [PubMed]
22. Jiang, H.M.; Cai, R.L.; Zang, Z.M.; Yang, W.C.; Wang, B.; Zhu, G.; Yuan, J.; She, Z.G. Azaphilone derivatives with anti-inflammatory activity from the mangrove endophytic fungus *Penicillium sclerotiorum* ZJHJJ-18. *Bioorg. Chem.* **2022**, *122*, 105721. [CrossRef] [PubMed]
23. Liu, H.X.; Liu, Z.M.; Chen, Y.C.; Tan, H.B.; Zhang, W.G.; Zhang, W.M. Polyketones from the endophytic fungus *Cytospora rhizophorae*. *Nat. Prod. Res.* **2021**, *37*, 1053–1059. [CrossRef] [PubMed]
24. Liu, H.X.; Tan, H.B.; Wang, W.X.; Zhang, W.G.; Chen, Y.C.; Liu, S.N.; Liu, Z.M.; Li, H.H.; Zhang, W.M. Cytorhizophins A and B, benzophenone-hemiterpene adducts from the endophytic fungus *Cytospora rhizophorae†*. *Org. Chem. Front.* **2019**, *6*, 591–596. [CrossRef]
25. Auamcharoen, W.; Kijjoa, A.; Chandrapatya, A.; Pinto, M.M.; Silva, A.M.S.; Naengchomnong, W.; Herz, W. A new tetralone from *Diospyros cauliflora*. *Biochem. Syst. Ecol.* **2009**, *37*, 690–692. [CrossRef]
26. Machida, K.; Matsuoka, E.; Kasahara, T.; Kikuchi, M. Studies on the Constituents of *Juglans* Species. I. Structural Determination of (4S)- and (4R)-4-Hydroxy-α-tetralone Derivatives from the Fruit of *Juglans mandshurica* MAXIM. var. *sieboldiana* Makino. *Chem Pharm. Bull.* **2005**, *53*, 934–937. [CrossRef]
27. Chen, Y.; Yang, W.C.; Zou, G.; Chen, S.Y.; Pang, J.Y.; She, Z.G. Bioactive polyketides from the mangrove endophytic fungi *Phoma* sp. SYSUSK-7. *Fitoterapia* **2019**, *139*, 10436. [CrossRef]
28. Qiu, P.; Liu, Z.M.; Chen, Y.; Cai, R.L.; Chen, G.Y.; She, Z.G. Secondary Metabolites with α-Glucosidase Inhibitory Activity from the Mangrove Fungus *Mycosphaerella* sp. SYSU-DZG01. *Mar. Drugs* **2019**, *17*, 483. [CrossRef]
29. Ichikawa, K.; Sasada, R.; Chiba, K.; Gotoh, H. Effect of Side Chain Functional Groups on the DPPH Radical Scavenging Activity of Bisabolane-Type Phenols. *Antioxidants* **2019**, *8*, 65. [CrossRef]
30. Odame, F.; Hosten, E.C.; Betz, R.; Krause, J.; Frost, C.L.; Lobb, K.; Tshentu, Z.R. Synthesis, characterization, computational studies and DPPH scavenging activity of some triazatetracyclic derivatives. *J. Iran. Chem. Soc.* **2021**, *18*, 1979–1995. [CrossRef]

Disclaimer/Publisher's Note: The statements, opinions and data contained in all publications are solely those of the individual author(s) and contributor(s) and not of MDPI and/or the editor(s). MDPI and/or the editor(s) disclaim responsibility for any injury to people or property resulting from any ideas, methods, instructions or products referred to in the content.

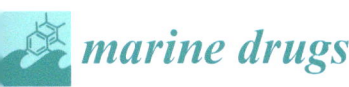

Article

Botryllin, a Novel Antimicrobial Peptide from the Colonial Ascidian *Botryllus schlosseri*

Nicola Franchi [1], Loriano Ballarin [2,*] and Francesca Cima [2]

[1] Department of Life Science, University of Modena and Reggio Emilia, 41125 Modena, Italy
[2] Department of Biology, University of Padova, 35131 Padova, Italy
* Correspondence: loriano.ballarin@unipd.it

Abstract: By mining the transcriptome of the colonial ascidian *Botryllus schlosseri*, we identified a transcript for a novel styelin-like antimicrobial peptide, which we named botryllin. The gene is constitutively transcribed by circulating cytotoxic morula cells (MCs) as a pre-propeptide that is then cleaved to mature peptide. The synthetic peptide, obtained from in silico translation of the transcript, shows robust killing activity of bacterial and unicellular yeast cells, causing breakages of both the plasma membrane and the cell wall. Specific monoclonal antibodies were raised against the epitopes of the putative amino acid sequence of the propeptide and the mature peptide; in both cases, they label the MC granular content. Upon MC degranulation induced by the presence of nonself, the antibodies recognise the extracellular nets with entrapped bacteria nearby MC remains. The obtained results suggest that the botryllin gene carries the information for the synthesis of an AMP involved in the protection of *B. schlosseri* from invading foreign cells.

Keywords: antimicrobial peptides; ascidians; *Botryllus*; haemocytes; tunicates

1. Introduction

The increasing and indiscriminate use of antibiotics in industrialised countries has led to such a wide diffusion of resistant pathogens [1], the World Health Organisation (WHO) stated that the problem cannot be neglected anymore, and coordinated and global efforts are required to overcome it [2]. Within this context, a promising approach can derive from the study of the antimicrobial peptides (AMPs), components of innate immunity, widely diffuse in invertebrates and vertebrates, showing a high degree of convergent evolution in terms of primary, secondary, and tertiary structure and biological roles [3]. They are a class of small proteins, a few dozen amino acids long and less than 10 kDa in molecular weight, containing structurally segregated hydrophilic (mostly cationic) and hydrophobic residues. The latter enable the interaction with microbial plasma membrane and alter the integrity of the phospholipid bilayer [4–9]. Therefore, they induce, directly or indirectly, the lysis of the target cells [6,9–11]; in addition, some of them permeabilise the plasma membrane and allow the entry of other AMPs with intracellular targets [12]. This assures an effective protection against microorganisms associated with weak or no microbial resistance [13,14]. AMPs can be broadly divided into linear (further subdivided into alpha-helix, all beta, beta hairpin, and non-regular) and cyclical peptides [3]. They play a fundamental role in the innate immune responses of multicellular organisms, exerting antiviral and antifungal activity, in addition to their antibacterial properties [9,11,15]. Furthermore, AMPs can modulate the activity of the immune system [16], hamper cancer development [17], shape the gut microbiota [18], and exert control on bacterial endosymbionts [19–22].

Marine invertebrates represent the largest biodiversity of multicellular eukaryotes. They are a rich source of natural products [23–25], including AMPs [25,26]. Tunicates (phylum Chordata) are considered the sister group of vertebrates [27]. Ascidians are the most abundant tunicate group, with 2300 of the 3000 known species included in this taxon. Many

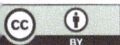

families of cytotoxic compounds from tunicates have been described [28]. They include alkaloids, polyketides, cyanobactines (cyclic peptides produced by symbiotic bacteria), and AMPs [25,29,30]. The last are mainly produced by circulating haemocytes. Styelins A and E of *Styela clava* contain 32 amino acids with an abundance of phenylalanine and various modified residues [31]. They are synthesised by cytotoxic granulocytes [31] and show similarities with the cecropins, described in Diptera and Lepidoptera [32]. Clavanins A-E and clavaspirin are histidine-rich, 23 amino-acid-long peptides also synthesised and released by circulating cytotoxic cells of *S. clava* [33,34]. The octapeptideplicatamide is an AMP synthesised by the haemocytes of the congeneric species *Styela plicata* [35]. Halocyamines A and B of *Halocynthia roretzi* are tetrapeptides produced by circulating cytotoxic cells [36]; their diphenol rings represent suitable substrates for the enzyme phenoloxidase (PO), which explains their cytotoxic activity. Indeed, PO, by oxidizing the polyphenol substrata produces reactive oxygen species and induces oxidative stress [37]. In *Ciona intestinalis* and *Ciona robusta*, two types of α-helix-AMPs are synthesised by cytotoxic haemocytes; the corresponding genes enhance their transcription upon the injection of nonself material in the body wall [38–41]. In some cases, AMPs are produced by symbiotic bacteria. For instance, didemnins are cyclic depsipeptides with antimicrobial activity isolated from species of the genus *Trididemnum*, with a molecular weight ranging from 0.94 to 1.1 kDa and synthesised by endosymbiotic α-proteobacteria of the genus *Tistrella* [42–44].

Botryllus schlosseri is a colonial ascidian living in shallow waters of all the seas and oceans. It represents a widely used model for studies of tunicate immunobiology [45]. As an invertebrate, it relies only on innate immunity for its defence, and circulating immunocytes are the main effectors of immune responses. The latter include phagocytes and cytotoxic morula cells (MCs) [46]. Phagocytes exert their immunosurveillance activity by ingesting foreign material having entered the circulation, whereas MCs induce inflammation and cytotoxicity upon the recognition of nonself molecules [45]. MCs are also the main source of various complement components [47–49] and influence the activity of phagocytes [45,50,51]. In this work, we report on the identification, by mining the *B. schlosseri* transcriptome, of a transcript for a putative styelin-like AMP that we named botryllin, which is actively transcribed by MCs. The synthetic peptide, obtained from in silico translation of the transcript, exerts a toxic activity towards bacterial and unicellular yeast cells. Specific antibodies raised against epitopes of the putative amino acid sequence of the propeptide and the mature peptide label the MC granular content. The same antibody, upon MC degranulation induced by the presence of foreign cells, recognises the extracellular traps nearby MC remains. Collectively, the obtained results suggest that the botryllin gene carries the information for the synthesis of a novel AMP involved in the protection of *B. schlosseri* from invading foreign cells.

2. Results

2.1. Botryllin Identification

By BLAST analysis of our B. schlosseri EST collection and 3′ RACE, we identified a transcript for a protein with similarity (33.3% identity) to *S. clava* styelins D and E, based on phylogenetic analysis. The protein was named botryllin, and the sequence of the transcript was deposited in Genbank under the accession number OP851480 and was confirmed by alignment with the *B. schlosseri* genome. The gene organisation and the transcript sequences are reported in Supplementary Figure S1. It codifies for a pre-propeptide of 158 amino acids, with a putative molecular weight of 18.11 kDa and a signal peptide of 23 residues. Analogously to styelins A–E from *S. clava* [32], the botryllin propeptide is likely split to the mature peptide of 37 amino acids that closely resembles the *S. clava* styelins (identity values ranging from 30 to 37.5%; Figure 1a). The deduced molecular weight of the mature peptide is 4.35 kDa, with a net positive charge, at pH 7.0, of 11.2.

According to CFSSP and PSIPRED prediction, 56.8% of the mature peptide has an alpha-helix secondary structure with a well-supported confidence of prediction (amino acids 4–10 and 22–35), whereas the prediction of a third alpha-helix domain (amino acids

14–16; 5.4% of the mature peptide) is not well supported (Figure 1b). PEP-FOLD3 predicted the 3D structure reported in Figure 1c. AMPA analysis supports its belonging to AMPs, with a mean antimicrobial value of 0.193, close to the value of Drosophila cecropin B.

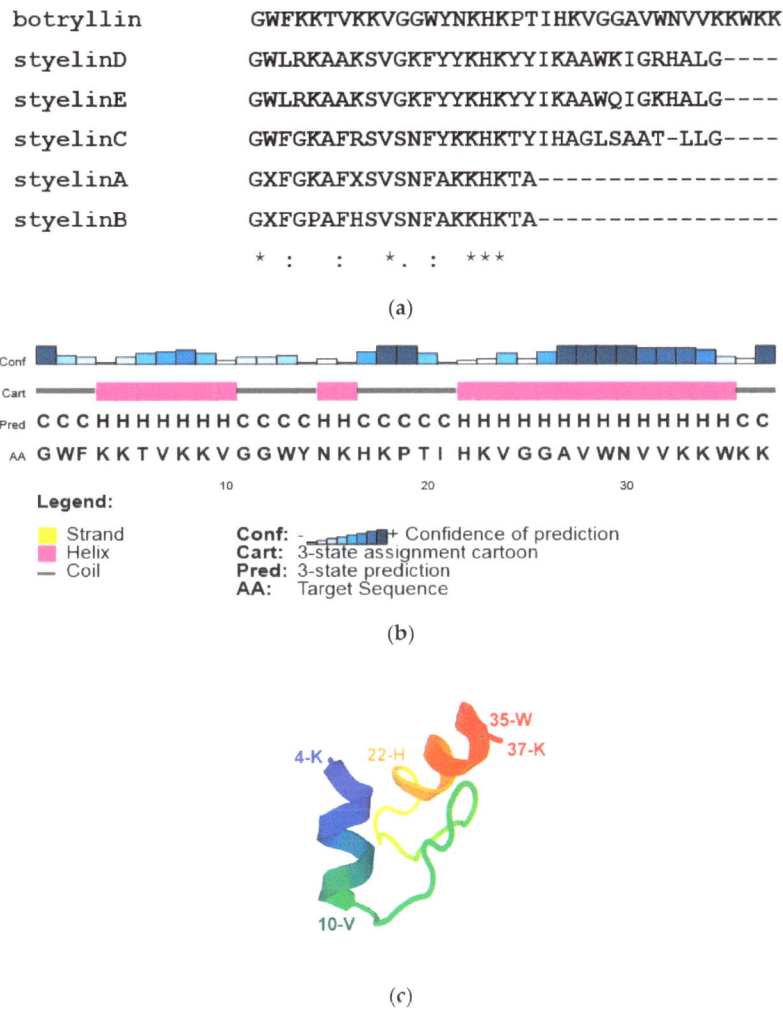

Figure 1. (a) Alignment of *B. schlosseri* botryllin and *S. clava* styelins. (b,c) Predicted structures of botryllin. (b) Secondary structure according to PSIPRED analysis. (c) 3D structure according to PEP-FOLD3.

2.2. Transcription Rate of the Botryllin Gene

Quantitative RT PCR analysis indicated no significant changes in the transcription rate of the botryllin gene up to 4 h of exposure to bacterial lipopolysaccharide (LPS; serotype 055:B5 from *E. coli*), *Bacillus clausii* cells, or zymosan particles from yeast cell walls for immune stimulation (data not shown).

2.3. Botryllin Has an Antimicrobial/Antimycotic Activity

The values of the minimal inhibitory concentration (MIC) and minimal bactericidal concentration (MBC) for the four bacterial strains and yeast cells are reported in Table 1. They suggest a real antimicrobial and antimycotic activity of the synthetic peptide, which is able to interfere with microorganism proliferation at relatively low concentrations, with the lowest value of MIC (3.1 µg mL^{-1}) for both the two Gram-positive species (B. clausii and *Staphylococcus epidermidis*). Only with the Gram-negative species *Escherichia coli*, the MIC value amounted to 50 µg mL^{-1}, whereas it resulted to 6.3 µg mL^{-1} in the case of *Proteus mirabilis* and *Saccharomyces cerevisiae* (Table 1).

Table 1. MIC and MBC values of botryllin on four bacterial strains and yeast cells.

Microorganism	MIC (µg mL^{-1})	MBC (µg mL^{-1})
Bacillus clausii	3.1	>50.0
Staphylococcus epidermidis	3.1	12.5
Escherichia coli	50.0	>50.0
Proteus mirabilis	6.3	>50.0
Saccharomyces cerevisiae	6.3	12.5

The peptide was also able to prevent bacterial and fungal growth when the microbial strains were re-suspended in Brain Heart Broth Infusion (BHI), indicating a potential biocidal activity. The highest potential bactericidal and fungicidal activities have been observed for *S. epidermidis* and *S. cerevisiae*, respectively, which showed the lowest value of MBC (12.5 µg mL^{-1}), whereas the MBC resulted higher than 50 µg mL^{-1} in all the other cases (Table 1).

The antimicrobial activity of botryllin was also assayed at various physico-chemical conditions, such as temperature, pH, and ionic strength, to determine the optimum and the resistance/decrease capability of the peptide (Table 2). In these experiments, *S. epidermidis* was chosen as a target strain for its sensitivity, as deduced on the basis of both MIC and MBC values. The predicted melting temperature (Tm) of botryllin, i.e., the temperature value at which half of its amino acids become destructured, resulted higher than 65 °C as the amino acid sequence has a Tm index of 3.44. In agreement with the prediction, the antimicrobial activity of the peptide was not influenced by heating up to 100 °C, with a MIC value of 12.5 µg mL^{-1} after heating for 2 h at 60 °C and 80 °C, and of 6.3 µg mL^{-1} after heating for 15 min at 100 °C. The peptide is more active at pH 7.0, 8.0, and 9.0 (MIC value: 12.5 µg mL^{-1}) with respect to lower pH. At pH 6.0, the MIC value was 50 µg mL^{-1} whereas at pH 5.0, the concentration required was higher than 50 µg mL^{-1}. No MIC was determined at pH 4.0, as bacteria were not able to grow in this acidic condition (Table 2). As for the effects of the increasing ionic strength in the medium, the presence of 150 mM NaCl did not affect the antimicrobial activity (MIC value: 12.5 µg mL^{-1}), whereas it was progressively decreased by increasing salt concentrations (25 and 50 µg mL^{-1} at 300 and 600 mM NaCl, respectively).

Table 2. MIC values of botryllin towards *S. epidermidis* at various temperatures, pH values, and ionic strength.

Temperature (°C)			pH				Ionic Strength [NaCl] (mM)		
60 (2 h)	80 (2 h)	100 (15 min)	6.0	7.0	8.0	9.0	150	300	600
12.5	12.5	6.3	50.0	12.5	12.5	12.5	12.5	25.0	50.0

2.4. Botryllin Increases the Mortality of Bacterial and Yeast Cells

After 20 h of incubation in the presence of 6.25 µg mL^{-1} synthetic botryllin, 3 of the 4 bacterial strains (*B. clausii*, *E. coli*, and *P. mirabilis*) showed a significant ($p < 0.05$) increase in cell mortality (more than 60%, around 50%, and less than 40%, respectively). No significant differences were observed in the case of *S. epidermidis*. At 25 µg mL^{-1} all the bacterial strains showed significant ($p < 0.05$) higher mortality than the controls: it amounted to more than 60% for *B. clausii* and *E. coli*, and to a value around 50% for *S. epidermidis* and *P. mirabilis* (Figure 2a–d,f). Yeast cells were also killed by synthetic botryllin, with a significant ($p < 0.05$) difference with respect to the controls at 25 µg mL^{-1} (around 30% of dead cells) (Figure 2e,g). The presence of anti-botryllin Ab2 antibody partially reduced the negative effect of botryllin (25 µg mL^{-1}) in the case of *B. clausii* and *E. coli*, whereas it completely inhibited the effect in the case of *S. epidermidis* and *P. mirabilis* and yeast cells (Figure 2a–e).

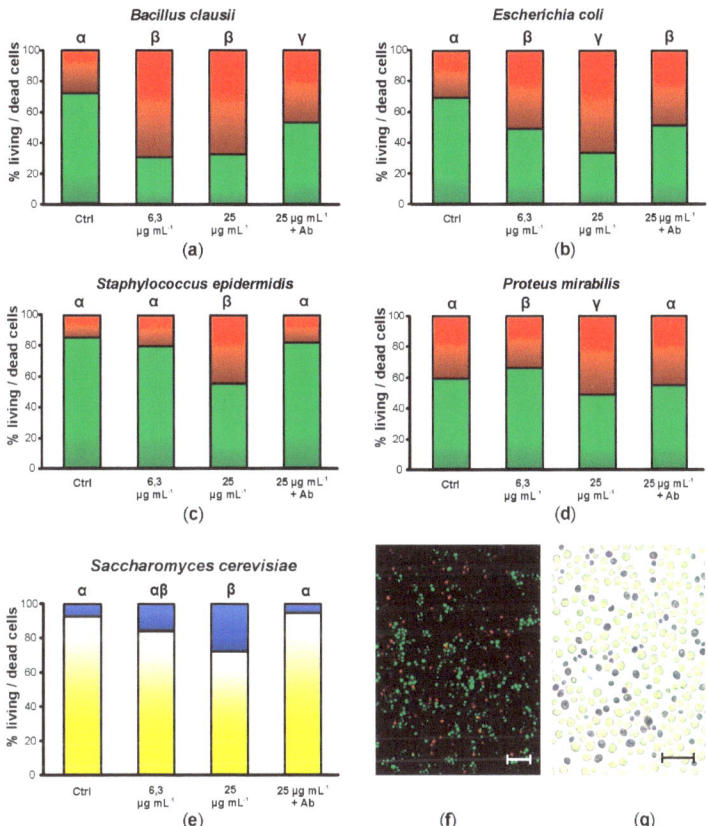

Figure 2. Mortality assay in the presence of botryllin. (**a–d**) Percentage of living (green) and dead (red) bacterial cells after 20 h of incubation in the presence of 6.3 and 25 µg mL^{-1} of synthetic botryllin, and 25 µg mL^{-1} of botryllin pre-incubated for 30 min with 10 µg mL^{-1} of anti-botryllin Ab2 antibody, as evaluated with the LIVE/DEAD BacLight Bacterial Viability kit; (**e**) percentage of living (yellow) and dead (blue) yeast cells after the treatments described above, evaluated with the Trypan Blue exclusion assay; (**f**) *S. epidermidis* cells labelled with the LIVE/DEAD after the exposure to 25 µg mL^{-1} of synthetic botryllin: dead cells appear red; (**g**) *S. cerevisiae* cells treated with Trypan Blue after the exposure to 25 µg mL^{-1} of synthetic botryllin: dead cells appear blue. Statistically significant ($p < 0.05$) differences in (**a–e**) are marked by different Greek letters on the top of the bars. Scale bars: 6 µm in (**f**), 30 µm in (**g**).

2.5. Botryllin Causes Irreversible Morphological Alterations of Microbial and Yeast Cells

Control microbial cells show a tight adhesion of the plasma membrane to the cell wall and a dense cytoplasm, with some paler regions corresponding to the nucleoid; some cells are dividing (Figure 3a,c and Figure 4a,e). The exposure to synthetic botryllin led to evident alterations to the cell morphology. At the concentration of 6.3 µg mL^{-1}, the peptide induced, in *B. clausii*, the detachment of the cell wall and the disassembly of the peptidoglycans that appear as a series of filaments protruding from the remains of the former. The plasma membrane appeared damaged with the consequent release of cytoplasmic material (Figure 3b). At 6.3 µg mL^{-1}, *S. epidermidis* cells showed the presence of numerous invaginations of the plasma membrane (Figure 3d), whereas at 25 µg mL^{-1} cell lysis was observed with disruption of the cell wall and the release of the cellular content (Figure 3e). At 6.3 µg mL^{-1}, *E. coli* cells underwent a general shrinkage of the cytoplasm with the increase of the periplasmic space, between the plasma membrane and the cell wall, and the condensation of the DNA, which appeared adherent to the plasma membrane (Figure 4b). At 25 µg mL^{-1}, the periplasmic space was generally increased, and many cells showed a damaged wall and the release of the cell content (Figure 4c,d). In *P. mirabilis*, a clear effect was observed at the concentration of the peptide of 25 µg mL^{-1} DNA condensed along the plasma membrane, the periplasmic space increased, and the cell wall lost its integrity (Figure 4f).

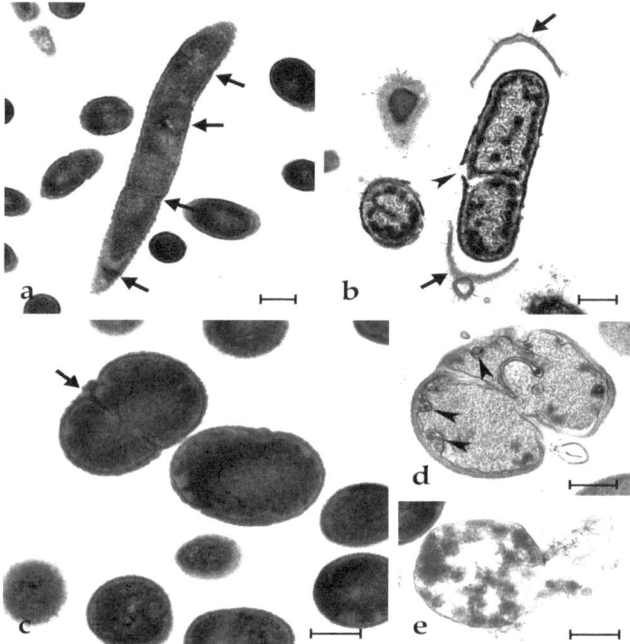

Figure 3. Transmission electron micrographs of *B. clausii* (**a,b**) and *S. epidermidis* (**c–e**) cells (**a,c**) Control (untreated) cells: arrows indicate cleavage furrows; (**b**) *B. clausii* cells after exposure to 25 µg mL^{-1} of synthetic botryllin. Arrows show the detachment of the cell wall and the arrowhead indicates the breakage of the plasma membrane; (**d,e**) *S. epidermidis* cells after the exposure to botryllin at the concentration of 6.3 and 25 µg mL^{-1}, respectively. Arrowheads in (**d**) indicate plasma membrane invaginations. Note in (**e**) the cell lysis after exposure to the highest peptide concentration Scale bars: 0.5 µm.

In the case of *S. cerevisiae*, control cells showed a normal budding activity (Figure 5a) which was not reported at 6.3 µg mL^{-1} of peptide. At this concentration, many vesicles appeared in the cytoplasm, which also resulted in less electron density than in controls; in addition, mitochondria showed an extensive altered morphology of cristae and an electron dense matrix (Figure 5b). At the peptide concentration of 25 µg mL^{-1}, the cytoplasm shrunk, and the plasma membrane detached from the cell wall, a giant vacuole appeared in the cytoplasm, mitochondria disappeared, and the nucleus fragmented in a series of electron dense spots of condensed chromatin (Figure 5c).

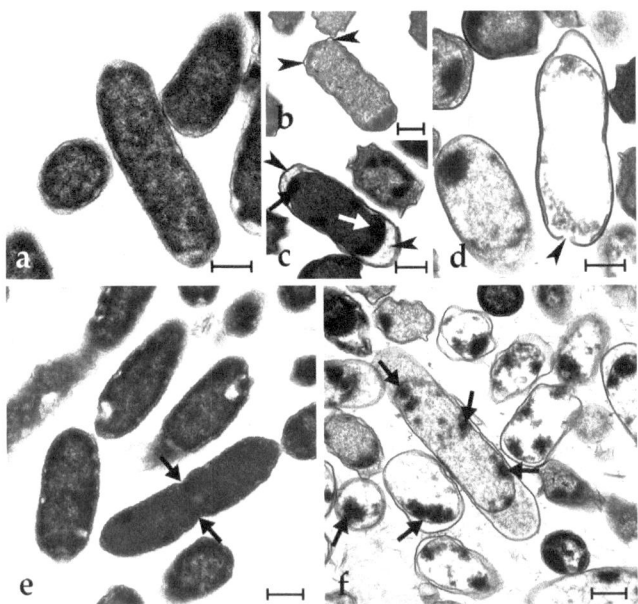

Figure 4. Transmission electron micrographs of *E. coli* (**a–d**) and *P. mirabilis* (**e,f**) cells. (**a,e**) Control (untreated) cells: arrows indicate a cleavage furrow; (**b–d**) *E. coli* cells after exposure to 6.3 (**b**) and 25 (**c,d**) µg mL^{-1} of synthetic botryllin. Arrowheads indicate the enlargement of the periplasmic space whereas arrow marks condensed DNA adherent to the plasma membrane; (**f**) *P. mirabilis* cells after the exposure to botryllin at the concentration of 25 µg mL^{-1}. Arrows indicate unusual DNA condensation along the periphery of the cell. Scale bars: 0.5 µm.

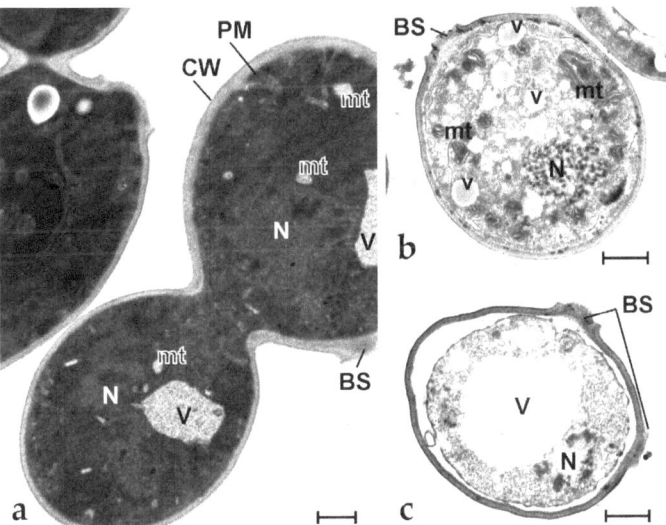

Figure 5. Transmission electron micrographs of *S. cerevisiae* cells. (**a**) Control (untreated) dividing cells; (**b,c**) Yeast cells after exposure to 6.3 µg mL^{-1} of synthetic botryllin. BS: budding scar; CW: cell wall; mt: mitochondrion; N: nucleus; V: vacuole; v: small vesicle. Scale bars: 1 µm.

2.6. Botryllin Is Synthesised by MC, Stored Inside Their Granules and Released upon MC Degranulation

In situ hybridization (ISH) analysis indicates that MCs are the only cells transcribing the *botryllin* gene (Figure 6a,b). The monoclonal anti-botryllin antibodies Ab1, Ab2, and Ab3 stained the granular content of MCs, indicating that the protein is stored inside MC granules (Figure 6c). The antibodies stained no other haemocyte type or tissue. This is further supported by observations under the TEM showing labelling inside the granules of MCs and of granular amoebocytes, the latter considered the MC precursors [46] (Figure 7a–d). Upon the exposure to microbial cells, MCs change their morphology and undergo degranulation: they release in the environment material that is recognised by the three antibodies and contributes to the formation of extracellular traps (ETs) found around MCs (Figure 6d,e). Electron microscopic analysis clearly indicates that immunopositivity to antibodies against the mature peptide (Ab1) is located in the fibrillary material released by MCs (Figure 7e), clearly indicating that active botryllin is a constituent of the extracellular traps formed by degranulating MCs.

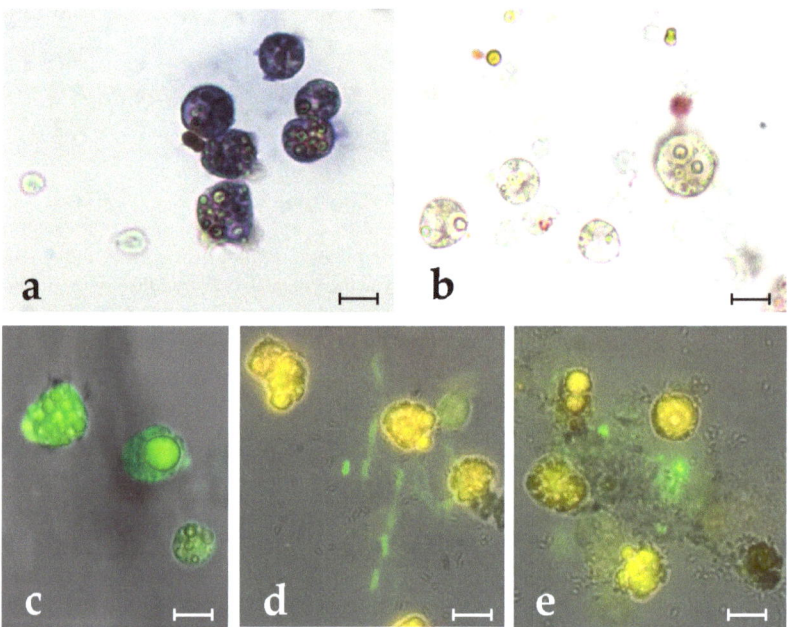

Figure 6. (**a,b**) ISH on *Botryllus* haemocytes with botryllin riboprobe. (**a**) Antisense probe positive cells, represented by MCs, stain blue; (**b**) Sense probe: MCs appear unstained (**c–e**) Immunofluorescence of haemocyte smears incubated with anti-botryllin Ab1 (**c,d**) and Ab3 (**e**) antibodies. (**c**) Immunopositive (green fluorescence) control MCs; (**d,e**) Immunopositive (green fluorescence) fibrillary material, forming extracellular traps, released in the presence of microbial cells (*S. epidermidis*), by MCs that appear unlabelled by the anti-botryllin antibody and only show the typical yellow autofluorescence of their vacuolar polyphenolic content. Scale bars: 10 µm.

2.7. B. clausii-Conditioned Medium (CM) Has Biocidal Activity That Is Inhibited by Anti-Botryllin Antibodies

B. clausii-derived CM significantly ($p < 0.05$) enhanced the fraction of dead *B. clausii* cells with respect to control. Analogously, the addition of synthetic botryllin at the concentration of 25 µg mL^{-1} led to a significant ($p < 0.05$) decrease of live cells. This increase was prevented by the addition of the anti-botryllin Ab2 or Ab3 antibodies, but not by preimmune mouse serum (Figure 8).

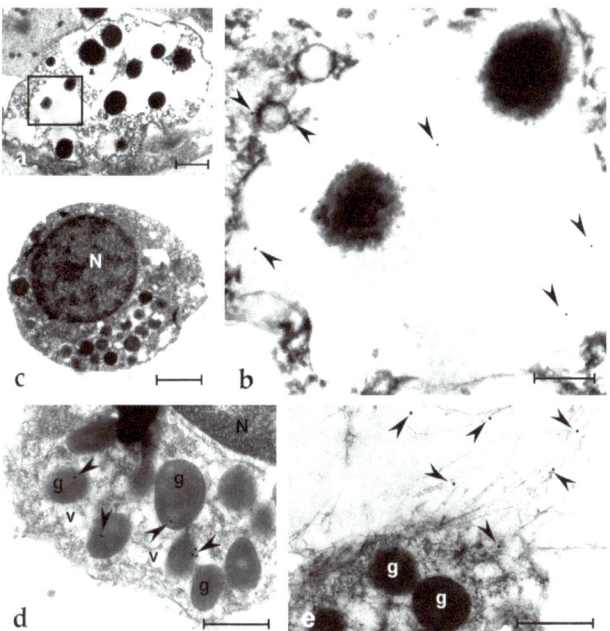

Figure 7. TEM micrographs of *Botryllus* haemocytes treated with the Ab1 anti-botryllin antibody; immunogold technique. (**a**) MC with large granules containing electron-dense material. An enlargement of the squared region is shown in (**b**), where some gold spherules (arrowheads) are visible. (**c**) A granular amoebocyte, precursor of MC, with the electron-dense granules; (**d**) Detail of a cytoplasmic region of a granular amoebocytes with labelled granules (arrowheads); (**e**) Immunopositive (arrowheads) extracellular fibrillary material released by MCs. g: granule; N: nucleus; v: small vesicle. Scale bars: 2 µm in (**a**), 0.5 µm in (**b**,**d**,**e**); 1 µm in (**c**).

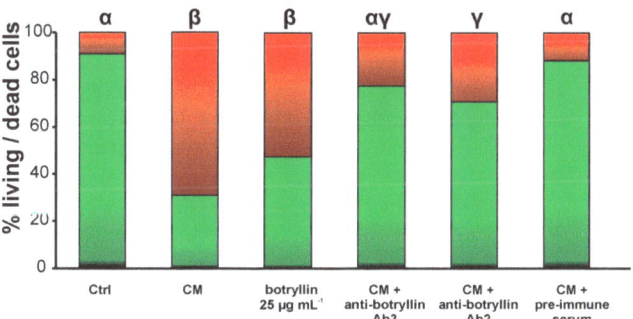

Figure 8. Percentage of living (green) and dead (red) *B. clausii* cells after 20 h of incubation in the presence of CM from *B. clausii*-exposed haemocytes, botryllin (25 µg mL^{-1}), CM plus anti-botryllin Ab2 or Ab3 antibodies, CM plus pre-immune mouse serum. Cell mortality was evaluated with the LIVE/DEAD BacLight Bacterial Viability kit. Significant ($p < 0.05$) differences among the various conditions are expressed with different letters.

3. Discussion

AMPs represent a widespread component of innate immunity and an ancient defence strategy assuring the survival of organisms by preventing the entry and the spreading of potentially pathogenic microorganisms. Since they interact directly with the plasma membrane of the foreign cells, the development of a resistance by microorganisms is quite rare [9,11,15,52]. This led to an increasing interest in this class of molecules for their possible application in the biomedical field, which is currently hampered by their potential cytotoxicity, the high costs of production, and limited information on their bacteriostatic and bactericidal activity [3,53].

The colonial ascidian B. schlosseri is a reliable organism for the study of tunicate innate immunity, and various humoral factors involved in the protection from foreign cells have been identified so far, including the enzyme PO [54–56], a rhamnose-binding lectin with opsonic properties [57,58] and various complement components modulating the immune responses [47–49,59].

Two main immunocyte types are present in the B. schlosseri haemolymph: phagocytes and MCs [46,60]. The latter are the most abundant circulating haemocytes [46] and the first circulating cells sensing the presence of nonself [61]. They are large cells (≥ 10 μm in diameter), with the cytoplasm filled with many granules, uniform in size (around 2 μm in diameter) and containing the enzyme PO, responsible for the cytotoxic activity characterising these cells, and its polyphenol substrata [46]. As a consequence of the nonself recognition, MCs release cytokines, recruiting other immunocytes at the infection site, and undergo degranulation, with the release of their granular content [45]. The enzyme PO, acting on the polyphenol substrata, produces reactive oxygen species that induce a condition of oxidative stress in the nearby cells, responsible for the cytotoxic activity of MCs [55,62–64]. Among the released granular material, the protein p102 forms a network of amyloid fibres that contribute to the formation of extracellular traps able to prevent the spreading of microbes inside the colonial circulation [65].

In the present work, we identified, in the B. schlosseri transcriptome, a transcript for a peptide showing similarity with styelins D and E from S. clava [31,32,66], a solitary ascidian belonging to the clade Styelidae that includes also the genus Botryllus. Investigating the available transcriptomes and genome of B. schlosseri, we identified three similar sequences from only one transcriptome. They differ in a few nucleotides, both at the coding sequences and untranslated regions. The high sequence variability found in B. schlosseri was already noticed (e.g., [57]). This, together with a still highly fragmented genome, does not allow us to ascertain whether the above sequences are the result of a recent gene duplication or, more likely, are attributable to isoforms and not to different paralogous genes. Future studies will be aimed at the resolution of this problem.

The primary sequence of the mature peptide was obtained by in silico translation of the identified transcript, and the obtained amino acid sequence was compared with those of styelins. Our peptide, which we named botryllin, and styelins share a high percentage of identity (higher than 30%) and the full conservation of some amino acids and the KHK motif. The synthetic peptide was constructed on the mature peptide sequence and used for functional analyses.

We studied the MIC and the MBC of the synthetic peptide towards two Gram-positive and two Gram-negative bacteria species. In agreement with the computer prediction, botryllin shows in vitro antimicrobial activity against the target bacterial cells, as well as towards baker's yeast cells. TEM analysis clearly indicates that synthetic botryllin induces severe morphological alterations in the tested microorganisms, ultimately leading to their death. However, it is conceivable that botryllin, analogously to styelin [67], has a broader spectrum of antimicrobial activity against a wide range of marine microorganisms that were not tested in the present study as they cannot be reared under laboratory conditions. In addition, similarly to styelins [66], various amino acids can be post-translationally modified so to further enhance the antimicrobial activity of the peptide. To verify this point, the biochemical purification of botryllin from the haemolymph of large colonies of B. schlosseri is required, and this will be a goal of our future research.

To evaluate the possible use of botryllin in a biotechnological or pharmaceutical context, we considered the resistance to denaturation at different temperatures and pHs. Thermal and pH stability are important, for instance, in treatments to get safe food without altering its taste, nutritional value, or colour [68,69]. Botryllin appears to be a stable molecule at different pHs and in a wide range of temperatures. This suggests a possible use of botryllin, once synthesised in large amounts in the laboratory, as a novel antibacterial compound in the pharmaceutical, medical, or veterinary fields, with a possible use in acid environments, such as the gastric lumen, where other AMPs can be denatured [67]. Its salt tolerance, as resulted from the experiments carried out at different ionic strengths, suggests its possible use as a new component of antifouling paints to be used in seawater without risks for the marine environment. Furthermore, the tolerance of botryllin to elevated salt concentrations can be exploited in those human pathologies, such as cystic fibrosis, characterised by high salt concentrations in the liquids moistening the lung cavities. The latter reduce defence responses and enhance the colonization of salt-resistant bacteria, such as *Pseudomonas aeruginosa* and *Staphylococcus aureus*, which can represent a serious risk for the life of patients [70]. However, studies on the cytotoxicity of botryllin towards mammalian cells and tissues are lacking, and this will be another aim of our future research.

Results obtained with the CM indicate that molecules with biocidal activity are released by haemocytes upon the recognition of microbes or, likely, also soluble nonself molecules. The significant decrease of the CM cytotoxic activity in the presence of anti-botryllin antibodies suggests that botryllin is present in the material(s) released by haemocytes.

ISH clearly indicates that botryllin is synthesised by MCs, the only immunocytes type actively transcribing the botryllin gene. The peptide is initially synthesised as a pre-propeptide of 158 amino acids, provided with a signal peptide of 23 residues, whereas the mature peptide results to 37 amino acids long, with a 3D structure including two short alpha helices. Immunocytochemical analysis indicates that it is stored inside MC granules; as stated above, upon the exposure to nonself, MCs degranulate and release their granular content, botryllin included. The absence of significant changes in the transcription level upon haemocyte exposure to nonself suggests that the increase in the molecule concentration in the infection sites is obtained by its release from the storage sites (MC granules), rather than through an increase in gene transcription. In addition, the labelling of MC granules by the Ab3 antibody, recognizing a propeptide epitope not included in the mature peptide, suggests that MC granules host the propeptide. Since the Ab3 antibody recognizes also the extracellular traps, we can suppose that its conversion to the mature peptide occurs in the extracellular environment, once the MC granular content has been released, through enzymatic proteolysis. In agreement with this hypothesis, we recently demonstrated the presence of the peptidase furin inside MC granules [65].

MC degranulation is usually associated with cytotoxicity and local cell death due to the contemporary release of the enzyme PO that, upon the oxidation of polyphenol substrata, produces reactive oxygen species (ROS; [63]). Interestingly, styelins (and probably botryllin) are DOPA-containing polypeptides [66] that can represent natural substrates of PO. This suggests that botryllin could exert its antimicrobial activity through both the alteration of the microbial plasma membrane, as reported for the majority of AMPs, and the production of ROS when oxidized by PO. Once released, botryllin is entangled in the net of amyloid material derived from the MC granular content [65] and becomes a constituent of the extracellular traps in order to increase the local concentration of AMP that helps in facing foreign cells and preventing their spreading in the circulation.

MCs are the effector cells of the allorejection reaction between contacting incompatible colonies [62,64]. As a consequence of the recognition of some still unknown content of the haemolymph plasma diffusing from the alien colony through the partially-fused tunics, they move towards the ampullae (the peripheral, sausage-like, blind endings of the circulation), facing the alien colony. Then, they migrate into the tunic and degranulate, contributing to the formation of the melanic, necrotic spots characterising the reaction [45,64]. It is conceivable that, as in the case of the recognition of microbes, botryllin is released also during the allorejection-associated degranulation, acting as a possible substrate for PO. This aspect, not yet investigated, suggests a possible role of the peptide in the protection from microbial invasion in the course of the allorejection reaction, during which the epithelium of the facing ampullar tips appear highly altered with the appearance of large fenestrations [71]. Future efforts will, therefore, also be aimed at investigating the possible role of botryllin in the allorejection reaction of B. schlosseri.

4. Materials and Methods

4.1. Animals

Colonies of B. schlosseri, collected near the marine station of the Department of Biology University of Padova, in Chioggia (Southern part of the Lagoon of Venice), were attached to glass slides, transferred in aerated aquaria at a constant temperature of 19 °C and 12 h:12 h of light:dark. They were fed with unicellular algae (Dunaliella sp., Tetraselmis sp.).

4.2. Haemocyte Collection

The peripheral vessel of colonies, previously blotted dry, was punctured with a fine tungsten needle; flowing haemolymph was collected with a glass micropipette and transferred in a 1.5-mL vial. It was spun at 780× g at 4 °C for 10 min, and the supernatant was discarded. Pelleted haemocytes were re-suspended in filtered seawater (FSW) to the final concentration of 5×10^6 cells mL^{-1}.

4.3. Primer Design, RNA Extraction, cDNA Synthesis, Cloning, and Sequencing

Total RNA was isolated from colonies of B. schlosseri and haemocytes with the RNA NucleoSpin RNA XS (Macherey–Nagel, Düren, Germany) kit, and its quality was determined by the $A_{260/280}$ ratio and visualised in Midori green (Nippon GeneticsEurope Gmbh, Düren, Germany)-stained 1.5% agarose gels. The first strand of cDNA was reverse transcribed from 1 µg of total RNA at 42 °C for 1 h in a 20 µL reaction mixture containing 1 µL of ImPromII Reverse Transcriptase (Promega, Madison, WI, USA) and 0.5 µg oligo(dT)-Anchor primer or random primers (Promega, Madison, WI, USA).

The primers reported in Table 3 were used for PCR reactions in a 25 µL reaction volume containing 1 µL of cDNA from B. schlosseri colonies, 2.5 µL of 10× incubation buffer (PCRBIO Classic Taq, PCR BIOSYSTEMS, London, UK) with 15 mM MgCl$_2$, 0.25 µM of each primer, 10 mM of each of the deoxynucleotide triphosphates, and 2 units of Taq polymerase. PCR was performed on a MyCycler (BioRad; Hercules, CA, USA) thermocycler with the following conditions: 94 °C for 2 min, then 40 cycles of 94 °C for 30 s, 55–60 °C for 30 s, 72 °C for 60 s, and 72 °C for 10 min. Amplicons were separated by electrophoresis on 1.5% agarose gel, and the corresponding bands were purified with the ULTRAPrep Agarose Gel Extraction Mini Prep kit (AHN Biotechnologie, Nordhausen Germany), ligated in pGEM-T Easy Vector (Promega, Madison, WI, USA), and cloned in DH-5α E. coli cells. Positively screened clones were Sanger sequenced at Eurofins Genomics (Ebersberg, Germany) on an ABI 3730XL Applied Biosystems apparatus (Life Technologies Europe BV, Monza, Italy). The 3′-rapid amplification of the cDNA ends (RACE) was performed using the 2nd Generation of the 5′/3′RACE Kit (Roche, Basel, Switzerland) In order to obtain the 3′ sequence of botryllin cDNA, the same forward primers used for RT-PCR and probe synthesis (Table 3) were used for nested PCR with anchor reverse primer according to the manufacturer's instructions.

Table 3. Primers used in the present work.

Primer	Sequence
Botryllin forward	CTGGTTTCTCCAATAACG
Botryllin reverse1	CAAGGTCATATTGGTGGCTA
Botryllin reverse2	GTCGAAGCTGTGCAAGACAT
Botryllin-qRT PCR For	GGTCGGGGGATGGTATAAT
Botryllin-qRT PCR Rev	ACCATCGTATTCGTCCCG
BsEF1-alpha qPCR For	GCCGCCATACTCTGAAGC
BsEF1-alpha qPCR Rev	GTCCAACTGGCACTGTTCC
Botryllin ISH For	GGTCGGGGGATGGTATAAT
Botryllin ISH Rev	CAAGGTCATATTGGTGGCTA

4.4. Three-Dimensional Structure of Botryllin

After in silico translation of the identified transcript with Expasy (https://web.expasy.org/translate/ (accessed on 23 October 2022)), the secondary structure of the peptide was predicted using CFSSP (http://www.biogem.org/tool/chou-fasman (accessed on 25 October 2022)) and PSIPRED (http://bioinf.cs.ucl.ac.uk/psipred (accessed on 25 October 2022)). The sequence was submitted to PEP-FOLD3 (https://bioserv.rpbs.univ-paris-diderot.fr/services/PEP-FOLD3 (accessed on 23 October 2022)) for the prediction of the 3D structure. AMPA (antimicrobial sequence scanning system; http://tcoffee.crg.cat/apps/ampa/do (accessed on 4 November 2022)) was used to evaluate the possible antimicrobial activity of the identified peptide.

4.5. Quantitative Real-Time PCT (qRT-PCR)

After the exposure to LPS (Sigma Aldrich, St. Louis, MO, USA), *B. clausii* or zymosan (Sigma Aldrich, St. Louis, MO, USA), haemocytes were collected, and their mRNA was extracted as reported before. Relative qRT-PCR was carried out, according to the method reported in Franchi and Ballarin [47], to estimate the relative variation of mRNA for botryllin. In this case, unexposed cells were considered as the reference control. Forward and reverse specific primers for the above-reported transcripts and for the elongation factor 1α (EF1α) were designed and reported in Table 3. All the designed primers contained parts of contiguous exons to exclude contamination by genomic DNA; a qualitative PCR was also carried out before qRT-PCR. In addition, the analysis of the qRT-PCR dissociation curve gave no indications of the presence of contaminating DNA. The following cycling parameters were used: 10 min at 95 °C (denaturation), 15 s at 95 °C plus 1 min at 60 °C, 15 s at 95 °C for 45 times, 1 min at 60 °C. Each set of samples was run three times on an Applied Biosystem 7900 HT Fast Real-Time PCR System (Life Technologies Europe BV, Monza, Italy), and each plate contained cDNA from three different biological and control samples ($n = 3$). The $2^{-\Delta\Delta CT}$ method [72] was used to estimate the relative amount of mRNA. The amounts of transcripts under different conditions were normalised to EF1α to compensate for variations in the amounts of cDNA.

4.6. In Situ Hybridization (ISH)

Using the primers reported in Table 3, we produced the DIG-labelled antisense riboprobes, as previously described [48]. Collected haemocytes were left to adhere for 30 min on SuperFrost Plus (Menzel–Glaser, Braunschweig, Germany) glass slides. Cells were then incubated for 1 h in FSW in the presence or in the absence (control) of either LPS (1 mg mL^{-1}; serotype 055:B5 from *E. coli*), *B. clausii* (4×10^8 cells mL^{-1}), or zymosan (1 mg mL^{-1}). After washing in FSW, they were fixed for 30 min at 4 °C in 4% paraformaldehyde plus 0.1% glutaraldehyde in 0.4 M cacodylate buffer, containing 1.7% NaCl and 1% sucrose. They were then permeabilised in a solution of 0.1% Triton X in phosphate-buffered saline (PBS: 1.37 M NaCl, 0.03 M KCl, 0.015 M KH$_2$PO$_4$, 0.065 M Na$_2$HPO$_4$, pH 7.2) for 5 min, washed in PBS and pre-incubated in Hybridization Cocktail 50% formamide (Amresco, Solon, OH, USA) for 1 h at 60 °C, and hybridised in the same solution containing 1 µg mL^{-1} riboprobe, overnight, at the same temperature. Cells were then washed in saline sodium citrate (SSC: 0.3 M NaCl, 40 mM sodium citrate, pH 4.5), for 5 min, and in a solution of 50% formamide in SSC at 60 °C, for 30 min, followed by an additional washing in PBS containing 0.1% Tween 20 (PBST) at room temperature, for 5 min. Haemocyte monolayers were then incubated in 1% powdered milk in PBST for 1 h (to reduce unspecific staining), followed by 5% methanol for 30 min (to block endogenous peroxidases). Cells were finally incubated at 4 °C overnight in an anti-DIG-monoclonal antibody labelled with alkaline phosphatase (Fab fragment; Roche Diagnostics, Basel, Switzerland), diluted 1/3000 in PBST. Samples were then stained with a solution of 0.3% nitro-blue tetrazolium/5-bromo-4-chloro-3-indolyphosphate- p-toluidine (NBT/BCIP) in Na-Tris-Mg buffer (NTM: 0.05%MgCl$_2$ 1M, 0.05% NaCl 2M, 0.1% Tris-HCl 2M, pH 9.5) for 10 min and washed in PBS. Slides were then washed in distilled water and mounted in Eukitt (Electron Microscopy Sciences, Hatfield,

PA, USA) before their observation under the light microscope. DIG-labelled sense probes were used as negative controls.

4.7. Synthetic Peptide and Specific Antibodies

The synthetic peptide and the antibodies were produced by Abmart Inc. (Shanghai China). The synthetic peptide fully respected the sequence of 37 amino acids of the mature peptide. Three monoclonal antibodies were obtained by the same company by immunising BALB/c mice with the sequences of three highly immunogenic peptides from the pro peptide sequence (Table 4). Pre-immune mouse serum was obtained by collecting the supernatant of freshly collected mouse blood after its centrifugation for 10 min at 780× *g* at 4 °C.

Table 4. Peptides used for the production of monoclonal antibodies.

Epitopes	Sequence Location	Antibody
GWYNKHKPTIHK	N-terminus of the mature peptide	Ab1
VKGWGKDSDKEL	C-terminus of the mature peptide and beyond	Ab2
KEHDRDEYDGAL	part of the propeptide beyond the C-terminus of the mature peptide	Ab3

4.8. Immunocytochemistry

Exposed haemocytes were fixed as described above, washed in PBS, permeabilised in PBST, and incubated for 30 min to 1% Evans Blue (to quench autofluorescence). Cells were then incubated for 30 min in 10% goat serum in PBS (to reduce nonspecific staining) and with Ab1, Ab2, or Ab3, at the concentration of 10 µg mL^{-1}, for 1 h. After washing in PBS, haemocytes were incubated for 1 h in biotin-conjugated goat anti-mouse IgG antibody (Calbiochem, San Diego, CA, USA), 10 µg mL^{-1} in PBS, washed again, and exposed to FITC conjugated streptavidin (Sigma Aldrich, St. Louis, MO, USA). After a final washing, slides were mounted with FluorSave™ Reagent (Calbiochem, San Diego, CA, USA) and observed under an Olympus (Tokyo, Japan) CX31 light microscope (LM) equipped with an LED fluorescence module with an exciting wavelength of 450 nm (Amplified by Fluorescence Excitation of Radiation Transmitted, AFTER, Fraen Corp. s.r.l., Milan, Italy).

4.9. Minimal Inhibitory Concentration (MIC) and Minimal Bactericidal Concentration (MBC) Determination

For the evaluation of MIC and MBC, four bacterial strains were used: *B. clausii* SIN O/C, T, N/R, and *S. epidermidis* ATCC 700565 as Gram-positive and *E. coli* O4 and *P. mirabilis* ATCC 29906 as Gram-negative. With the exception of *B. clausii* (commercial *Enterogermina* Sanofi, Opella Healthcare Italy S.r.l., Origgio, Italy),they were gently provided by Prof. G Bertoloni, Department of Histology, Microbiology and Medical Biotechnologies, University of Padova, and Prof. R. Provvedi, Department of Biology, University of Padova. In addition baker's yeast (*S. cerevisiae*) was also used to evaluate the antimycotic activity of botryllin.

Bacteria were grown in sterile brain heart infusion (BHI; Honeywell-Fluka, Charlotte NC, USA), and the microbial concentration was assessed by the determination of the absorbance at 580 nm with a Beckman Coulter Life Science (Brea, CA, USA) DU 730 UV/Vis spectrophotometer.

For MIC assessment, 50 µL of synthetic botryllin (100 µg mL^{-1} in BHI) were serially diluted in the wells of a 96-well, flat-bottomed microplate, and 50 µL of bacterial or yeast suspension, at the concentration corresponding to 0.01 absorbance units, were added to each well. Cells were incubated for 20 h at 37 °C, and the absorbance at 580 nm of the cell suspensions was then determined with a Plate Reader photometer (Elettrofor Scientific Instruments, Borsea, (RO), Italy) to evaluate the microbial growth.

For the evaluation of MBC, the content of the wells with the absence of growth was collected, centrifuged at 10,000× *g*, re-suspended in 100 µL of BHI, and transferred to new wells of a 96-well, flat-bottomed microplate. It was incubated for 20 h at 37 °C, and the absorbance of the wells at 580 nm was finally read with the microplate reader.

4.10. Microbial Cell Mortality Assay

The mortality of the bacterial strains was evaluated using the LIVE/DEAD BacLight Bacterial Viability kit for microscopy (Molecular Probes, Eugene, OR, USA). Briefly, 100 µL of bacterial cells at the concentration corresponding to 0.01 absorbance units were incubated for 20 h at 37 °C with 0 (control), 6.3, and 25 µg mL^{-1} of synthetic botryllin in BHI, and with 25 µg mL^{-1} of synthetic botryllin pre-incubated for 30 min with 10 µg mL^{-1} of anti-botryllinAb2 antibody. In another series of experiments, *B. clausii* cells were incubated in the presence or in the absence (control) of CM (see below) or CM and anti-botryllin Ab2 or Ab3 antibodies (pre-immune mouse serum in controls). Then, cells were pelleted by centrifugation and re-suspended in 0.85% NaCl. An equal volume of solutions A and B of the Bacterial Viability kit were mixed together and added to the bacterial suspensions in the ratio of 3:1 (vol:vol). After 15 min of incubation, cells were pelleted as described above and re-suspended in 50 µL of 0.85% NaCl, and 5 µL of the resulting suspension were laid on a Superfrost^{TM} Plus (Thermo Scientific, Waltham, MA, USA) glass slide and observed under the light microscope equipped with fluorescence module. Live cells appeared green when the excitation light of 535 nm was used, whereas dead cells resulted in red when excited with blue light (450 nm). Images were acquired with a Lumenera Infinity 2 camera, and the percentage of living and dead cells was determined by analysing images with the Infinity Analyze 5.0.0 software (Lumenera Corporation, Teledyne Technologies Inc., Thousand Oaks, CA, USA).

The effects of the synthetic peptide on yeast mortality were evaluated with the Trypan Blue exclusion assay [73]. Yeast cells, previously exposed to 6.3 and 25 µg mL^{-1} of synthetic botryllin in BHI, and with 25 µg mL^{-1} of synthetic botryllin pre-incubated with 10 µg mL^{-1} of anti-botryllin Ab2 antibody, were incubated in a 0.4% solution of Trypan Blue for 5 min and observed under the light microscope. Dead cells resulted as blue-stained.

4.11. Temperature, pH and Salinity Stability Assays

We used *S. epidermidis* for the evaluation of the effects of variations of physico-chemical parameters on the antibacterial activity of botryllin by evaluating the MIC values. The synthetic peptide, prepared as described above, was exposed at 60 and 80 °C for 4 h and at 100 °C for 15 min. It was then cooled at room temperature and used for MIC assay. In addition, the Tm of botryllin, i.e., the temperature value at which half of its amino acids result as destructured, was predicted with the software Tm Predictor (http://tm.life.nthu.edu.tw (accessed on 14 September 2022)).

To evaluate the effects of pH, the peptide was diluted in BHI prepared with 0.1 M Na-acetate buffer at pH 4.0 and 5.0; with 0.1 M phosphate buffer at pH 6.0, 7.0, and 8.0; and with 0.1 M Tris-HCl at pH 9.0.

The effects of the ionic strength on antimicrobial activity were assayed by MIC determination of the peptide diluted in BHI containing 150, 300, and 600 mM NaCl.

4.12. Electron Microscopy

Microbial and yeast cells, previously incubated with the synthetic peptide for 20 h at 37 °C, were pelleted by centrifugation; fixed in 2% glutaraldehyde in 0.2 M Na-cacodylate buffer, pH 7.2, for 2 h at 4 °C; dehydrated in an increasing ethanol series; and embedded in Epon (Fluka). Ultrathin sections (60–70 nm) were stained with uranyl acetate and lead citrate. They were finally observed under a FEI TECNAI 12 transmission electron microscope (TEM), at 75 kV, equipped with a TIETZ high-resolution digital camera.

For immunocytochemical analyses, samples were dehydrated in increasing ethanol concentrations and embedded in London Resin White (LRW, Polyscience, Warrington, PA, USA). Ultrathin sections, once collected on copper grids, were incubated for 10 min in 10% goat serum, washed in PBS, incubated overnight in the primary antibody (Ab1) at the concentration reported above, washed again, and treated for 1 h with goat anti-mouse IgG antibody (10 µg mL^{-1}) conjugated with colloidal gold spherules (15 nm in diameter). Grids were then washed in PBS and in distilled water and stained with uranyl acetate and lead citrate. Sections were finally observed under the TEM, as reported above.

4.13. Preparation of Conditioned Medium (CM)

B. schlosseri haemocytes, collected as described above, were incubated for 30 min in FSW in the presence or in the absence (control) of 2×10^9 *B. clausii* spores (*Enterogermina* Sanofi, Opella Healthcare Italy S.r.l., Origgio, Italy). They were then centrifuged at 2000× g for 5 min, the supernatant was collected, and 1% (vol:vol) of Protease Inhibitor Mix (GE Healthcare Europe GmbH, Freiburg, Germany) was added before its storage at −20 °C until use as CM in microbial cell mortality assay, as described above.

4.14. Statistical Analysis

All the experiments were repeated with three different colonies ($n = 3$). Each experiment was carried out in triplicate. The fraction of labelled cells was compared with the chi square test, whereas qRT-PCT data were analysed with the one-way ANOVA followed by the Duncan's test for multiple comparisons with DSAASTAT v. 1.1 2011 [74]. Differences were considered statistically significant when $p < 0.05$.

Supplementary Materials: The following supporting information can be downloaded at: https://www.mdpi.com/article/10.3390/md21020074/s1. Figure S1. (a) Gene organisation of botryllin (b) Nucleotide and amino acid sequences of the pre-propeptide transcript. The signal peptide and the mature peptide are boxed red and green, respectively.

Author Contributions: Conceptualisation, L.B., F.C. and N.F.; supervision, F.C. and N.F.; investigation, methodology, data curation, formal analysis, F.C. and N.F.; writing—original draft preparation and editing, L.B. All authors have read and agreed to the published version of the manuscript.

Funding: This research was supported by grants from the Italian MIUR through the Department of Biology, University of Padova, PRID BIRD183771/18 to LB and DOR 2020 to FC.

Institutional Review Board Statement: Not applicable.

Data Availability Statement: All data generated or analysed during this study are included in this published article. The sequence of the botryllin transcript has been deposited in GenBank as described in Material and Methods.

Acknowledgments: The authors wish to thank Z. Romanyuk, E. Gelsi, T. Holtz, and E. Morbiato who worked to this project for their bachelor thesis, and I. Olivi, who worked part of the project for her master thesis.

Conflicts of Interest: The authors declare no conflict of interest. The funders had no role in the design of the study; in the collection, analyses, or interpretation of data; in the writing of the manuscript; or in the decision to publish the results.

References

1. Gould, I.M. Stewardship of antibiotic use and resistance surveillance: The international scene. *J. Hosp. Infect.* **1999**, *43*, S253–S260. [CrossRef] [PubMed]
2. O'Neill, J. *Review on Antimicrobial Resistance. Tackling Drug-Resistant Infections Globally: Final Report and Recommendations*; HM Government and Wellcome Trust: London, UK, 2016.
3. Giuliani, A.; Pirri, G.; Nicoletto, S.F. Antimicrobial peptides: An overview of a promising class of therapeutics. *Cent. Eur. J. Biol.* **2007**, *2*, 1–33. [CrossRef]
4. Bierbaum, G.; Sahl, H.G. Induction of autolysis of staphylococci by the basic peptide antibiotics Pep 5 and nisin and their influence on the activity of autolytic enzymes. *Arch. Microbiol.* **1985**, *141*, 249–254. [CrossRef] [PubMed]
5. Westerhoff, H.V.; Juretić, D.; Hendler, R.W.; Zasloff, M. Magainins and the disruption of membrane-linked free-energy transduction. *Proc. Natl. Acad. Sci. USA* **1989**, *86*, 6597–6601. [CrossRef]
6. Matsuzaki, K. Why and how are peptide-lipid interactions utilized for self-defense? Magainins and tachyplesins as archetypes. *Biochim. Biophys. Acta* **1999**, *1462*, 1–10. [CrossRef]

7. Yang, L.; Weiss, T.M.; Lehrer, R.I.; Huang, H.W. Crystallization of antimicrobial pores in membranes: Magainin and protegrin. *Biophys J.* **2000**, *79*, 2002–2009. [CrossRef]
8. Kragol, G.; Lovas, S.; Varadi, G.; Condie, B.A.; Hoffmann, R.; Otvos, L., Jr. The antibacterial peptide pyrrhocoricin inhibits the ATPase actions of DnaK and prevents chaperone-assisted protein folding. *Biochemistry* **2001**, *40*, 3016–3026. [CrossRef]
9. Lazzaro, B.P.; Zasloff, M.; Rolff, J. Antimicrobial peptides: Application informed by evolution. *Science* **2020**, *368*, eaau5480. [CrossRef]
10. Shai, Y. Mechanism of the binding, insertion and destabilization of phospholipid bilayer membranes by alpha-helical antimicrobial and cell non-selective membrane-lytic peptides. *BiochimBiophys Acta* **1999**, *1462*, 55–70.
11. Huan, Y.; Kong, Q.; Mou, H.; Yi, H. Antimicrobial peptides: Classification, design, application and research progress in multiple fields. *Front. Microbiol.* **2020**, *11*, 582779. [CrossRef]
12. Rabel, D.; Charlet, M.; Ehret-Sabatier, L.; Cavicchioli, L.; Cudic, M.; Otvos, L., Jr.; Bulet, P. Primary structure and in vitro antibacterial properties of the *Drosophila melanogaster* attacin C pro-domain. *J. Biol. Chem.* **2004**, *279*, 14853–14859. [CrossRef] [PubMed]
13. Fjell, C.D.; Hiss, J.A.; Hancock, R.E.; Schneider, G. Designing antimicrobial peptides: Form follows function. *Nat. Rev. Drug Discov.* **2011**, *11*, 37–51. [CrossRef] [PubMed]
14. Bahar, A.A.; Ren, D. Antimicrobial peptides. *Pharmaceuticals* **2013**, *6*, 1543–1575. [CrossRef] [PubMed]
15. Zasloff, M. Antimicrobial peptides of multicellular organisms. *Nature* **2002**, *415*, 389–395. [CrossRef] [PubMed]
16. Hancock, R.E.; Sahl, H.G. Antimicrobial and host-defense peptides as new anti-infective therapeutic strategies. *Nat. Biotechnol.* **2006**, *24*, 1551–1557. [CrossRef] [PubMed]
17. Deslouches, B.; Di, Y.P. Antimicrobial peptides with selective antitumor mechanisms: Prospect for anticancer applications. *Oncotarget.* **2017**, *8*, 46635–46651. [CrossRef] [PubMed]
18. Bevins, C.L.; Salzman, N.H. Paneth cells, antimicrobial peptides and maintenance of intestinal homeostasis. *Nat. Rev. Microbiol.* **2011**, *9*, 356–368. [CrossRef]
19. Login, F.H.; Balmand, S.; Vallier, A.; Vincent-Monégat, C.; Vigneron, A.; Weiss-Gayet, M.; Rochat, D.; Heddi, A. Antimicrobial peptides keep insect endosymbionts under control. *Science* **2011**, *334*, 362–365. [CrossRef]
20. Franzenburg, S.; Walter, J.; Künzel, S.; Wang, J.; Baines, J.F.; Bosch, T.C.; Fraune, S. Distinct antimicrobial peptide expression determines host species-specific bacterial associations. *Proc. Natl. Acad. Sci. USA* **2013**, *110*, E3730–E3738. [CrossRef]
21. Cullen, T.W.; Schofield, W.B.; Barry, N.A.; Putnam, E.E.; Rundell, E.A.; Trent, M.S.; Degnan, P.H.; Booth, C.J.; Yu, H.; Goodman, A.L. Gut microbiota. Antimicrobial peptide resistance mediates resilience of prominent gut commensals during inflammation. *Science* **2015**, *347*, 170–175. [CrossRef]
22. Arnold, M.F.F.; Shabab, M.; Penterman, J.; Boehme, K.L.; Griffitts, J.S.; Walker, G.C. Genome-wide sensitivity analysis of the microsymbiont *Sinorhizobiummelitoti* to symbiotically important, defensin-like host peptides. *mBio* **2017**, *8*, e01060-17. [CrossRef] [PubMed]
23. Leal, M.C.; Puga, J.; Serôdio, J.; Gomes, N.C.M.; Calado, R. Trends in the discovery of new marine natural products from invertebrates over the last two decades—Where and what are we bioprospecting? *PLoS ONE* **2012**, *7*, e30580. [CrossRef] [PubMed]
24. Datta, D.; Talapatra, S.; Swarnakar, S. Bioactive compounds from marine invertebrates for potential medicines—An overview. *Int. Lett. Nat. Sci.* **2015**, *34*, 42–61. [CrossRef]
25. Romano, G.; Almeida, M.; Varela Coelho, A.; Cutignano, A.; Gonçalves, L.G.; Hansen, E.; Khnykin, D.; Mass, T.; Ramšak, A.; Rocha, M.S.; et al. Biomaterials and bioactive natural products from marine invertebrates: From basic research to innovative applications. *Mar. Drugs* **2022**, *20*, 219. [CrossRef]
26. Tincu, J.A.; Taylor, S.W. Antimicrobial peptides from marine invertebrates. *Antimicrob. Agents Chemother.* **2004**, *48*, 3645–3654. [CrossRef]
27. Delsuc, F.; Brinkmann, H.; Chourrout, D.; Philippe, H. Tunicates and not cephalochordates are the closest living relatives of vertebrates. *Nature* **2006**, *439*, 965–968. [CrossRef] [PubMed]
28. Casertano, M.; Menna, M.; Imperatore, C. The ascidian-derived metabolites with antimicrobial properties. *Antibiotics* **2020**, *9*, 510. [CrossRef]
29. Kwan, J.C.; Donia, M.S.; Han, A.W.; Hirose, E.; Haygood, M.G.; Schmidt, E.W. Genome streamlining and chemical defense in a coral reef symbiosis. *Proc. Natl. Acad. Sci. USA* **2012**, *109*, 20655–20660. [CrossRef]
30. Schmidt, E.W.; Donia, M.S.; McIntosh, J.A.; Fricke, W.F.; Ravel, J. Origin and variation of tunicate secondary metabolites. *J. Nat Prod.* **2012**, *75*, 295–304. [CrossRef]
31. Lehrer, R.I.; Andrew Tincu, J.; Taylor, S.W.; Menzel, L.P.; Waring, A.J. Natural peptide antibiotics from tunicates: Structures, functions and potential uses. *Integr. Comp. Biol.* **2003**, *43*, 313–322. [CrossRef]
32. Zhao, C.; Liaw, L.; Lee, I.H.; Lehrer, R.I. cDNA cloning of three cecropin-like antimicrobial peptides (styelins) from the tunicate, *Styela clava*. *FEBS Lett.* **1997**, *412*, 144–148. [CrossRef] [PubMed]
33. Lee, I.H.; Zhao, C.; Nguyen, T.; Menzel, L.; Waring, A.J.; Sherman, M.A.; Lehrer, R.I. Clavaspirin, an antibacterial and haemolytic peptide from *Styela Clava*. *J. Pept. Res.* **2001**, *58*, 445–456. [PubMed]
34. Menzel, L.P.; Lee, I.H.; Sjostrand, B.; Lehrer, R.I. Immunolocalization of clavanins in *Styela clava* hemocytes. *Dev. Comp. Immunol.* **2002**, *26*, 505–515. [CrossRef] [PubMed]

35. Tincu, J.A.; Menzel, L.P.; Azimov, R.; Sands, J.; Hong, T.; Waring, A.J.; Taylor, S.W.; Lehrer, R.I. Plicatamide, an antimicrobial octapeptide from *Styela plicata* hemocytes. *J. Biol. Chem.* **2003**, *278*, 13546–13553. [CrossRef] [PubMed]
36. Azumi, K.; Yokosawa, H.; Ishii, S. Halocyamines: Novel antimicrobial tetrapeptide-like substances isolated from the hemocytes of the solitary ascidian *Halocynthia Roretzi*. *Biochemistry* **1990**, *29*, 159–165. [CrossRef] [PubMed]
37. Ballarin, L. Ascidian cytotoxic cells: State of the art and research perspectives. *ISJ-Invertebr. Surviv. J.* **2012**, *9*, 1–6.
38. Fedders, H.; Michalek, M.; Grötzinger, J.; Leippe, M. An exceptional salt-tolerant antimicrobial peptide derived from a novel gene family of haemocytes of the marine invertebrate *Ciona intestinalis*. *Biochem. J.* **2008**, *416*, 65–75. [CrossRef]
39. Fedders, H.; Leippe, M. A Reverse search for antimicrobial peptides in *Ciona intestinalis*: Identification of a gene family expressed in hemocytes and evaluation of activity. *Dev. Comp. Immunol.* **2008**, *32*, 286–298. [CrossRef]
40. Fedders, H.; Podschun, R.; Leippe, M. The antimicrobial peptide Ci-MAM-A24 is highly active against multidrug-resistant and anaerobic bacteria pathogenic for humans. *Int. J. Antimicrob. Agents* **2010**, *36*, 264–266. [CrossRef]
41. Di Bella, M.D.; Fedders, H.; Leippe, M.; De Leo, G. A preliminary study on antimicrobial peptides in the naturally damaged tunic of *Ciona intestinalis* (Tunicata). In *Science Against Microbial Pathogens: Communicating Current Research and Technological Advances*, Méndez-Vilas, A., Ed.; Formatex Research Center: Badajoz, Spain, 2011; pp. 1003–1007.
42. Tsukimoto, M.; Nagaoka, M.; Shishido, Y.; Fujimoto, J.; Nishisaka, F.; Matsumoto, S.; Harunari, E.; Imada, C.; Matsuzaki, T. Bacterial production of the tunicate-derived antitumor cyclic depsipeptidedidemnin B. *J. Nat. Prod.* **2011**, *74*, 2329–2331 [CrossRef]
43. Xu, Y.; Kersten, R.D.; Nam, S.J.; Lu, L.; Al-Suwailem, A.M.; Zheng, H.; Fenical, W.; Dorrestein, P.C.; Moore, B.S.; Qian, P.Y. Bacterial biosynthesis and maturation of the didemnin anti-cancer agents. *J. Am. Chem. Soc.* **2012**, *134*, 8625–8632. [CrossRef] [PubMed]
44. Ramesh, C.; Tulasi, B.R.; Raju, M.; Thakur, N.; Dufossé, L. Marine natural products from tunicates and their associated microbes *Mar. Drugs* **2021**, *19*, 308. [CrossRef] [PubMed]
45. Franchi, N.; Ballarin, L. Immunity in Protochordates: The tunicate perspective. *Front. Immunol.* **2017**, *8*, 674. [CrossRef] [PubMed]
46. Ballarin, L.; Cima, F. Cytochemical properties of *Botryllus schlosseri* haemocytes: Indications for morpho-functional characterisation *Eur. J. Histochem.* **2005**, *49*, 255–264.
47. Franchi, N.; Ballarin, L. Preliminary characterization of complement in a colonial tunicate: C3, Bf and inhibition of C3 opsonic activity by compstatin. *Dev. Comp. Immunol.* **2014**, *46*, 430–438. [CrossRef]
48. Franchi, N.; Ballarin, L. Morula cells as key hemocytes of the lectin pathway of complement activation in the colonial tunicate *Botryllus schlosseri*. *Fish Shellfish Immunol.* **2017**, *63*, 157–164.
49. Peronato, A.; Franchi, N.; Ballarin, L. Insights into the complement system of tunicates: C3a/C5aR of the colonial ascidian *Botryllus schlosseri*. *Biology* **2020**, *9*, 263. [CrossRef]
50. Menin, A.; Del Favero, M.; Cima, F.; Ballarin, L. Release of phagocytosis-stimulating factor (s) by morula cells in a colonial ascidian. *Mar. Biol.* **2005**, *148*, 225–230. [CrossRef]
51. Menin, A.; Ballarin, L. Immunomodulatory molecules in the compound ascidian *Botryllus schlosseri*: Evidence from conditioned media. *J. Invertebr. Pathol.* **2008**, *99*, 275–280. [CrossRef]
52. Vizioli, J.; Salzet, M. Antimicrobial peptides from animals: Focus on invertebrates. *Trends Pharmacol. Sci.* **2002**, *23*, 494–496 [CrossRef]
53. Jenssen, H.; Hamill, P.; Hancock, E.W.R. Peptide antimicrobial agents. *Clin. Microbiol. Rev.* **2006**, *19*, 491–511. [CrossRef] [PubMed]
54. Ballarin, L.; Cima, F.; Sabbadin, A. Phenoloxidase in the colonial ascidian *Botryllus schlosseri* (Urochordata: Ascidiacea). *Anim. Biol.* **1994**, *3*, 41–48.
55. Ballarin, L.; Cima, F.; Sabbadin, A. Phenoloxidase and cytotoxicity in the compound ascidian *Botryllus schlosseri*. *Dev. Comp. Immunol.* **1998**, *22*, 479–492. [CrossRef]
56. Frizzo, A.; Guidolin, L.; Ballarin, L.; Sabbadin, A. Purification and partial characterisation of phenoloxidase from the colonial ascidian *Botryllus schlosseri*. *Mar. Biol.* **1999**, *135*, 483–488. [CrossRef]
57. Gasparini, F.; Franchi, N.; Spolaore, B.; Ballarin, L. Novel rhamnose-binding lectins from the colonial ascidian *Botryllus schlosseri*. *Dev. Comp. Immunol.* **2008**, *32*, 1177–1191. [CrossRef]
58. Franchi, N.; Schiavon, F.; Carletto, M.; Gasparini, F.; Bertoloni, G.; Tosatto, S.C.E.; Ballarin, L. Immune roles of a rhamnose-binding lectin in the colonial ascidian *Botryllus schlosseri*. *Immunobiology* **2011**, *216*, 725–736. [CrossRef]
59. Peronato, A.; Drago, L.; Rothbaecher, U.; Macor, P.; Ballarin, L.; Franchi, N. Complement system and phagocytosis in a colonial protochordate. *Dev. Comp. Immunol.* **2020**, *103*, 103530. [CrossRef]
60. Ballarin, L.; Cima, F.; Sabbadin, A. Histoenzymatic staining and characterization of the colonial ascidian *Botryllus schlosseri* hemocytes. *Boll. Zool.* **1993**, *60*, 19–24. [CrossRef]
61. Ballarin, L.; Franchini, A.; Ottaviani, E.; Sabbadin, A. Morula cells as the main immunomodulatory haemocytes in ascidians: Evidences from the colonial species *Botryllus schlosseri*. *Biol. Bull.* **2001**, *201*, 59–64. [CrossRef]
62. Ballarin, L.; Cima, F.; Sabbadin, A. Morula cells and histocompatibility in the colonial ascidian *Botryllus schlosseri*. *Zool. Sci.* **1995**, *12*, 757–764. [CrossRef]
63. Ballarin, L.; Cima, F.; Floreani, M.; Sabbadin, A. Oxidative stress induces cytotoxicity during rejection reaction in the compound ascidian *Botryllus schlosseri*. *Comp. Biochem. Physiol.* **2002**, *133C*, 411–418. [CrossRef] [PubMed]

64. Cima, F.; Sabbadin, A.; Ballarin, L. Cellular aspects of allorecognition in the compound ascidian *Botryllus schlosseri*. *Dev. Comp. Immunol.* **2004**, *28*, 881–889. [CrossRef] [PubMed]
65. Franchi, N.; Ballarin, L.; Peronato, A.; Cima, F.; Grimaldi, A.; Girardello, R.; de Eguileor, M. Functional amyloidogenesis in immunocytes from the colonial ascidian *Botryllus schlosseri*: Evolutionary perspective. *Dev. Comp. Immunol.* **2019**, *90*, 108–120. [CrossRef] [PubMed]
66. Taylor, S.W.; Craig, A.G.; Fischer, W.H.; Park, M.; Lehrer, R.I. Styelin D, an extensively modified antimicrobial peptide from ascidian hemocytes. *J. Biol. Chem.* **2000**, *275*, 38417–38426. [CrossRef] [PubMed]
67. Lee, I.H.; Cho, Y.; Lehrer, R.I. Styelins, broad-spectrum antimicrobial peptides from the solitary tunicate, *Styela clava*. *Comp. Biochem. Physiol.* **1997**, *118B*, 515–521. [CrossRef]
68. Awuah, G.B.; Ramaswamy, H.S.; Economides, A. Thermal processing and quality: Principles and overview. *Chem. Eng. Process.* **2007**, *46*, 584–602. [CrossRef]
69. Lappe, R.; Cladera-Olivera, F.; Dominguez, A.P.M.; Brandelli, A. Kinetics and thermodynamics of thermal inactivation of the antimicrobial peptide cerein 8A. *J. Food Eng.* **2009**, *91*, 223–227. [CrossRef]
70. Goldman, M.J.; Anderson, G.M.; Stolzenberg, E.D.; Kari, U.P.; Zasloff, M.; Wilson, J.M. Human beta-defensin-1 is a salt-sensitive antibiotic in lung that is inactivated in cystic fibrosis. *Cell* **1997**, *88*, 553–560. [CrossRef]
71. Sabbadin, A.; Zaniolo, G.; Ballarin, L. Genetic and cytological aspects of histocompatibility in ascidians. *Boll. Zool.* **1992**, *59*, 167–173. [CrossRef]
72. Livak, K.J.; Schmittgen, T.D. Analysis of relative gene expression data using real-time quantitative PCR and the 2(-Delta Delta C(T)) method. *Methods* **2001**, *25*, 402–408. [CrossRef]
73. Gorman, A.; Mc Carty, J.; Finucane, D.; Reville, W.; Catter, T. Morphological assessment of apoptosis. In *Techniques in Apoptosis—A User's Guide*; Catter, T.G., Martin, S.J., Eds.; Portland Press Ltd.: London, UK, 1996; pp. 1–20.
74. Onofri, A. Routine statistical analyses of field experiments by using an Excel extension. In Proceedings of the 6th National Conference of Italian Biometric Society, Pisa, Italy, 20–22 June 2007; pp. 93–96.

Disclaimer/Publisher's Note: The statements, opinions and data contained in all publications are solely those of the individual author(s) and contributor(s) and not of MDPI and/or the editor(s). MDPI and/or the editor(s) disclaim responsibility for any injury to people or property resulting from any ideas, methods, instructions or products referred to in the content.

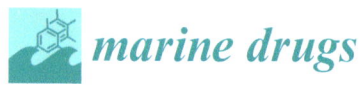

Article

Anti-Diabetic Activity of a Novel Exopolysaccharide Produced by the Mangrove Endophytic Fungus *Penicillium janthinellum* N29

Zhuling Shao [1], Yingying Tian [2], Shan Liu [1], Xiao Chu [1] and Wenjun Mao [1,3,*]

[1] Key Laboratory of Marine Drugs of Ministry of Education, Shandong Provincial Key Laboratory of Glycoscience and Glycotechnology, School of Medicine and Pharmacy, Ocean University of China, Qingdao 266003, China
[2] Marine Biomedical Research Institute of Qingdao, Qingdao 266237, China
[3] Laboratory for Marine Drugs and Bioproducts, National Laboratory for Marine Science and Technology (Qingdao), Qingdao 266237, China
* Correspondence: wenjunm@ouc.edu.cn

Abstract: Marine microorganisms often produce exopolysaccharides with novel structures and diverse biological activities due to their specific marine environment. The novel active exopolysaccharides from marine microorganisms have become an important research area in new drug discovery, and show enormous development prospects. In the present study, a homogeneous exopolysaccharide from the fermented broth of the mangrove endophytic fungus *Penicillium janthinellum* N29, designated as PJ1-1, was obtained. The results of chemical and spectroscopic analyses showed that PJ1-1 was a novel galactomannan with a molecular weight of about 10.24 kDa. The backbone of PJ1-1 was composed of →2)-α-D-Man$p$-(1→, →4)-α-D-Man$p$-(1→, →3)-β-D-Gal$f$-(1→ and →2)-β-D-Gal$f$-(1→ units with partial glycosylation at C-3 of →2)-β-D-Gal$f$-(1→ unit. PJ1-1 had a strong hypoglycemic activity in vitro, evaluated using the assay of α-glucosidase inhibition. The anti-diabetic effect of PJ1-1 in vivo was further investigated using mice with type 2 diabetes mellitus induced by a high-fat diet and streptozotocin. The results indicated that PJ1-1 markedly reduced blood glucose level and improved glucose tolerance. Notably, PJ1-1 increased insulin sensitivity and ameliorated insulin resistance. Moreover, PJ1-1 significantly decreased the levels of serum total cholesterol, triglyceride and low-density lipoprotein cholesterol, enhanced the level of serum high-density lipoprotein cholesterol and alleviated dyslipidemia. These results revealed that PJ1-1 could be a potential source of anti-diabetic agent.

Keywords: mangrove endophytic fungus; exopolysaccharide; structure; anti-diabetic activity

1. Introduction

Diabetes mellitus is a kind of endocrine metabolic disease, and its incidence has recently increased because of changes in diet, unhealthy lifestyles and environmental factors [1]. Type 2 diabetes mellitus (T2DM) is the most common type of diabetes around the world and accounts for about 90% of diabetes patients [2]. T2DM is characterized by hyperglycemia that will lead to a series of complications, including hyperlipidemia, diabetic nephropathy and liver impairment [3]. Diabetic complications can cause serious damage to human health and even threaten life [4,5]. Anti-diabetes drugs, such as metformin, rosiglitazone, sulfonylurea, acarbose and miglitol, have been widely used in the therapy of diabetes [6]. However, the drugs possess some side effects, such as hepatotoxicity and adverse gastrointestinal symptoms [7]. In order to meet the growing demand for anti-diabetic drugs, it is crucial to search for natural sources of anti-diabetic agents.

Polysaccharides have attracted considerable attention due to their unique structures and biological activities. It has been noted that they have potential anti-diabetic activity [8]. Sun et al. found that the exopolysaccharide EPS-III produced by *Cordyceps militaris* effectively inhibited α-glucosidase activity, and it could reduce plasma glucose concentration, improve glucose tolerance and repair dyslipidemia in STZ-induced diabetic mice [9]. The polysaccharides isolated from *Gomphidiaceae rutilus* increased insulin sensitivity and reduced blood glucose level [10]. Ye et al. revealed that the polysaccharides from *Enteromorpha prolifera* improved oral glucose tolerance metric and relieved insulin resistance in T2DM mice [11]. Shan et al. reported that the fucoidan from *Fucus vesiculosus* possessed a potent inhibitory effect on α-glucosidase activity [12]. The stimulatory activity of polysaccharides from algae on insulin secretion in vitro was also found [13]. So far, investigation into the anti-diabetic properties of the exopolysaccharides from mangrove endophytic fungi has rarely been reported.

Mangrove forests are considered to be dynamic ecotones or transition zones between terrestrial and marine habitats, and are biodiversity spots for marine fungi [14]. Mangrove fungi constitute the second largest ecological group of marine fungi due to their complex and special environment [15]. However, few reports have correlated the structure and biological activity of exopolysaccharides from mangrove endophytic fungi. In this study, a homogenous exopolysaccharide which possessed an obvious hypoglycemic activity in vitro was first isolated from the liquid culture broth of the mangrove endophytic fungus *Penicillium janthinellum* N29. The structure of the exopolysaccharide was characterized by a combination of chemical and spectroscopic methods, and its anti-diabetic effect in vivo was investigated.

2. Results and Discussion

2.1. Structural Characteristics of the Exopolysaccharide PJ1-1

The crude exopolysaccharide was obtained from the culture medium of the mangrove endophytic fungus *P. janthinellum* N29. The yield of the crude exopolysaccharide was about 6.25 g/L. The exopolysaccharide was fractionated using a Q Sepharose Fast Flow column into three fractions. The fraction eluted with distilled water was the most abundant and was further purified on a Sephacryl S-100/HR column. A major fraction, designated PJ1-1, was obtained. PJ1-1 displayed a single and symmetrical peak in the high-performance gel permeation chromatography (HPGPC) chromatogram (Figure 1A); thus, PJ1-1 was a homogeneous polysaccharide. The molecular weight of PJ1-1 was estimated to be about 10.24 kDa by reference to a calibration curve made by pullulan standards. The total sugar content of PJ1-1 was 97.45%. No protein was detected in PJ1-1. The ultraviolet (UV) spectrum analysis of PJ1-1 showed that no absorption peak appeared at 280 nm, further illustrating that PJ1-1 did not contain protein [16]. Reversed-phase high-performance liquid chromatography (HPLC) analysis showed that PJ1-1 consisted of mannose (52.71%) and galactose (47.29%) (Figure 1B). The sugar configuration analysis using HPLC indicated that both the mannose and galactose in PJ1-1 were in the D-configuration (Figure 1C).

Methylation analysis can provide important information regarding the linkage pattern of sugar residues. The identification and the proportion of the methylated alditol acetate of PJ1-1 are listed in Table 1. The mannose part of PJ1-1 showed three ion peaks. 1,5-Di-O-acetyl-2,3,4,6-tetra-O-methyl mannitol was detected, indicating the presence of the terminal unit Man*p*-(1→, 1,2,5-Tri-O-acetyl-3,4,6-tri-O-methyl mannitol and 1,4,5-tri-O-acetyl-2,3,6-tri-O-methyl mannitol were attributed to →2)-Man*p*-(1→ and →4)-Man*p*-(1→ residues, respectively. The galactose part of PJ1-1 had four ion peaks. 1,4-Di-O-acetyl-2,3,5-tri-O-methyl-galactitol was detected, indicating the presence of the terminal unit Gal*f*-(1→. 1,2,4-Tri-O-acetyl-3,5,6-di-O-methyl galactitol likely originating from →2)-Gal*f*-(1→ residue, while 1,3,4-tri-O-acetyl-2,5,6-di-O-methyl galactitol could represent →3)-Gal*f*-(1→ residue. 1,2,3,4-Tetra-O-acetyl-5,6-O-methyl galactitol could be from →2,3)-Gal*f*-(1→ residue. The presence of →2,3)-Gal*f*-(1→ suggested that PJ1-1 contained partial branches at C-2 of →3)-Gal*f*-(1→ or C-3 of →2)-Gal*f*-(1→ residues. The linkage patterns of the mannose and galactose units were further confirmed by NMR analysis.

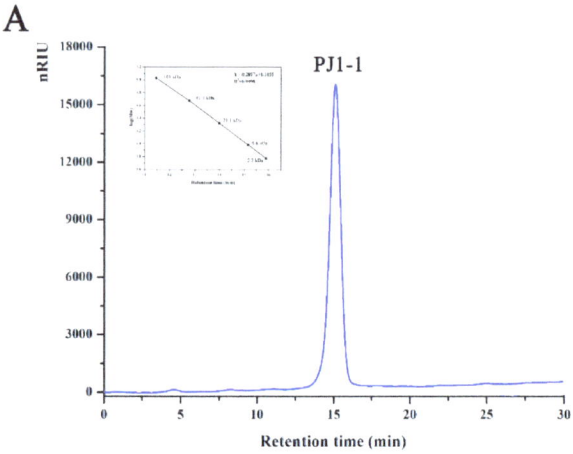

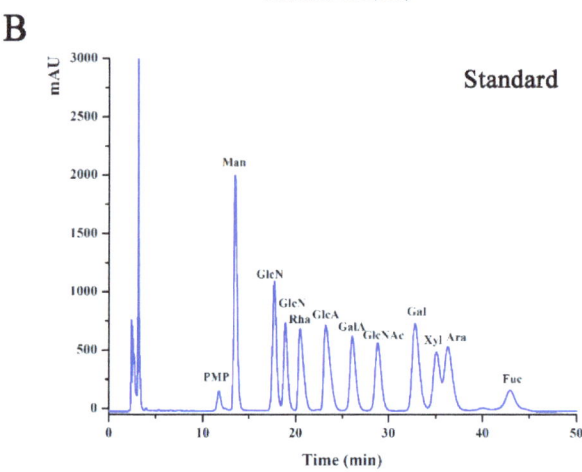

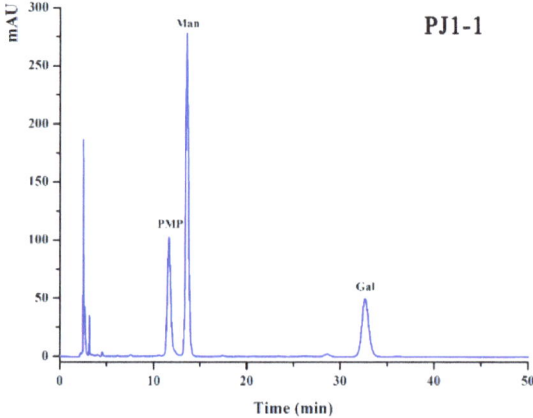

Figure 1. Cont.

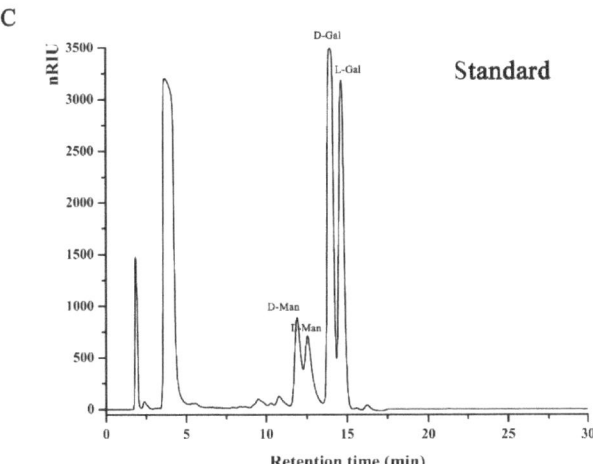

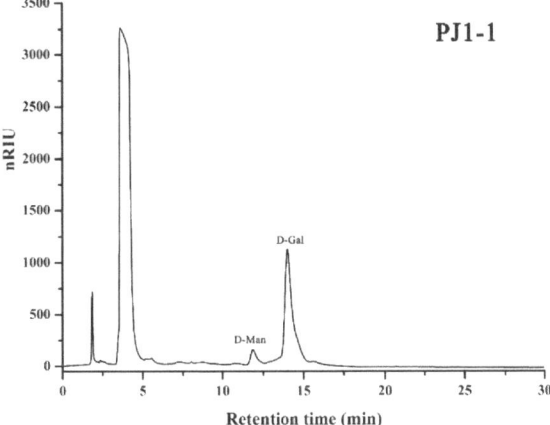

Figure 1. High-performance gel permeation chromatography and high-performance liquid chromatography chromatograms of PJ1-1. (**A**) High-performance gel permeation chromatography chromatogram on a Shodex OHpak SB-803 HQ column and the standard curve of molecular weight; (**B**) high-performance liquid chromatography chromatogram for the monosaccharide composition analysis (Man: D-mannose, GlcN: D-glucosamine, Rha: L-rhamnose, GlcA: D-glucuronic acid, GalA: D-galacturonic acid, Glc: D-glucose, Gal: D-galactose, Xyl: D-xylose, Ara: L-arabinose, Fuc: L-fucose); and (**C**) high-performance liquid chromatography chromatogram for the sugar configuration determination (D-Man: D-mannose, L-Man: L-mannose, D-Gal: D-galactose, L-Gal: L-galactose).

Table 1. Result of methylation analysis of PJ1-1.

Methylated Alditol Acetate	Molar Percent Ratio	Linkage Pattern
1,5-Di-O-acetyl-2,3,4,6-tetra-O-methyl mannitol	8.11	Manp-(1→
1,4-Di-O-acetyl-2,3,5,6-tri-O-methyl galactitol	7.50	Galf-(1→
1,2,5-Tri-O-acetyl-3,4,6-tri-O-methyl mannitol	29.45	→2)-Manp-(1→
1,4,5-Tri-O-acetyl-2,3,6-tri-O-methyl mannitol	15.15	→4)-Manp-(1→
1,2,3,4-Tetra-O-acetyl-5,6-O-methyl galactitol	11.48	→2,3)-Galf (1→
1,2,4-Tri-O-acetyl-3,5,6-di-O-methyl galactitol	13.01	→2)-Galf-(1→
1,3,4-Tri-O-acetyl-2,5,6-di-O-methyl galactitol	15.30	→3)-Galf-(1→

In order to further investigate the structure of PJ1-1, NMR spectra analysis of PJ1-1 was carried out (Figure 2). In the ^{1}H NMR spectrum of PJ1-1, 7 anomeric proton signals, which occurred at 5.29, 5.25, 5.23, 5.20, 5.16, 5.12 and 5.08 ppm, had relative integrals of 1.92:0.75:0.85:0.49:0.99:0.53:1. Other proton signals were located in the region of 4.20–3.60 ppm, which were attributed to H2–H6 of the sugar residues. In the anomeric region of the ^{13}C NMR spectrum of PJ1-1, 7 anomeric carbon signals appeared at 99.76, 102.19, 103.79, 106.25, 107.87, 108.67 and 109.31 ppm. The chemical displacement of heterocarbon (C1) corresponds to α-type and β-type glucoside structures in the ^{13}C NMR spectra at 90–104 ppm and 105–110 ppm, respectively [17]. The anomeric carbon signals at 106.25, 107.87, 108.67 and 109.31 ppm illustrated the presence of β-galactofuranose residues in PJ1-1 because only the anomeric carbon signals of β-D-galactofuranose and α-L-arabinofuranose could move to more than 105 ppm in the low field [18]. The signals at 99.76, 102.19 and 103.79 ppm were attributed to α-mannopyranose units [19,20]. The C2–C6 signals were distributed in the region of 60–90 ppm. The chemical shifts at 81.42 and 89.53 ppm might have been the C2–C4 signals of β-D-galactofuranose as the chemical shifts of C2–C6 would not exceed 80 ppm in common hexopyranose [21].

The ^{1}H–^{1}H correlated spectroscopy (COSY) and ^{1}H–^{1}H total correlation spectroscopy (TOCSY) afforded a variety of proton correlations with the sugar units. The C–H correlations were assigned from the ^{1}H–^{13}C heteronuclear single quantum coherence spectroscopy (HSQC) of PJ1-1. The H-1 of A at 5.29 ppm was related with the C-1 at 102.19 ppm, and A was assigned to →2)-α-D-Man$p$-(1→ unit due to the downfield shift of C-2 (79.67 ppm) in comparison with that of the parent α-D-Man$p$ [22]. The H-1 of B at 5.25 ppm corresponded to the C-1 at 108.67 ppm. B was attributed to →2,3)-β-D-Gal$f$-(1→ unit because the signals of the down-field chemical shifts of C-2 at 89.53 ppm and C-3 at 75.87 ppm [23]. The H-1 of C at 5.23 ppm was related to the C-1 at 106.25 ppm. C was assigned to the →2)-β-D-Gal$f$-(1→ unit because the C-2 shift of C changed to low displacement at 89.53 ppm [24]. The H-1 signal of D at 5.20 ppm was correlated to the anomeric carbon signal at 107.87 ppm, and D was assigned to the β-D-Gal$f$-(1→ unit [25]. The H-1 signal of E at 5.16 ppm was related to the C-1 signal at 99.76, and E was attributed to the →4)-α-D-Man$p$-(1 → unit due to the correlated signals H-4/C-4 (3.82/74.78 ppm). The H-1 signal of F at 5.12 ppm was correlated to the C-1 signal at 103.79 ppm, and F was assigned to the α-D-Man$p$-(1→ unit [26]. G was assigned to the →3)-β-D-Gal$f$-(1 → unit due to the shift of the C-3 changing to low displacement at 79.78 ppm. By combining the data from the ^{1}H–^{1}H COSY, ^{1}H–^{1}H TOCSY and ^{1}H–^{13}C HSQC spectra, the assignment of the main proton and carbon signals of the seven sugar residues could be completed (Table 2).

Table 2. ^{1}H and ^{13}C chemical shifts of PJ1-1.

Sugar Residues	Chemical Shifts (ppm) [a]					
	H1/C1	H2/C2	H3/C3	H4/C4	H5/C5	H6/C6
→2)-α-D-Man$p$-(1→	5.29/102.19	4.15/79.67	4.01/71.64	3.71/71.39	3.66/68.35	3.76/62.48
→2,3)-β-D-Gal$f$-(1→	5.25/108.67	4.17/89.53	4.10/75.87	3.87/81.42	3.98/61.98	-/-
→2)-β-D-Gal$f$-(1→	5.23/106.25	4.17/89.53	4.03/71.64	3.87/81.42	3.78/61.98	-/-
β-D-Gal$f$-(1→	5.20/107.87	4.15/79.90	4.01/71.56	3.73/82.30	-/-	-/-
→4)-α-D-Man$p$-(1→	5.16/99.76	4.10/71.56	3.87/71.97	3.82/74.78	3.72/68.47	3.65/64.28
α-D-Man$p$-(1→	5.12/103.79	3.92/71.56	4.01/71.64	3.75/67.96	3.72/64.30	3.92/62.58
→3)-β-D-Gal$f$-(1→	5.08/109.31	4.18/82.61	4.07/79.78	3.77/83.67	3.72/64.30	-/-

[a] Spectra were performed on an Agilent DD2 500 MHz NMR spectrometer. Chemical shifts are referenced to internal acetone at 2.225 ppm for ^{1}H and 31.07 ppm for ^{13}C. Man$p$: mannopyranose, Gal$f$: galactofuranose.

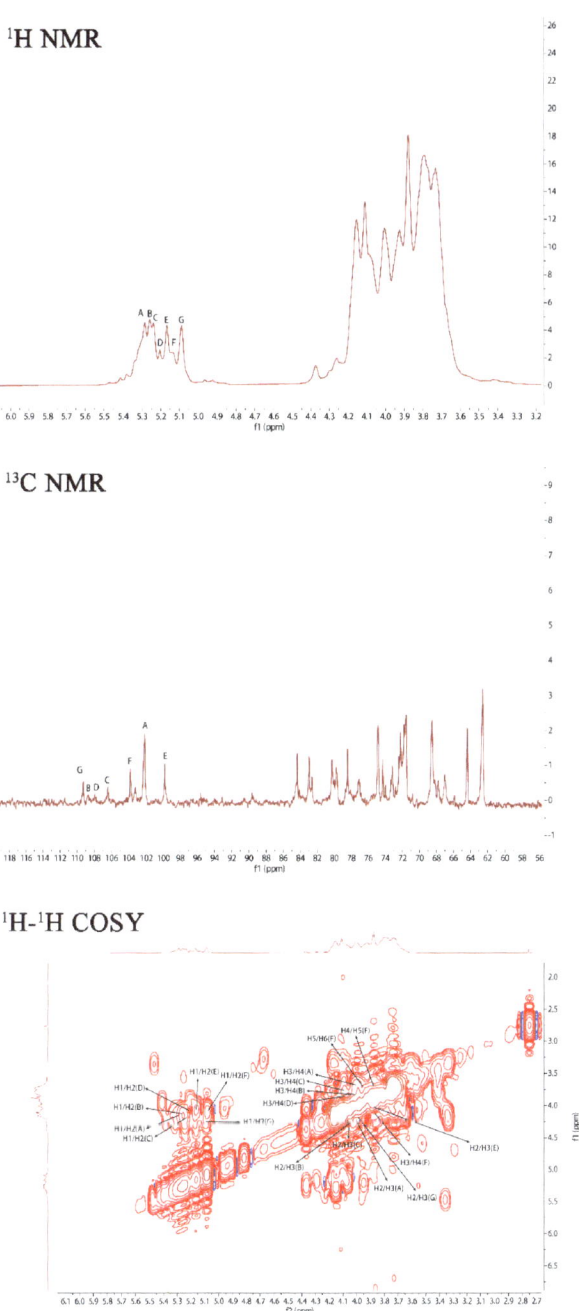

Figure 2. Cont.

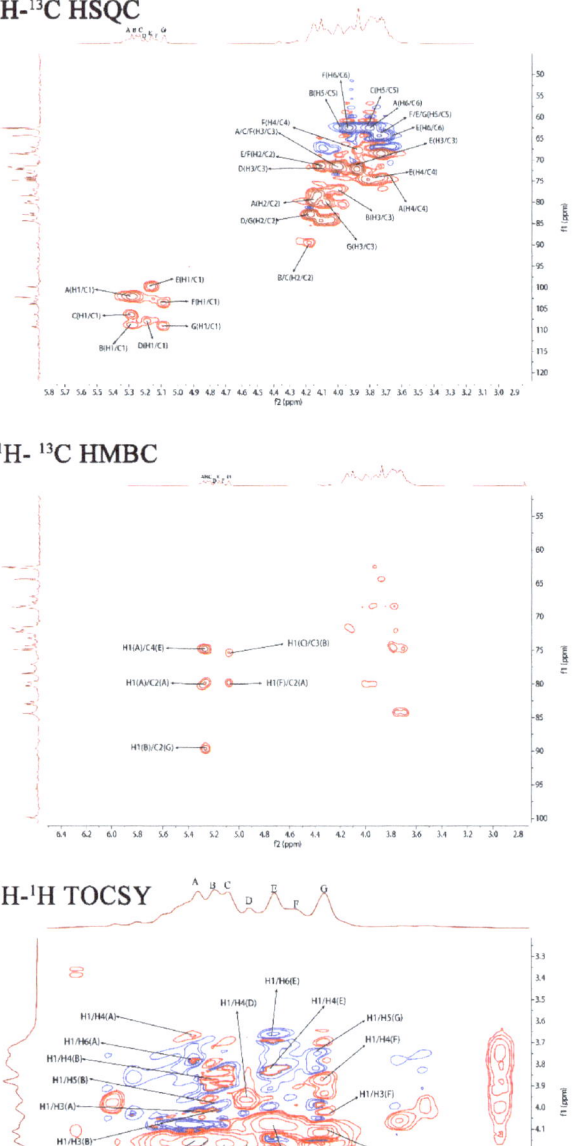

Figure 2. Cont.

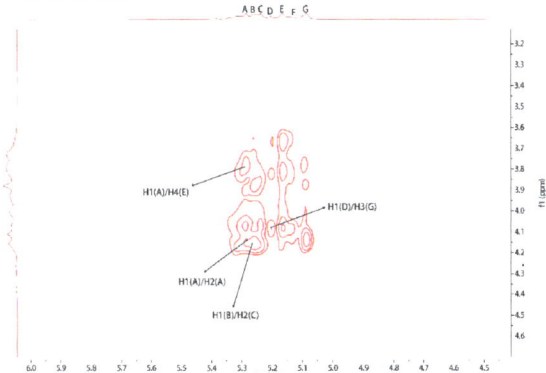

Figure 2. NMR spectra of PJ1-1. Spectra were performed on an Agilent DD2 500 MHz NMR spectrometer using acetone as internal standard. A: →2)-α-D-Manp-(1→; B: →2,3)-β-D-Galf-(1→; C: →2)-β-D-Galf-(1→; D: β-D-Galf-(1→; E: →4)-α-D-Manp-(1→; F: α-D-Manp-(1→; and G: →3)-β-D-Galf-(1→. Manp: mannopyranose, Galf: galactofuranose.

The repeating sequences in PJ1-1 were obtained using ^{1}H–^{1}H nuclear Overhauser enhancement spectroscopy (NOESY) and ^{1}H–^{13}C heteronuclear multiple bond correlation spectroscopy (HMBC). In the ^{1}H–^{13}C HMBC spectrum, the cross signal H-1(B)/C-2(C) proved that the C-1 of the →2,3)-β-D-Galf-(1→ unit was linked to the O-2 position of the →2)-β-D-Galf-(1→ unit. The cross signal H-1(A)/C-2(A) illustrated that the C-1 of the →2)-α-D-Manp-(1→ unit was attached to the O-2 position of the →2)-α-D-Manp-(1→ unit. The cross signal H-1(A)/C-4(E) showed that the C-1 of the →2)-α-D-Manp-(1→ unit was linked to the O-4 position of the →4)-α-D-Manp-(1→ unit. The related signal H-1(F)/C-2(A) indicated that the C-1 of the α-D-Manp-(1→ unit was attached to the O-2 position of the →2)-α-D-Manp-(1→ unit. The cross signal H-1(G)/C-3(B) proved that the C-1 of the →3)-β-D-Galf-(1→ unit was linked to the O-3 position of the →2,3)-β-D-Galf-(1→ unit. Furthermore, the cross signal H-1 (G)/C-3 (B) revealed the characteristics of the side chain. In the ^{1}H–^{1}H NOESY spectrum, the related signal H-1(D)/H-3(G) proved that the C-1 of the β-D-Galf-(1→ unit was linked to the O-3 position of the →3)-β-D-Galf-(1→ unit. The cross signals H-1(A)/H-4(E), H-1(A)/H-2(A) and H-1(B)/H-2(C) further proved the presence of sequences →2)-α-D-Manp-(1→4)-α-D-Manp-(1→, →2)-α-D-Manp-(1→2)-α-D-Manp-(1→ and →2,3)-β-D-Galf-(1→2)-β-D-Galf-(1→.

Based on the above analyses, it was concluded that the backbone of PJ1-1 was constituted by the →2)-α-D-Manp-(1→, →4)-α-D-Manp-(1→, →3)-β-D-Galf-(1→ and →2)-β-D-Galf-(1→ units with partial branches at C-3 of the →2)-β-D Galf (1) unit. The branches were mainly composed of the →3)-β-D-Galf-(1→ unit. An in-depth spectroscopic investigation on the fine structure of the side chains in PJ1-1 is required. The possible major disaccharides in PJ1-1 was shown in Figure 3.

So far, reports on the structural characterization of exopolysaccharides from the mangrove endophytic fungus have been seldom found. The exopolysaccharide Fw-1 from the mangrove-associated fungus *Fusarium oxysporum* contained a backbone of (1→6)-linked β-D-galactofuranose residue, and the branches were constituted by terminal α-D-glucopyranose residue, or short chains containing (1→2)-linked α-D-glucopyranose, (1→2)-linked β-D-mannopyranose and terminal β-D-mannopyranose residues. The side chains were connected to the C-2 of the galactofuranose residue of the backbone [27]. The backbone of the exopolysaccharide As1-1 from the mangrove endophytic fungus *Aspergillus* sp. Y16 mainly consisted of a (1→2)-linked α-D-mannopyranose unit, substituted at C-6 by the (1→6)-linked α-D-mannopyranose, (1→)-linked β-D-galactofuranose and (1→)-linked β-D-mannopyranose units [28]. PJ1-1 possessed different structural characteristics from the exopolysaccharides from these mangrove endophytic fungi. The exopolysaccharide PJ1-1 from the mangrove endophytic fungus *P. janthinellum* N29 constituted the →2)-α-D-Man*p*-(1→, →4)-α-D-Man*p*-(1→, →2)-β-D-Gal*f*-(1→ and →3)-β-D-Gal*f*-(1→ units. The branch which contained the →3)-β-D-Gal*f*-(1→unit was at C-3 of the →2)-β-D-Gal*f*-(1→ unit. The exopolysaccharides with galactofuranose units are often produced by mangrove endophytic fungi, and can be very useful chemotaxonomic markers [29]. Our result also demonstrated that the galactofuranose units may be a characteristic component of the exopolysaccharides from mangrove endophytic fungi. The generality extent of the structural characteristics in the exopolysaccharides from other mangrove endophytic fungi must be further investigated.

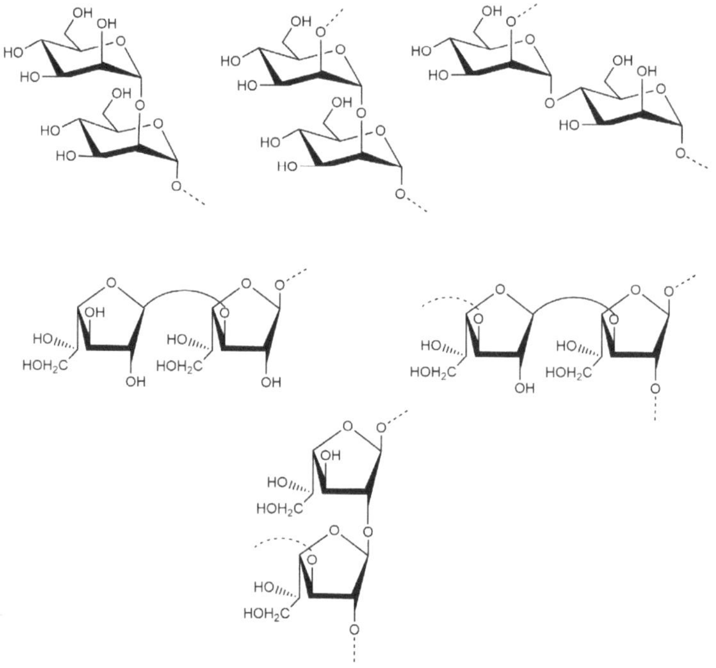

Figure 3. Possible structures of the main repeating disaccharides in PJ1-1.

2.2. Influence of PJ1-1 on α-Glucosidase Activity In Vitro

α-Glucosidase is a glycoside hydrolase found in the small intestine that may rapidly hydrolyze dietary starches and cause a rise in blood glucose level. Thus, the inhibition of α-glucosidase activity is an efficient strategy to reduce hyperglycemia in diabetic individuals. In the present study, the inhibition effect of PJ1-1 on α-glucosidase activity was investigated using acarbose as a reference. As shown in Figure 4, the inhibitory effect of PJ1-1 on α-glucosidase activity was in a concentration-dependent manner. The α-glucosidase activity was effectively inhibited by PJ1-1, and the inhibitory rate was about 70.52% at 5 mg/mL. Additionally, the inhibitory effect of PJ1-1 on α-glucosidase activity was slightly lower than that of acarbose. The data indicated that PJ1-1 could be a potential hypoglycemic polysaccharide. Thus, the anti-diabetic activity of PJ1-1 in vivo was further explored using T2DM mice induced by high-fat diet and STZ.

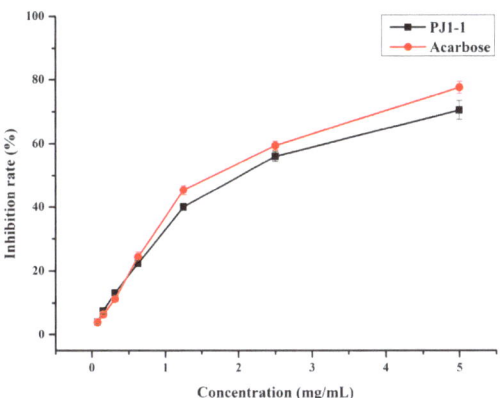

Figure 4. Inhibitory effect of PJ1-1 on α-glucosidase activity in vitro.

2.3. Antidiabetic Activity In Vivo of PJ1-1

A combination of high-fat diet and low-dose streptozotocin (STZ) treatment has been extensively utilized to produce an experimental mice model with T2DM [30]. Feeding a high-fat diet to mice can result in blood glucose and serum lipid metabolic disorders, as well as insulin resistance, which are similar to the early symptoms of human T2DM. STZ injection is used to kill a portion of the islet β-cells. In this study, mice with T2DM induced by a high-fat diet and STZ were used to study the anti-diabetic effect of PJ1-1 in vivo.

2.3.1. Effects of PJ1-1 on Body Weight and Fasting Blood Glucose Level

The influence of PJ1-1 on body weight is shown in Figure 5A. By comparison with the normal control (NC) group, the body weight in the model control (MC) group obviously reduced. However, after treatment with PJ1-1, the body weights significantly elevated compared with the MC group ($p < 0.01$). These results indicated that PJ1-1 could effectively improve the loss of body weight in high-fat-diet- and STZ-induced T2DM mice.

Table 3. Effect of PJ1-1 on fasting blood glucose level in the type 2 diabetes mellitus mice.

	Fasting Blood Glucose Level (mmol/L) [a]					
	NC	MC	PC	PJ1-1-H	PJ1-1-M	PJ1-1-L
0 week	5.25 ± 0.18	18.21 ± 0.77 [##]	20.15 ± 2.15 [##]	20.67 ± 2.08 [##]	21.02 ± 2.66 [##]	22.14 ± 1.92 [##]
1 week	5.19 ± 0.18	21.47 ± 1.10 [##]	21.18 ± 2.15	21.28 ± 2.11	21.06 ± 2.21	20.89 ± 1.51
2 week	5.27 ± 0.32	21.50 ± 1.10 [##]	21.12 ± 1.60	18.62 ± 1.04 [**]	19.59 ± 1.73	20.12 ± 1.54
3 week	5.19 ± 0.18	21.77 ± 0.89 [##]	18.18 ± 0.99 [**]	16.60 ± 1.62 [**]	16.33 ± 1.75 [**]	18.82 ± 1.37 [**]
4 week	5.10 ± 0.25	22.13 ± 0.76 [##]	14.40 ± 0.90 [**]	15.32 ± 1.44 [**]	16.77 ± 1.47 [**]	17.62 ± 0.97 [**]
5 week	5.19 ± 0.32	21.75 ± 1.36 [##]	9.75 ± 1.34 [**]	12.58 ± 0.77 [**]	15.42 ± 1.58 [**]	16.91 ± 1.71 [**]

[a] Values are mean ± SD ($n = 6$). [##] $p < 0.01$ vs. the normal control group; [**] $p < 0.01$ vs. the model control group.

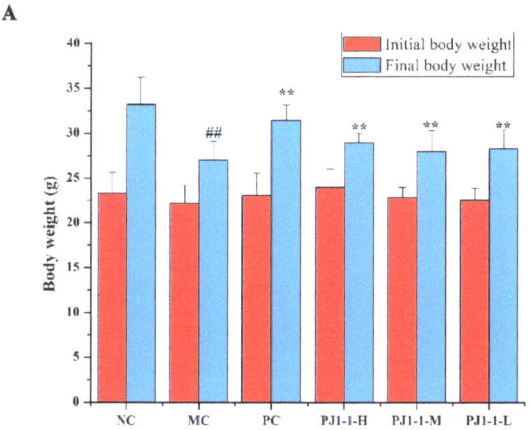
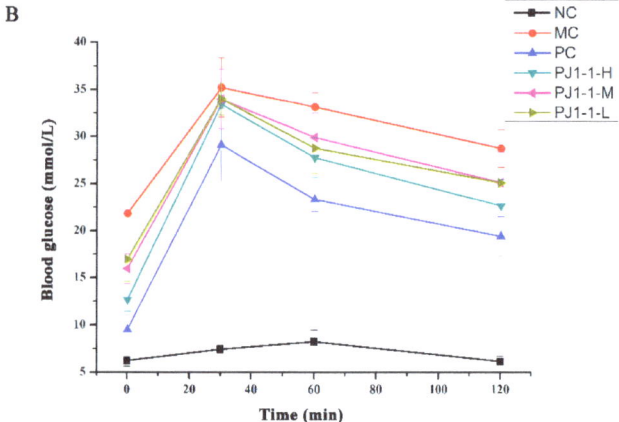
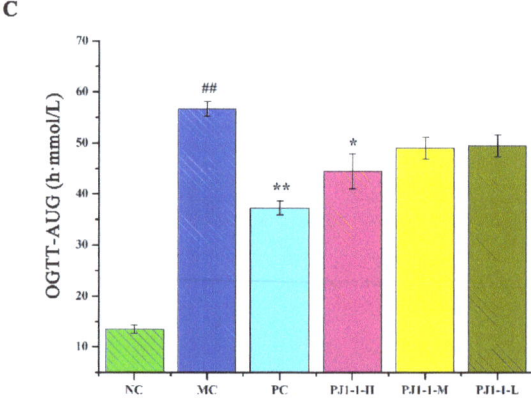

Figure 5. Effects of PJ1-1 on body weight and glucose tolerance in the type 2 diabetes mellitus mice. (**A**) Body weight; (**B**) oral glucose tolerance tests; and (**C**) oral glucose tolerance tests -area under the curve. ## $p < 0.01$ vs. the normal control group; * $p < 0.05$ vs. the model control group, ** $p < 0.01$ vs. the model control group.

Hyperglycemia is a major symptom of diabetes; thus, reducing fasting blood glucose (FBG) is the main target of treating diabetes. FBG is a fundamental indicator of blood glucose balance. The effect of PJ1-1 on the level of FBG was investigated using the T2DM mice, and the results are listed in Table 3. The level of FBG in the NC group was stable at 5.10–5.27 mmol/L throughout the administration period. However, the level of FBG in the MC group substantially increased compared with the NC group ($p < 0.01$), illustrating that the blood glucose balance was disordered because of the high-fat diet and STZ treatment. After treatment with PJ1-1 for one week, the levels of FBG in the PJ1-1 groups continued to increase. However, from the third to fifth weeks, the levels of FBG in the PJ1-1 groups significantly decreased in comparison with the MC group ($p < 0.01$). In the fifth week, compared with the MC group, the levels of FBG in the high dose of PJ1-1 (PJ1-1-H) group, middle dose of PJ1-1 (PJ1-1-M) group and low dose of PJ1-1 (PJ1-1-L) group decreased by 42.16%, 29.10% and 22.26%, respectively. The decreasing effect of PJ1-1 on the level of FBG was dose-dependent. The level of FBG in the positive control (PC) group showed a 55.17% decrease in the fifth week. These data indicated that PJ1-1 could effectively improve blood glucose balance.

2.3.2. Effect of PJ1-1 on Glucose Tolerance

The influence of PJ1-1 on the glucose tolerance in the T2DM mice was evaluated using the assays of oral glucose tolerance tests (OGTT) and OGTT-area under the curve (OGTT-AUC). As shown in Figure 5B, after 30 min of administration, the blood glucose levels increased rapidly and reached the highest value in all groups, and then gradually decreased. The blood glucose level in the NC group returned to normal at 120 min, but the glucose level in the MC group remained at a high level of about 28.77 mmol/L. These results indicated that glucose tolerance was impaired seriously in the T2DM mice. However, by comparison with the MC group, the blood glucose levels in the three PJ1-1 groups markedly reduced at 120 min, especially in the PJ1-1-H group. The glucose level in the PJ1-1-H group decreased to 22.67 mmol/L, illustrating that a certain concentration of PJ1-1 could improve glucose tolerance. The blood glucose level in the PC group reduced to 19.44 mmol/L at 120 min. As shown in Figure 5C, compared with the NC group, the OGTT-AUC increased by 76.14% ($p < 0.01$) in the MC group, indicating that the glucose tolerance of the T2DM mice was retrograded severely. However, the level of OGTT-AUC in the PJ1-1-H group significantly reduced compared with the MC group ($p < 0.05$). In addition, it was obvious that rosiglitazone treatment induced a significant decrease in the level of OGTT-AUC in comparison with the MC group. These results indicated that PJ1-1 possessed a better ability to stimulate glucose metabolism, and improved glucose tolerance in the T2DM mice.

2.3.3. Effect of PJ1-1 on Insulin Resistance

Insulin is a potent anabolic agent, promoting the cellular uptake, storage and synthesis of nutrients, while blocking nutrient breakdown and release into the circulation. Insulin secretion deficiency and insulin resistance are typical features of T2DM, which result in hyperglycemia and impaired glucose metabolism [31]. Here, the assays of the fasting insulin content, the quantitative insulin sensitivity check index (QUICKI), the index of homeostasis model assessment of insulin resistance (HOMA-IR) and the index of homeostasis model assessment β (HOMA-β) were used for the evaluation of insulin resistance.

As shown in Figure 6, after treatment with a high-fat diet and STZ, compared with the NC group, the fasting insulin content and HOMA-IR index in the MC group obviously increased, while the QUICKI and HOMA-β indexes obviously decreased, indicating that the diabetic mice occurred insulin resistance. However, compared with the MC group, the fasting insulin content in the PJ1-1-H group significantly decreased ($p < 0.05$). The fasting insulin content in the PJ1-1 m and PJ1-1-L groups also reduced, although these data were not significantly different compared with that of the MC group. The fasting insulin content in the PC group markedly diminished compared with the MC group ($p < 0.01$). It was also noted that PJ1-1 could markedly increase the QUICKI index compared with the MC group. The indexes of QUICKI in the PJ1-1-H, PJ1-1 m and PJ1-1-L groups increased by 12.80%, 7.69% and 7.66%, respectively. For the PC group, the index of QUICKI increased by 20.51%. Additionally, PJ1-1 significantly decreased the HOMA-IR index in a dose-dependent manner compared with the MC group, but PJ1-1 did not exhibit a noticeable effect on the HOMA-β index in comparison with the MC group. The QUICKI index is a critical indicator that measures insulin sensitivity in mice. The higher the content, the greater the carbohydrate breakdown efficiency. HOMA-IR reflects the hypoglycemic efficiency of insulin in mice due to the feedback loop between the blood glucose output and insulin secretion. The responsiveness of the liver and peripheral tissues to insulin reduced as the HOMA-IR score rose. These results indicated that PJ1-1 could effectively increase insulin sensibility, ameliorate insulin resistance and improve the hypoglycemic efficiency of insulin in the T2DM mice.

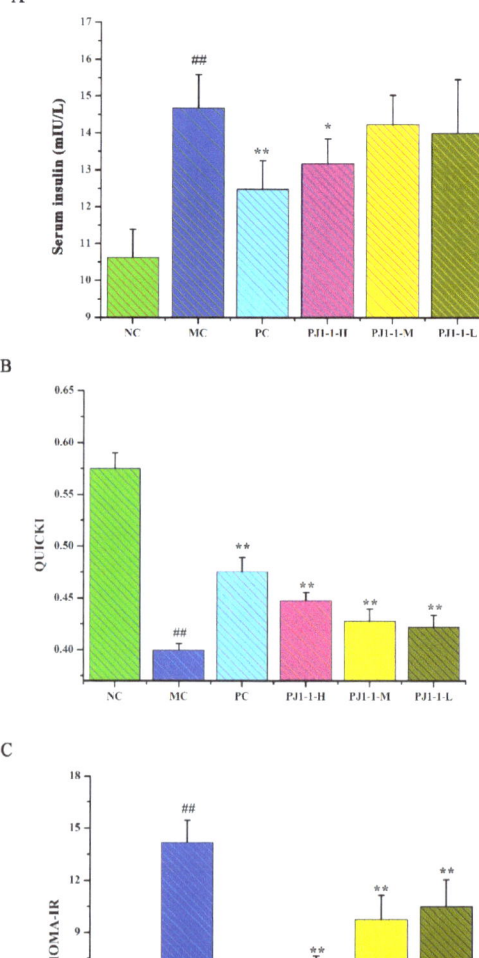

Figure 6. Cont.

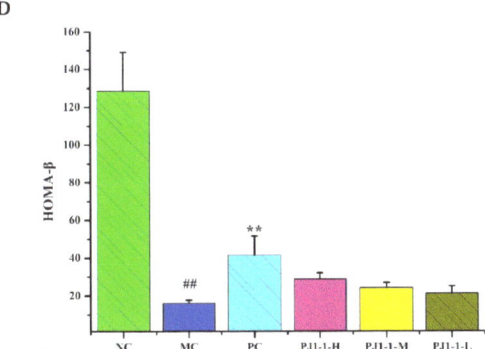

Figure 6. Influence of PJ1-1 on insulin resistance in the type 2 diabetes mellitus mice. (**A**) Fasting insulin content; (**B**) quantitative insulin sensitivity check index; (**C**) index of homeostasis model assessment of insulin resistance; and (**D**) index of homeostasis model assessment β. ## $p < 0.01$ vs. the normal control group; * $p < 0.05$ vs. the model control group, ** $p < 0.01$ vs. the model control group.

2.3.4. Influences of PJ1-1 on Lipid Metabolism

Dyslipidemia is one of the risk factors of T2DM and causes a disruption in lipid metabolism. Hyperlipidemia is an early event in the development of cardiovascular disease in T2DM patients. Dysregulation of lipid metabolism can result in systemic disruption of insulin and glucose metabolism [32]. As shown in Figure 7, compared with the NC group, the total cholesterol (TC), triglyceride (TG) and low-density lipoprotein-cholesterin (LDL-C) levels in the MC group significantly increased ($p < 0.01$) and the high-density lipoprotein–cholesterin (HDL-C) level markedly reduced ($p < 0.01$). After treatment with PJ1-1 for 5 weeks, the TG level significantly decreased in the PJ1-1-H group ($p < 0.01$) compared with the MC group. Moreover, PJ1-1 markedly increased the TC levels in a dose-dependent manner compared with the MC group. The LDL-C levels effectively diminished in the PJ1-1-H ($p < 0.01$) and PJ1-1 m ($p < 0.05$) groups, while the HDL-C level significantly increased in the PJ1-1-H group ($p < 0.05$). In addition, it was obvious that rosiglitazone treatment induced a significant decrease in the levels of TG, TC and LDL-C, and resulted in an increase in the HDL-C level in comparison with the MC group. These results suggested that PJ1-1 ameliorated dyslipidemia in the T2DM mice and promoted lipid metabolism by decreasing TG, TC and LDL-C levels and increasing HDL-C level.

The above results demonstrated that PJ1-1 possesses an obvious anti-diabetic activity in vivo. PJ1-1 significantly improved blood glucose balance and glucose tolerance. In addition, PJ1-1 increased insulin sensitivity and ameliorated insulin resistance. Furthermore, PJ1-1 obviously reduced the serum TG, TC and LDL-C levels, increased HDL-C level and repaired dyslipidemia. Hyperglycemia is a major symptom of diabetes that can cause a series of complications. T2DM is characterized by the increasing death of β-cells and resultant insulin secretion impairment. Insulin resistance pertains to low-efficiency glucose utilization that renders insulin insensitivity in an organism. The obvious features of insulin resistance include high levels of blood glucose and serum insulin. Moreover, T2DM is frequently accompanied by aberrant lipid metabolism [33]. The present data revealed that PJ1-1 had the potential to develop into a novel anti-diabetic agent for prevention and therapy of T2DM. The anti-diabetic activity of PJ1-1 could be associated with its structural characteristics. The presence of α-(1→4) glycosidic linkages of polysaccharides has been reported to be critical for α-glucosidase inhibitory activity [34]. Gao et al. found that the polysaccharide ARLP-W from *Anoectochilus roxburghi*, which contained glycosidic linkages of β-1, 4-Man$p$, could decrease the level of hyperglycaemia, protect the islets, improve insulin resistance and increase the β-cell area in T2DM mice [35]. Liu et al. reported that the polysaccharides which possessed a β-D-(1→6)- glycosidic bond improved the insulin level and decreased the blood glucose level in streptozotocin-induced diabetic mice [36].

However, it is difficult to reach a conclusion on the relationship between the structure and antidiabetic activity of the polysaccharides. The generality extent of the relationship requires further investigation.

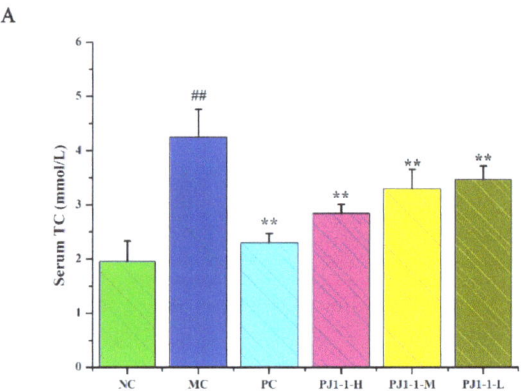

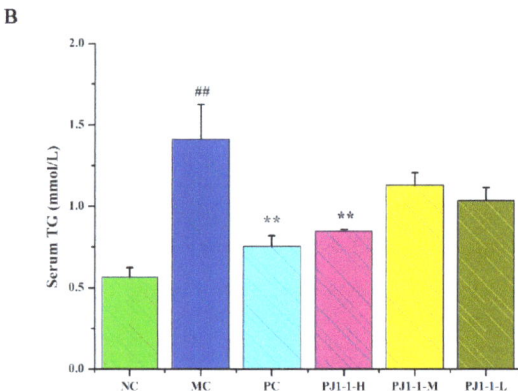

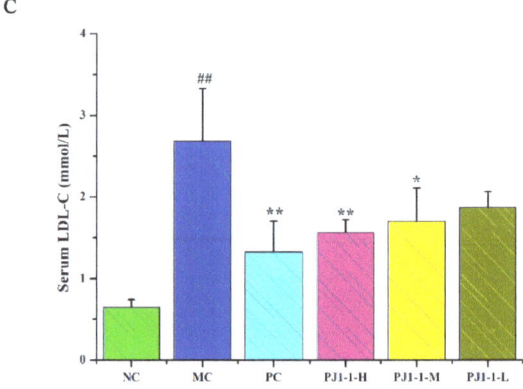

Figure 7. *Cont.*

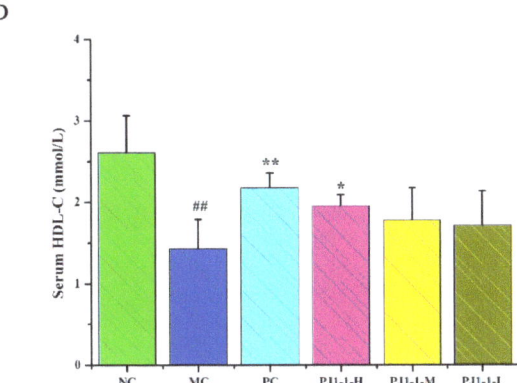

Figure 7. Effect of PJ1-1 on lipid metabolism in the type 2 diabetes mellitus mice. (**A**) Total cholesterol level; (**B**) triglyceride level; (**C**) low-density lipoprotein-cholesterin level; and (**D**) high-density lipoprotein–cholesterin level. ## $p < 0.01$ vs. the normal control group; * $p < 0.05$ vs. the model control group, ** $p < 0.01$ vs. the model control group.

3. Materials and Methods

3.1. Materials

p-Nitrophenyl-α-D-glucopyranoside, α-glucosidase (EC 3.2.1.20, from Saccharomyces cerevisiae), 1-phenyl-3-methyl-5-pyrazolone and monosaccharide standards (D-mannose, L-rhamnose, D-glucose, D-glucuronic acid, D-galacturonic acid, N-acetyl-β-D-glucosamine, D-glucose, D-galactose, D-xylose, L-arabinose, and L-fucose) were obtained from Sigma–Aldrich (St. Louis, MO, USA). Pullulan standards (Mw: 5.9, 9.6, 21.1, 47.1, and 107 kDa) were obtained from Showa Denko K.K. (Tokyo, Japan). Q Sepharose Fast Flow and Sephacryl S-100/HR were obtained from GE Healthcare Life Sciences (Piscataway, NJ, USA). Bicinchoninic acid (BCA) protein assay kit and glucose assay kit with o-toluidine were obtained from Beyotime Biotechnology (Shanghai, China). STZ and rosiglitazone were obtained from Aladdin Chemical Co., Ltd. (Shanghai, China). Mouse insulin enzyme-linked immunosorbent assay (ELISA) kit was obtained from Solarbio Biotechnology (Beijing, China). The assay kits for TC, TG, HDL-C and LDL-C were obtained from Nanjing Jiancheng Bioengineering Institute (Nanjing, China).

3.2. Animals

Four-week-old male C57BL/6J mice (18–22 g, SPF grade) were obtained from Charles River Laboratories (Beijing, China) and housed under standard feeding circumstances with a 12 h light/dark cycle and free access to food and water. Animal experiments were permitted by the institutional animal care and use committee of Ocean University of China (OUC-SMP-20220403).

3.3. Strains and Culture Conditions

The fungus *P. janthinellum* N29 was isolated from a piece of fresh tissue from the inner part of the medicinal mangrove *Acanthus ilicifolius* collected from the South China Sea. It was identified according to a molecular biological protocol by DNA amplification and sequencing of the ITS region. The sequence data have been submitted to GenBank with the accession number MW178203. *P. janthinellum* N29 was grown in potato dextrose agar medium containing glucose (20 g/L), sea salt (15 g/L) and potato starch (200 g/L), at pH 7.0 at 28 °C for 15 days on a reciprocal shaker. Finally, 150 L of liquid culture broth was obtained.

3.4. Preparation of the Exopolysaccharide PJ1-1

The exopolysaccharide from the fermentation broth of the fungus *P. janthinellum* N29 was isolated according to the method reported previously [37]. The fermentation broth was centrifuged (8000× *g*, 10 min) to separate the mycelia and supernatant. The supernatant was concentrated to one-third of its original volume with a rotary evaporator under reduced pressure at 55 °C. Subsequently, 4 volumes of 95% ethanol were added (*v*/*v*) and kept at 4 °C for 24 h. The precipitate was collected via centrifugation (3600× *g*, 10 min) and dialyzed in a cellulose membrane tubing (flat width 44 mm, molecular weight cut off 3500) against distilled water for 48 h. The retained fraction was concentrated and lyophilized and a crude polysaccharide was obtained. The crude polysaccharide was fractionated on a Q Sepharose Fast Flow column (60 cm × 30 mm) by eluting with a step-wise gradient of 0, 0.025 and 0.4 mol/L NaCl at a flow rate of 1.0 mL/min. The eluates were collected by an auto-collector, and the total sugar content was detected using the phenol–sulfuric acid method [38]. According to the profile of the gradient elution, the fraction PJ1 eluted with distilled water was the most abundant and was further purified on a Sephacryl S-100 column (95 cm × 25 mm) eluting with 0.2 mol/L NH_4HCO_3 at a flow rate of 0.2 mL/min Major fractions were collected, freeze-dried and designated as PJ1-1.

3.5. Composition Analysis

Total sugar content was measured using the phenol–sulfuric acid method with mannose as the standard [38]. Protein was analyzed using the BCA protein assay kit [39]. Purity and molecular weight of PJ1-1 were assessed using HPGPC [40]. The assay was performed on an Agilent 1260 Infinity HPLC instrument (Agilent Technologies, Santa Clara, CA, USA) fitted with a Shodex OHpak SB-803 HQ column (8.0 mm × 300 mm, Showa Denko K.K. Tokyo, Japan) and a refractive index detector (Agilent RID-10A Series). The molecular weight was estimated by reference to a calibration curve made by pullulan standards (M_w 107, 47.1, 21.1, 9.6 and 5.9 kDa).

Monosaccharide composition was determined with reversed-phase HPLC after precolumn derivatization [41]. Briefly, PJ1-1 (5 mg) was hydrolyzed with 2 mol/L trifluoroacetic acid at 105 °C for 4 h. After that, the excess acid was removed with methanol using a nitrogen blower three times. The dry hydrolysate was dissolved in 1.5 mL of distilled water and centrifuged (4500× *g*, 10 min). Subsequently, the supernatant solution (160 µL) was derivatized with 160 µL of 0.3 mol/L NaOH, 400 µL of 0.5 mol/L PMP solution (in methanol) and 210 µL of distilled water at 70 °C for 60 min. After cooling down to room temperature, 160 µL of 0.3 mol/L HCl solution was added to terminate the reaction, followed by extraction with 0.8 mL of chloroform three times. The supernatant was filtered through a 0.45 µm membrane, and 10 µL of the resulting solution was injected into the Eclipse XDB-C18 column (4.6 mm × 250 mm, 5 µm). The chromatogram was performed on an Agilent 1260 Infinity HPLC instrument fitted with an Agilent XDB-UV detector (254 nm) The mobile phase was a mixture of 0.1 mol/L KH_2PO_4 in water (pH 6.7)–acetonitrile (83:17) The flow rate was 1.0 mL/min, and column temperature was 30 °C.

Sugar configuration was measured as described by Tanaka et al. [42]. PJ1-1 was degraded with 2 mol/L trifluoroacetic acid at 105 °C for 4 h. Then, the hydrolysate was heated with l-cysteine methyl ester in pyridine at 60 °C for 1 h. The o-tolyl isothiocyanate solution was added to the mixture, and was further heated at 60 °C for 1 h. The reaction mixture was analyzed on an Agilent 1260 Infinity HPLC instrument fitted with an Eclipse XDB-C18 column and an Agilent XDB-UV detector (254 nm, Agilent Technologies, Santa Clara, CA, USA).

3.6. Methylation Analysis

Methylation analysis of PJ1-1 was carried out according to the previously described method with some modification [43]. PJ1-1 (10 mg) was dried in a vacuum-drying oven (55 °C) for 24 h and then dissolved in 2 mL of anhydrous dimethyl sulfoxide with stirring for 12 h under nitrogen protection. Afterwards, 1 mL of iodomethane was added to the reaction system in the dark, N$_2$ was used to drive out the air, and the reaction continued for another 1 h. The completion of methylation was confirmed by Fourier-transform infrared (FTIR) spectroscopy. The completely methylated product was re-dissolved in 2 mL of trifluoroacetic acid (2 mol/L) and sealed at 105 °C for 6 h, and then reduced with NaBH$_4$ and acetylated to convert into alditol acetates by reacting with acetic anhydride–pyridine at 100 °C for 2 h. The acetylated product was dissolved in chloroform (4 mL) and washed with distilled water three times. Thereafter, the partially methylated alditol acetates were analyzed on a TRACE 1300-ISQ instrument (Thermo Scientific, Waltham, MA, USA) equipped with a DB-225 fused silica capillary column (0.25 mm × 30 m, 0.25 µm, Agilent Technologies, Santa Clara, CA, USA).

3.7. Spectroscopy Analysis

^{1}H NMR and ^{13}C NMR spectra were performed at 25 °C on an Agilent DD2 500M NMR spectrometer (Agilent Technologies, Santa Clara, CA, USA). Polysaccharide (60 mg) was deuterium-exchanged by lyophilization three times with 99.9% D$_2$O and then was dissolved in 0.5 mL of 99.9% D$_2$O and transferred into NMR tube. Chemical shift was expressed as δ (ppm) relative to acetone (^{1}H: 2.225 ppm, ^{13}C: 31.07 ppm). ^{1}H–^{1}H COSY, ^{1}H–^{1}H TOCSY, ^{1}H–^{13}C HSQC, ^{1}H–^{1}H NOESY and ^{1}H–^{13}C HMBC experiments were also carried out. Spectra were processed and analyzed using MestReNova (V12.0.3, Mestrelab Research, Santiago de Compostela, Spain). For the FTIR spectrum, the polysaccharide was ground with KBr, pressed into a 1 mm transparent sheet and then determined on a Nicolet Nexus 470 spectrometer (Thermo Fisher Scientific, Waltham, MA, USA) with a scan range of 400–4000 cm^{-1}. UV spectrum was recorded on a UV-2802 PC spectrophotometer (UNICO Shanghai Instrument Co., Ltd., Shanghai, China) between 190 and 400 nm.

3.8. α-Glucosidase Inhibitory Assay

The α-glucosidase inhibitory activity was measured as per the reported method with some modifications [44]. Summarily, the α-glucosidase (750 U) was dissolved in 0.01 mol/L PBS (2 mL, pH 6.8) and shaken for 5 min. The obtained α-glucosidase solution was applied to enzyme inhibition assays with an enzyme activity of 0.2 U/mL. A total of 90 µL of PJ1-1 with different concentrations (0.08, 0.16, 0.32, 0.64, 1.25, 2.50 and 5.00 mg/mL), 100 µL of α-glucosidase (0.5 U/mL) and 20 µL of p-nitrophenol-α-D-glucopyranoside substrate were prepared with 0.01 mol/L PBS (pH 6.8). The mixture solution was shaken vigorously and followed by incubation at 37 °C for 30 min. A total of 100 µL of 0.2 mol/L Na$_2$CO$_3$ was added to terminate the whole reaction. Acarbose was used as positive control. The absorbance was recorded at 405 nm using a microplate reader (Biotek ELx808, BioTek Instruments, Inc. Winooski, VT, USA). The α-glucosidase inhibitory rate was calculated as follows:

$$\text{Inhibition rate (\%)} = 100 - \frac{A_{test} - A_{test\ blank}}{A_{control} - A_{control\ blank}} \times 100$$

A$_{test}$: PJ1-1 or acarbose. A$_{test\ blank}$: PJ1-1 or acarbose, no α-glucosidase. A$_{control}$: no PJ1-1 or acarbose. A$_{control\ blank}$: no α-glucosidase and PJ1-1 or acarbose. The half inhibitory concentration value (IC$_{50}$) was the concentration of the α-glucosidase inhibitor concentration which inhibited the α-glucosidase activity by 50%.

3.9. In Vivo Experiment

3.9.1. Animal Experimental Design

Four-week-old male C57BL/6J mice (18 ± 2 g) were housed in a room with a 12 h light/dark cycle, a temperature of 24–26 °C and a relative humidity of 50–70% with free access to food and water. After a one-week environmental adaptation period, six mice were randomly separated as the NC group and fed a normal diet. The other mice were fed a high-fat diet (10% lard oil, 20% saccharose, 2.5% cholesterol, 0.5% sodium cholate and 67% normal diet) for 6 weeks with sufficient food and water, and then were subjected to intraperitoneal injection of STZ at a dose of 30 mg/kg on day 1–3. After 3 days of STZ treatment, the FBG levels of the mice were measured using a glucose assay kit. The mice with FBG $\geq$ 11.1 mmol/L were regarded as diabetic and then used in the subsequent analysis.

The diabetic mice were randomly divided into five groups ($n = 6$ per group): MC group, PC group, PJ1-1-L group (100 mg/kg/day), PJ1-1 m group (200 mg/kg/day) and PJ1-1-H group (400 mg/kg/day). For the next 35 days, the mice in the PJ1-1 groups were treated with PJ1-1 (100, 200, or 400 mg/kg) via intragastric administration once a day, and the mice in the NC and MC groups were administrated with corresponding volumes of saline. Meanwhile, the mice in the PC group were treated with rosiglitazone at a dose of 200 mg/kg via intragastric administration once a day. The body weight and FBG level of the mice were measured once a week. Their water and food intake was monitored once every 3 days. After 12 h of the final administration, the mice were sacrificed via cervical dislocation. The body weights of mice were measured, and the blood samples were taken from the orbital sinus and centrifuged (4000× g, 10 min) to gain the serum samples, which were stored at −80 °C until analysis.

3.9.2. FBG and OGTT

All mice were fasted for 12 h every weekend and their FBG levels were measured using a glucose assay kit with o-toluidine [45]. After 35 days of intragastric administration, the 12 h fasted mice in all groups were intragastrically administered glucose (2.0 g/kg). The blood glucose levels were measured sequentially at 0, 30, 60 or 120 min. AUC was calculated according to the following formula:

$$\text{AUC} = 0.25 \times (G_{0h} + G_{0.5h}) + 0.25 \times (G_{0.5h} + G_{1.0h}) + 0.5 \times (G_{0h} + G_{2.0h}).$$

3.9.3. Assays of Fasting Insulin Content and Related Indexes

Fasting insulin content of serum was measured using an ELISA kit according to the manufacturer's instructions [46]. Additionally, the HOMA-IR index was calculated using the formula: HOMA-IR = FBG content (mmol/L) × fasting insulin content (mIU/L)/22.5. The HOMA-β index was calculated using the formula: HOMA-β = 20 × fasting insulin content (mIU/L)/[FBG (mmol/L) − 3.5]. QUICKI was measured using the following equation: 1/(lg FBG content (mmol/L) + lg fasting insulin content (mIU/L)) [47].

3.9.4. Determination for Lipid Metabolic Parameter Levels

The levels of the sera TC, TG, LDL-C and HDL-C were tested using commercial enzymatic kits following the instructions on the kits [48].

3.10. Statistical Analysis

Data analyses were performed using Origin 2021b. The results were expressed as the mean ± standard deviation. The mean values among treatment groups were statistically analyzed by one-way analysis of variance (ANOVA) test. Turkey's test was used to compare the results. $p < 0.05$ was considered statistically significant.

4. Conclusions

The exopolysaccharide PJ1-1 from the mangrove endophytic fungus *Penicillium janthinellum* N29 is a galactomannan comprising the →2)-α-D-Man$p$-(1→, →4)-α-D-Man$p$-(1→, →3)-β-D-Gal$f$-(1→ and →2)-β-D-Gal$f$-(1→ units. The branches consist of →3)-β-D-Gal$f$-(1→ units located at C-3 of the →2)-β-D-Gal$f$-(1→ unit. Compared to the MC group, PJ1-1 possessed a better ability to stimulate glucose metabolism, and improved the hypoglycemic efficiency of insulin and lipid metabolism in the T2DM mice. These data illustrated that PJ1-1 might be a potential anti-diabetic agent. Further investigation on the anti-diabetic mechanism of PJ1-1 is underway. Continuous studies will promote the development of anti-diabetic agents from marine microorganism.

Author Contributions: Z.S.: methodology, investigation, writing—original draft. Y.T.: methodology, investigation. S.L.: investigation. X.C.: investigation. W.M.: supervision, funding acquisition, writing—review and editing. All authors have read and agreed to the published version of the manuscript.

Funding: This investigate was supported by the National Key Research and Development Program of China (2018YFC0310900), the National Natural Science Foundation of China (41476108) and the Marine S&T Fund of Shandong Province for Pilot National Laboratory for Marine Science and Technology (Qingdao) (2018SDKJ0401).

Institutional Review Board Statement: The study was permitted by the Animal Care and Use Committee of Ocean University of China (OUC-SMP-20220403, approved on 3 April 2022).

Informed Consent Statement: Not applicable.

Data Availability Statement: Data presented in this study are available on request.

Conflicts of Interest: The authors declare no conflict of interest.

References

1. Patel, B.K.; Patel, K.H.; Moochhala, S.M. Gut microbiota intervention strategies using active components from medicinal herbs to evaluate clinical efficacy of type 2 diabetes—A review. *CTD* **2023**, *3*, e170. [CrossRef]
2. Ogurtsova, K.; da Rocha Fernandes, J.; Huang, Y.; Linnenkamp, U.; Guariguata, L.; Cho, N.H.; Cavan, D.; Shaw, J.; Makaroff, L. IDF Diabetes Atlas: Global estimates for the prevalence of diabetes for 2015 and 2040. *Diabetes Res. Clin. Pract.* **2017**, *128*, 40–50. [CrossRef]
3. Bello, N.A.; Pfeffer, M.A.; Skali, H.; McGill, J.B.; Rossert, J.; Olson, K.A.; Weinrauch, L.; Cooper, M.E.; de Zeeuw, D.; Rossing, P. Retinopathy and clinical outcomes in patients with type 2 diabetes mellitus, chronic kidney disease, and anemia. *BMJ Open Diabetes Res.* **2014**, *2*, e11. [CrossRef] [PubMed]
4. Hou, X.; Yi, C.; Zhang, Z.; Wen, H.; Sun, Y.; Xu, J.; Yang, T. Repair and mechanism of oligopeptide SEP-3 on oxidative stress liver injury induced by sleep deprivation in mice. *Mar. Drugs* **2023**, *21*, 139. [CrossRef] [PubMed]
5. Ma, Q.; Li, Y.; Li, P.; Wang, M.; Wang, J.; Tang, Z.; Wang, T.; Luo, L.; Wang, C.; Zhao, B. Research progress in the relationship between type 2 diabetes mellitus and intestinal flora. *Biomed. Pharmacother.* **2019**, *117*, 109138. [CrossRef] [PubMed]
6. Wińska, K.; Mączka, W.; Gabryelska, K.; Grabarczyk, M. Mushrooms of the genus *Ganoderma* used to treat diabetes and insulin resistance. *Molecules* **2019**, *24*, 4075. [CrossRef]
7. Rosas-Ramírez, D.; Escandón-Rivera, S.; Pereda-Miranda, R. Morning glory resin glycosides as α-glucosidase inhibitors: In vitro and in silico analysis. *Phytochemistry* **2018**, *148*, 39–47. [CrossRef]
8. Wang, L.; Chen, C.; Zhang, B.; Huang, Q.; Fu, X.; Li, C. Structural characterization of a novel acidic polysaccharide from *Rosa roxburghii* Tratt fruit and its α-glucosidase inhibitory activity. *Food Funct.* **2018**, *9*, 3974–3985. [CrossRef]
9. Sun, H.; Yu, X.; Li, T.; Zhu, Z. Structure and hypoglycemic activity of a novel exopolysaccharide of *Cordyceps militaris*. *Int. J. Biol. Macromol.* **2021**, *166*, 496–508. [CrossRef]
10. Yang, S.; Qu, Y.; Zhang, H.; Xue, Z.; Liu, T.; Yang, L.; Sun, L.; Zhou, Y.; Fan, Y. Hypoglycemic effects of polysaccharides from *Gomphidiaceae rutilus* fruiting bodies and their mechanisms. *Food Funct.* **2020**, *11*, 424–434. [CrossRef]
11. Ye, H.; Shen, Z.; Cui, J.; Zhu, Y.; Li, Y.; Chi, Y.; Wang, J.; Wang, P. Hypoglycemic activity and mechanism of the sulfated rhamnose polysaccharides chromium (III) complex in type 2 diabetic mice. *Bioorg. Chem.* **2019**, *88*, 102942. [CrossRef]
12. Shan, X.; Liu, X.; Hao, J.; Cai, C.; Fan, F.; Dun, Y.; Zhao, X.; Liu, X.; Li, C.; Yu, G. In vitro and in vivo hypoglycemic effects of brown algal fucoidans. *Int. J. Biol. Macromol.* **2016**, *82*, 249–255. [CrossRef] [PubMed]
13. Xue, Z.; Sun, X.M.; Chen, C.; Zhang, X.Y.; Chen, X.L.; Zhang, Y.Z.; Xu, F. A novel alginate lyase: Identification, characterization, and potential application in alginate trisaccharide preparation. *Mar. Drugs* **2022**, *20*, 159. [CrossRef]
14. Barros, J.; Seena, S. Fungi in freshwaters: Prioritising aquatic hyphomycetes in conservation goals. *Water* **2022**, *14*, 605. [CrossRef]
15. Gonçalves, M.F.; Esteves, A.C.; Alves, A. Marine fungi: Opportunities and challenges. *Encyclopedia* **2022**, *2*, 559–577. [CrossRef]
16. Chen, G.; Kan, J. Characterization of a novel polysaccharide isolated from *Rosa roxburghii* Tratt fruit and assessment of its antioxidant in vitro and in vivo. *Int. J. Biol. Macromol.* **2018**, *107*, 166–174. [CrossRef]
17. Zhou, S.; Huang, G.; Chen, G. Extraction, structural analysis, derivatization and antioxidant activity of polysaccharide from Chinese yam. *Food Chem.* **2021**, *361*, 130089. [CrossRef]
18. Zhu, R.; Zhang, X.; Wang, Y.; Zhang, L.; Zhao, J.; Chen, G.; Ning, C. Characterization of polysaccharide fractions from fruit of *Actinidia arguta* and assessment of their antioxidant and antiglycated activities. *Carbohyd. Polym.* **2019**, *210*, 73–84. [CrossRef] [PubMed]
19. Li, S.; Pan, C.; Xia, W.; Zhang, W.; Wu, S. Structural characterization of the polysaccharide moiety of an aqueous glycopeptide from mannatide. *Int. J. Biol. Macromol.* **2014**, *67*, 351–359. [CrossRef]
20. Ljpkind, G.M.; Shashkov, A.S.; Nifant'ev, N.E.; Kochetkov, N.K. Computer-assisted analysis of the structure of regular branched polysaccharides containing 2, 3-disubstituted rhamnopyranose and mannopyranose residues on the basis of ^{13}C NMR data. *Carbohyd. Res.* **1992**, *237*, 11–22. [CrossRef] [PubMed]

21. Chen, Y.; Mao, W.; Yan, M.; Liu, X.; Wang, S.; Xia, Z.; Xiao, B.; Cao, S.; Yang, B.; Li, J. Purification, chemical characterization, and bioactivity of an extracellular polysaccharide produced by the marine sponge endogenous fungus *Alternaria* sp. SP-32. *Mar. Biotechnol.* **2016**, *18*, 301–313. [CrossRef] [PubMed]
22. Liu, L.; Xu, J.; Na, R.; Du, R.; Ping, W.; Ge, J.; Zhao, D. Purification, characterization and partial biological activities of exopolysaccharide produced by *Saccharomyces cerevisiae* Y3. *Int. J. Biol. Macromol.* **2022**, *206*, 777–787. [CrossRef]
23. Zhou, D.; Li, P.; Dong, Z.; Wang, T.; Sun, K.; Zhao, Y.; Wang, B.; Chen, Y. Structure and immunoregulatory activity of β-D-galactofuranose-containing polysaccharides from the medicinal fungus *Shiraia bambusicola*. *Int. J. Biol. Macromol.* **2019**, *129*, 530–537. [CrossRef] [PubMed]
24. Wang, N.; Jia, G.; Wang, C.; Chen, M.; Xie, F.; Nepovinnykh, N.; Goff, H.D.; Guo, Q. Structural characterisation and immunomodulatory activity of exopolysaccharides from liquid fermentation of *Monascus purpureus* (Hong Qu). *Food Hydrocolloid.* **2020**, *103*, 105636. [CrossRef]
25. Luo, D.; Wang, Z.; Zhou, R.; Cao, S. A polysaccharide from *Umbilicaria yunnana*: Structural characterization and anti-inflammation effects. *Int. J. Biol. Macromol.* **2020**, *151*, 870–877. [CrossRef] [PubMed]
26. Zhang, Y.; Zeng, Y.; Cui, Y.; Liu, H.; Dong, C.; Sun, Y. Structural characterization, antioxidant and immunomodulatory activities of a neutral polysaccharide from *Cordyceps militaris* cultivated on hull-less barley. *Carbohyd. Polym.* **2020**, *235*, 115969. [CrossRef]
27. Chen, Y.; Mao, W.; Tao, H.; Zhu, W.; Yan, M.; Liu, X.; Guo, T.; Guo, T. Preparation and characterization of a novel extracellular polysaccharide with antioxidant activity, from the mangrove-associated fungus *Fusarium oxysporum*. *Mar. Biotechnol.* **2015**, *17*, 219–228. [CrossRef]
28. Chen, Y.; Mao, W.; Tao, H.; Zhu, W.; Qi, X.; Chen, Y.; Li, H.; Zhao, C.; Yang, Y.; Hou, Y. Structural characterization and antioxidant properties of an exopolysaccharide produced by the mangrove endophytic fungus *Aspergillus* sp. Y16. *Bioresour. Technol.* **2011**, *102*, 8179–8184. [CrossRef]
29. Prathyusha, A.; Mohana Sheela, G.; Berde, C.V.; Bramhachari, P. *Current Perspectives on the Novel Structures and Antioxidant Properties of Mangrove Endophytic Fungal Exopolysaccharides, Advances in Endophytic Fungal Research*; Springer: Cham, Switzerland, 2019; pp. 233–242.
30. Srinivasan, K.; Viswanad, B.; Asrat, L.; Kaul, C.; Ramarao, P. Combination of high-fat diet-fed and low-dose streptozotocin-treated rat: A model for type 2 diabetes and pharmacological screening. *Pharmacol. Res.* **2005**, *52*, 313–320. [CrossRef]
31. Saltiel, A.R. Insulin signaling in health and disease. *J. Clin. Investig.* **2021**, *131*, 142241. [CrossRef]
32. Vichaibun, V.; Khananurak, K.; Sophonnithiprasert, T. Comparative analysis of plasma total antioxidant capacity in patients with hyperglycemia and hyperglycemia plus dyslipidemia. *Diabetes Metab. Synd.* **2019**, *13*, 90–94. [CrossRef] [PubMed]
33. Liu, Y.; Chen, D.; You, Y.; Zeng, S.; Hu, Y.; Duan, X.; Chen, D. Structural characterization and antidiabetic activity of a glucopyranose-rich heteropolysaccharide from *Catathelasma ventricosum*. *Carbohyd. Polym.* **2016**, *149*, 399–407. [CrossRef] [PubMed]
34. Wang, Q.; Wu, X.; Shi, F.; Liu, Y. Comparison of antidiabetic effects of saponins and polysaccharides from *Momordica charantia* L. in STZ-induced type 2 diabetic mice. *Biomed. Pharmacother.* **2019**, *109*, 744–750. [CrossRef] [PubMed]
35. Hsu, W.K.; Hsu, T.H.; Lin, F.Y.; Cheng, Y.K.; Yang, J.P. Separation, purification, and α-glucosidase inhibition of polysaccharides from *Coriolus versicolor* LH1 mycelia. *Carbohyd. Polym.* **2013**, *92*, 297–306. [CrossRef] [PubMed]
36. Gao, H.; Ding, L.; Liu, R.; Zheng, X.; Xia, X.; Wang, F.; Qiu, Y. Characterization of *Anoectochilus roxburghii* polysaccharide and its therapeutic effect on type 2 diabetic mice. *Int. J. Biol. Macromol.* **2021**, *179*, 259–269. [CrossRef]
37. Yan, M.; Mao, W.; Liu, X.; Wang, S.; Xia, Z.; Cao, S.; Li, J.; Qin, L.; Xian, H. Extracellular polysaccharide with novel structure and antioxidant property produced by the deep-sea fungus *Aspergillus versicolor* N$_2$bc. *Carbohydr. Polym.* **2016**, *147*, 272–281. [CrossRef]
38. Dubois, M.; Gilles, K.A.; Hamilton, J.K.; Rebers, P.T.; Smith, F. Colorimetric method for determination of sugars and related substances. *Anal. Chem.* **1956**, *28*, 350–356. [CrossRef]
39. Glyk, A.; Heinisch, S.L.; Scheper, T.; Beutel, S. Comparison of colorimetric methods for the quantification of model proteins in aqueous two-phase systems. *Anal. Biochem.* **2015**, *477*, 35–37. [CrossRef] [PubMed]
40. Mao, W.; Li, H.; Li, Y.; Zhang, H.; Qi, X.; Sun, H.; Chen, Y.; Guo, S. Chemical characteristic and anticoagulant activity of the sulfated polysaccharide isolated from *Monostroma latissimum* (Chlorphyta). *Int. J. Biol. Macromol.* **2009**, *44*, 70–74. [CrossRef]
41. Qin, L.; He, M.; Yang, Y.; Fu, Z.; Tang, C.; Shao, Z.; Zhang, J.; Mao, W. Anticoagulant-active sulfated arabinogalactan tan from *Chaetomorpha linum*: Structural characterization and action on coagulation factors. *Carbohydr. Polym.* **2020**, *242*, 116394. [CrossRef]
42. Tanaka, T.; Nakashima, T.; Ueda, T.; Tomii, K.; Kouno, I. Facile discrimination of aldose enantiomers by reversed-phase HPLC. *Chem. Pharm. Bull.* **2007**, *55*, 899–901. [CrossRef] [PubMed]
43. Harris, P.J.; Henry, R.J.; Blakeney, A.B.; Stone, B.A. An improved procedure for the methylation analysis of oligosaccharides and polysaccharides. *Carbohydr. Res.* **1984**, *127*, 59–73. [CrossRef]
44. Ni, M.; Hu, X.; Gong, D.; Zhang, G. Inhibitory mechanism of vitexin on α-glucosidase and its synergy with acarbose. *Food Hydrocolloid.* **2020**, *105*, 105824. [CrossRef]
45. Usoltseva, R.V.; Anastyuk, S.D.; Shevchenko, N.M.; Surits, V.V.; Silchenko, A.S.; Isakov, V.V.; Zvyagintseva, T.N.; Thinh, P.D.; Ermakova, S.P. Polysaccharides from brown algae *Sargassum duplicatum*: The structure and anticancer activity in vitro. *Carbohyd. Polym.* **2017**, *175*, 547–556. [CrossRef] [PubMed]

46. Arasteh, A.; Aliyev, A.; Khamnei, S.; Delazar, A.; Mesgari, M.; Mehmannavaz, Y. Crocus sativus on serum glucose, insulin and cholesterol levels in healthy male rats. *J. Med. Plants Res.* **2010**, *4*, 397–402.
47. Wu, L.; Yuan, A.; Tian, X.; Cao, J.; Qi, X.; Wei, Y.; Shen, S. Cell-membrane-coated cationic nanoparticles disguised as macrophages for the prevention and treatment of type 2 diabetes mellitus. *ACS Appl. Mater. Inter.* **2022**, *14*, 50499–50506. [CrossRef]
48. Xiong, W.; Gu, L.; Wang, C.; Sun, H.; Liu, X. Anti-hyperglycemic and hypolipidemic effects of *Cistanche tubulosa* in type 2 diabetic db/db mice. *J. Ethnopharmacol.* **2013**, *150*, 935–945. [CrossRef]

Disclaimer/Publisher's Note: The statements, opinions and data contained in all publications are solely those of the individual author(s) and contributor(s) and not of MDPI and/or the editor(s). MDPI and/or the editor(s) disclaim responsibility for any injury to people or property resulting from any ideas, methods, instructions or products referred to in the content.

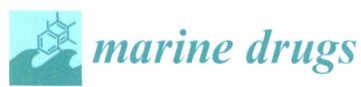

Article

Semi-Synthesis and Biological Evaluation of 25(*R*)-26-Acetoxy-3*β*,5*α*-Dihydroxycholest-6-One

Mireguli Maimaitiming [1,2,†], Ling Lv [1,2,†], Xuetao Zhang [1,2], Shuli Xia [1,2], Xin Li [1,2], Pingyuan Wang [1,2,*], Zhiqing Liu [1,2,*] and Chang-Yun Wang [1,2,*]

[1] Institute of Evolution & Marine Biodiversity, School of Medicine and Pharmacy, College of Food Science and Engineering, Ocean University of China, Qingdao 266003, China
[2] Laboratory for Marine Drugs and Bioproducts, Qingdao National Laboratory for Marine Science and Technology, Qingdao 266237, China
* Correspondence: wangpingyuan@ouc.edu.cn (P.W.); liuzhiqing@ouc.edu.cn (Z.L.); changyun@ouc.edu.cn (C.-Y.W.)
† These authors contributed equally to this work.

Abstract: Previously, we identified a series of steroids (**1–6**) that showed potent anti-virus activities against respiratory syncytial virus (RSV), with IC_{50} values ranging from 3.23 to 0.19 μM. In this work, we first semi-synthesized and characterized the single isomer of **5**, 25(*R*)-26-acetoxy-3*β*,5*α*-dihydroxycholest-6-one, named as (25*R*)-**5**, in seven steps from a commercially available compound diosgenin (**7**), with a total yield of 2.8%. Unfortunately, compound (25*R*)-**5** and the intermediates only showed slight inhibitions against RSV replication at the concentration of 10 μM, but they possessed potent cytotoxicity activities against human bladder cancer 5637 (HTB-9) and hepatic cancer HepG2 with IC_{50} values ranging from 3.0 to 15.5 μM without any impression of normal liver cell proliferation at 20 μM. Among them, the target compound (25*R*)-**5** possessed cytotoxicity activities against 5637 (HTB-9) and HepG2 with IC_{50} values of 4.8 μM and 15.5 μM, respectively. Further studies indicated that compound (25*R*)-**5** inhibited cancer cell proliferation through inducing early and late-stage apoptosis. Collectively, we have semi-synthesized, characterized and biologically evaluated the 25*R*-isomer of compound **5**; the biological results suggested that compound (25*R*)-**5** could be a good lead for further anti-cancer studies, especially for anti-human liver cancer.

Keywords: steroid; semi-synthesis; anti-RSV activity; anti-cancer activity; cytotoxicity; apoptosis

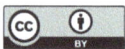

Citation: Maimaitiming, M.; Lv, L.; Zhang, X.; Xia, S.; Li, X.; Wang, P.; Liu, Z.; Wang, C.-Y. Semi-Synthesis and Biological Evaluation of 25(*R*)-26-Acetoxy-3*β*,5*α*-Dihydroxycholest-6-One. *Mar. Drugs* **2023**, *21*, 191. https://doi.org/10.3390/md21030191

Academic Editor: Haruhiko Fuwa

Received: 27 February 2023
Revised: 18 March 2023
Accepted: 18 March 2023
Published: 20 March 2023

Copyright: © 2023 by the authors. Licensee MDPI, Basel, Switzerland. This article is an open access article distributed under the terms and conditions of the Creative Commons Attribution (CC BY) license (https://creativecommons.org/licenses/by/4.0/).

1. Introduction

Steroids, containing a basic 17 carbon atom-formed perhydrocyclopentanophenanthrene skeleton, represent a polycyclic compound superfamily including sterol, bile acids sex hormones, molting hormones of insects, adrenal cortical hormones and other physiologically active substances [1]. Steroids widely exist in plants, animals, microorganisms and other living organisms and possess significant and distinct roles in the construction of cell membranes, cell stability and growth, proliferation, cell function and other cell biological processes [1–3]. Therefore, numerous steroid compounds play essential roles in the treatment of various human diseases including cancer, inflammation, infection metabolic diseases, cardiovascular diseases, heart diseases, neurological disorders and other human diseases [4–11]. Especially, the tetracyclic ring steroid plays a significant role in drug discovery [12,13]. Due to the wide application in human diseases' therapy and drug discovery programs, the identification of new bioactive steroids has attracted lots of attention from the pharmaceutical industry and academia.

In recent years, one of our research interests has been to discover novel bioactive steroids with anti-virus, anti-inflammatory, anti-oxidant and anti-cancer activities from marine organisms as chemical probes to influence biological systems or to act as lead compounds for further drug development [14–20]. Interestingly, a series of steroids (**1–6**

Figure 1) were isolated from the gorgonian *Echinogorgia rebekka* from the South China Sea, which showed potent anti-virus activities against respiratory syncytial virus (RSV), with IC_{50}s ranging from 0.19 to 3.23 µM [16]. As previously reported, RSV is a severe infectious disease that causes about 60,000 in-hospital deaths every year in children under the age of 5 [21]. Unfortunately, there are no licensed vaccines for RSV. The only FDA-approved drug, palivizumab, has failed to show sufficient efficacy and is accompanied by serious side-effects [21]. Therefore, novel and effective anti-RSV agents are still an urgent need. Meanwhile, our previously reported steroids (Figure 1) showed potent in vitro anti-RSV activities and were supposed to be an excellent anti-RSV lead for further drug development. However, an insufficient amount of these steroids (**1–6**, Figure 1) hampers the further exploration, which is a well-acknowledged challenge in this field [22]. Especially, compound **5**, first discovered from gorgonian *Acalycigorgia inermis* in 2000 by the Shin group, was isolated as inseparable C25-epimeric mixtures [23]. The anti-RSV activity of compound **5** was not studied previously, but it exhibited moderate anti-proliferation activity against the human leukemia cell line K-562, with a LC_{50} of 0.9 µg/mL [16,23]. In order to characterize it and to explore the anti-RSV studies of the single isomer of compound **5**, in this work, we semi-synthesized, characterized and biologically evaluated the 25*R*-isomer of compound **5** for the first time.

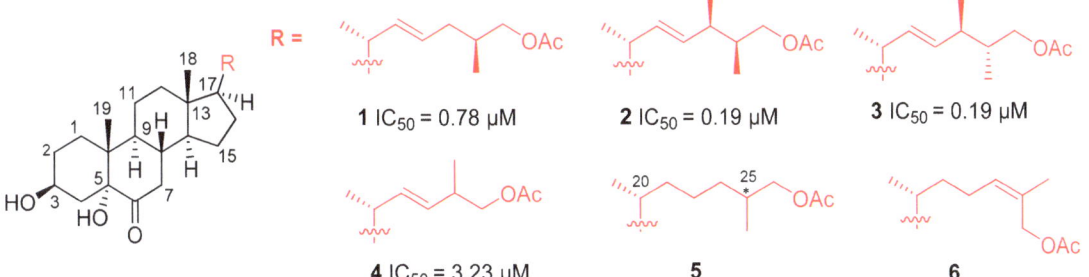

Figure 1. Chemical structures and anti-RSV activities of steroid compounds **1–6**.

2. Results and Discussion

2.1. Chemistry

The synthetic procedure of a single isomer of compound **5**, 25(*R*)-26-acetoxy-3β,5α-dihydroxycholest-6-one, namely (25*R*)-**5**, is shown in Scheme 1. As outlined in Scheme 1, intermediate **8**, containing three hydroxy groups, was prepared by the reduction of the commercially available nature product diosgenin (**7**) using Zn dust in the mixed solution of HCl and EtOH, with an excellent yield of 78% [24]. Protection of two hydroxy groups of intermediate **8** with the pivaloyl group resulted in compound **9**. Protection of the third hydroxy of intermediate **9** was accomplished under methanesulfonic anhydride in the presence of pyridine as the base, leading to compound **10** [24]. Deprotection and reduction of intermediate **10** with LiAlH$_4$ under the condition of reflux produced intermediate **11** with a yield of 91% [24,25]. Protection of the hydroxyl group on the linker terminal of compound **11** by acetyl chloride in the presence of Et$_3$N led to intermediate **12** with a moderate yield. Asymmetric dihydroxylation of compound **12** with the magnesium monoperoxyphthalate hexahydrate as the epoxidizing agent, followed by an epoxide opening in the presence of a catalytic amount of Bi(OTf)$_3$, provided compound **13** [26,27]. Finally, compound (25*R*)-**5** was obtained by specific mono-oxidation of the key intermediate **13** with *N*-bromosuccinimide in the mixture solution of acetic acid, acetone and water, with a yield of 47% [26].

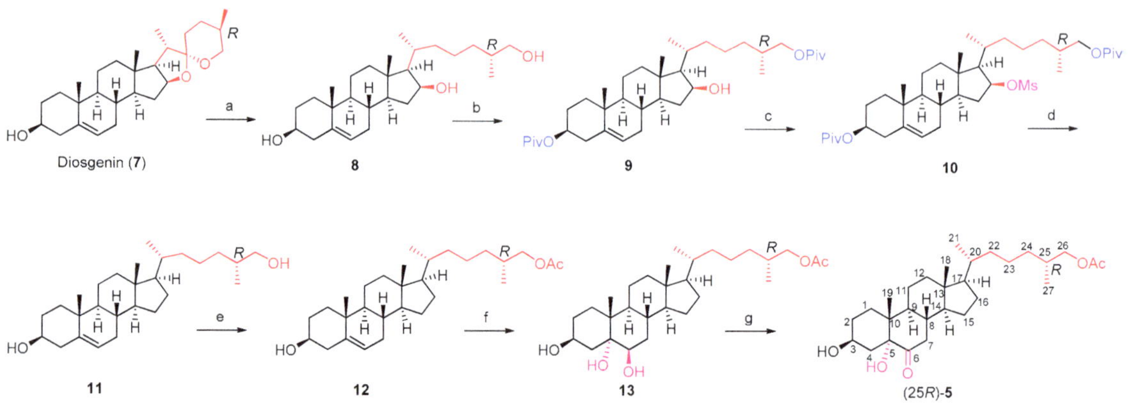

Scheme 1. Semi-synthesis of (25*R*)-**5**. Reagents and conditions: (**a**) Zn dust, HCl, EtOH, reflux, 1.5 h, 78%; (**b**) pivaloyl chloride, pyridine, THF, 0-rt, overnight, 49%; (**c**) methanesulfonic anhydride, pyridine, 0-rt, overnight, 99%; (**d**) LiAlH$_4$, Et$_2$O, reflux, 10 h, 91%; (**e**) acetyl chloride, Et$_3$N, DMAP, CH$_2$Cl$_2$, overnight, 42%; (**f**) (i) magnesium monoperoxyphthalate hexahydrate, acetone, reflux, 30 min; (ii) Bi(OTf)$_3$, acetone, rt, 1 h, 41%; (**g**) *N*-bromosuccinimide, acetic acid, acetone, H$_2$O, 0-rt, 1 h, 47%.

2.2. Characteristic Analysis

The high-resolution electron spray ionization mass (HRMS-ESI) of compound (25*R*)-**5** possessed [M + H]$^+$ peak at *m/z* 477.3578 and [M + Na]$^+$ peak at *m/z* 499.3401 (Figure S1), corresponding to the reported molecular formula of C$_{29}$H$_{48}$O$_5$ of compound **5** [16,23]. Further, the ^{1}H and ^{13}C NMR spectrometry analysis suggested that our semi-synthesized compound (25*R*)-**5** was a single isomer and the spectrum data (Table 1, Figures S2–S5) were identical to the reported data of compound **5** [23]. As shown in Table 1, the four methyl proton signals in the high-field region were observed at δ_H 0.91 (d, *J* = 6.7 Hz), 0.90 (d, *J* = 6.5 Hz), 0.79 (s) and 0.64 (s), together with the ^{13}C NMR signals at δ_C 18.6, 16.8, 14.0 and 12.0, respectively. The ^{1}H proton signal of the acetoxy group on the linker terminal of the compound was found at δ_H 2.05 (s), as well as the ^{13}C NMR signals at δ_C 171.4 and 21.0, respectively. The hydroxy group signals of compound **5** were not given in previous reports, we also did not find the two hydroxy group signals in the ^{1}H NMR spectrometry. Luckily, when we changed the solvent from CDCl$_3$ into DMSO-*d$_6$*, the two hydroxy group signals were observed clearly at δ_H 5.29 (s) and 4.35 (d, *J* = 5.6 Hz) (Figures S4 and S5). Additionally, the chemical shifts (Table 1, Figures S2 and S3) of the steroidal tetracyclic scaffold were all in agreement with reported and our previously identified data. The absolute configuration of compound (25*R*)-**5** was established on the basis of the configuration of previously confirmed compound **12** and detailed ^{1}H NMR spectroscopic data, especially the chirality of the C-25 position.

As shown in Figure 2 and Figure S6, compounds (25*R*)-**5** and **5** were analyzed by high-performance liquid chromatography (HPLC) to confirm that compound (25*R*)-**5** was one isomer of compound **5**. As expected, compound (25*R*)-**5** only showed one peak, with the retention time of 6.262 min; in contrast, compound **5** possessed two peaks, with the retention times of 6.255 and 6.944 min, respectively.

Table 1. ^{1}H NMR and ^{13}C NMR data of compound **5** and (25R)-**5**.

(25R)-**5**

Position	5 (CDCl$_3$, δ in ppm) [a]		(25R)-5 (CDCl$_3$, δ in ppm) [b]	
	^{1}H NMR	^{13}C NMR	^{1}H NMR	^{13}C NMR
1	1.70, m 1.54, brd	29.8	1.79–1.66, m 1.56–1.42, m	29.8
2	1.87, m 1.46, m	30.3	1.89–1.82, m 1.56–1.42, m	30.2
3	3.98, m	67.3	4.01–3.98, m	67.2
4	1.86–1.81, m 1.79, m	36.4	1.89–1.82, m 1.79–1.66, m	36.1
5		80.9		80.5
6		212.3		213.5
7	2.72, dd (13.2, 12.2) 2.12, dd (13.2, 4.4)	41.8	2.73, t (12.6) 2.10, dd (13.0, 4.6)	41.8
8	1.70, m	37.3	1.79–1.66, m	37.4
9	1.86–1.81, m	44.5	1.89–1.82, m	44.3
10		42.4		42.5
11	1.46, m 1.29, m	21.4	1.56–1.42, m 1.38–1.20, m	21.4
12	2.02, ddd (12.2, 3.4, 2.4) 1.23, ddd (12.8, 12.2, 3.4)	39.6	2.03–1.98, m 1.38–1.20, m	39.6
13		43.1		43.1
14	1.31, m	56.3	1.38–1.20, m	56.3
15	1.51, m 1.04, m	23.9	1.56–1.42, m 1.07–0.95, m	23.9
16	1.86–1.81, m 1.25, m	28.1	1.89–1.82, m 1.38–1.20, m	28.1
17	1.12, m	56.05 56.02	1.15–1.10, m	56.1
18	0.65, s	12.0	0.64, s	12.0
19	0.81, s	14.1	0.79, s	14.0
20	1.35, m	35.68 35.62	1.38–1.20, m	35.6
21	0.91, d (6.8)	18.6	0.90, d (6.5)	18.6
22	1.30, m 1.21, m	33.85 33.70	1.38–1.20, m	33.7
23	1.35, m 1.19, m	23.30 23.26	1.38–1.20, m	23.3
24	1.35, m 1.02, m	36.05 35.95	1.38–1.20, m 1.07–0.95, m	36.0
25	1.77, m	32.54 32.48	1.79–1.66, m	32.5
26	0.93, d (6.8), maj 0.92, d (6.8), maj	17.01 16.78	0.91, d (6.7)	16.8
27	3.96, dd (10.7, 7.3), min 3.95, dd (10.7, 7.3), maj 3.84, dd (10.7, 2.4), maj 3.83, dd (10.7, 1.9), min	69.59 69.45	3.93, dd, (10.6, 6.0) 3.83, dd, (10.7, 6.9)	69.6
OAc	2.06, s	171.3 (C) 21.0 (CH$_3$)	2.05, s	171.4 (C) 21.0 (CH$_3$)

[a] Data are taken from reference [19]. [b] NMR spectra were recorded on a BRUKER AVANCE NEO (^{1}H, 400 MHz; ^{13}C, 100 MHz) spectrometer. ^{1}H and ^{13}C NMR spectra were recorded with TMS as an internal reference.

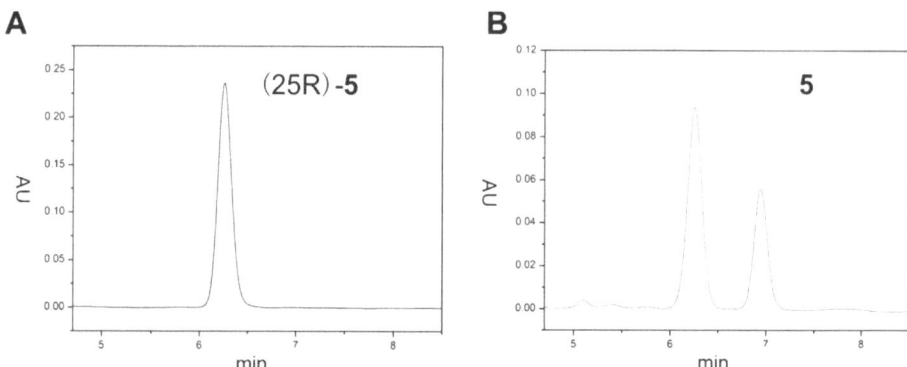

Figure 2. The HPLC chromatograms of compounds (25R)-**5** (**A**) and **5** (**B**). HPLC conditions: Waters Xbridge C18 (250 mm × 4.6 mm, 5 μm), flow rate 1.0 mL/min, UV detection at 203 nm and linear gradient from 90% MeOH in water to 100% MeOH in 20 min followed by 30 min of the last-named solvent. The horizontal axis is retention time (min, from 5 to 9 min is shown in these figures) and the axis of ordinate is relative intensity absorbance unit (AU).

2.3. Biological Studies

With compounds (25R)-**5** and the intermediates in hand, their anti-viral activities against RSV were evaluated by a quantitative reverse transcription PCR (RT-qPCR) method in Hep G2 cells, which is a standard method for the anti-viral activity analysis. Unfortunately, all of the tested compounds only showed a slight inhibition on RSV replication at the concentration of 10 μM (Table 2). Although these compounds were not good enough for further anti-RSV studies, they could be seen as good starting points for further structure optimization.

Table 2. Anti-RSV activities of compounds (25R)-**5**, **8**, **11**, **13** and **5** [a].

Compounds	8	11	13	(25R)-5	5	Remdesivir
Inhibition rate (%)	24.9 ± 2.6	22.2 ± 3.9	13.6 ± 2.1	29.4 ± 7.1	18.3 ± 3.8	91.8 ± 0.5

[a] The values are the mean ± SEM of at least three independent experiments. The inhibition rates (%) were calculated by comparing the untreated cells.

Considering the preliminary anti-proliferation activities against the human leukemia K-562 cell line of compound **5** in previous studies [16,23], we then turned to the exploration of the cytotoxicity activity of compound (25R)-**5**. Hence, the semi-synthesized compound (25R)-**5**, along with the more drug-like intermediates **8**, **11** and **13** during the synthesis of (25R)-**5**, were selected for the biological evaluation of proliferation inhibitory activities against nineteen human cancer and one normal liver cell lines using a CCK-8 assay. First, the anti-proliferation activity of compound (25R)-**5** was tested against the human leukemia K-562 cell line, but it only showed a weak inhibition activity at the concentration of 20 μM (Table 3). Meanwhile, all the three intermediates **8**, **11** and **13** did not exhibit any anti-proliferative activities against K-562 cancer cells at 20 μM. As listed in Table 3, similar results were also obtained with nine human cancer cell lines, including HeLa, TE-1, GBC-SD, MCF7, SF126, DU145, CAL-62, HOS and 293T. The intermediate **8** displayed moderate anti-proliferation activity against the human lung adenocarcinoma A549 cell line (53% inhibition rate at 20 μM, Table 3), whereas compound (25R)-**5** and intermediates **11** and **13** did not show an inhibition rate over 50%. This result suggested that the hydroxy group at the C-16 position and the double bond of compound **8** had an important role for the anti-proliferation activity against the A549 cell line. Similarly, the same structure–activity relationship (SAR) could also be observed in the human colorectal HCT 116 cancer cell line.

Furthermore, all the four compounds exhibited moderate growth inhibitory effects against human gastric MKN-45 and pancreatic PATU8988T cancer cell lines (~50% inhibition rates at 20 µM, Table 3). In Table 3, the four compounds displayed potent activities, with the best inhibition rates over 70% against human melanoma A-375, bladder cancer 5637 (HTB-9) and hepatic cancer HepG2 cell lines. More importantly, all the four compounds had no growth inhibitory effects against the normal human liver L-02 cell line (<10% inhibition rate at 20 µM, Table 3), indicating that these compounds could selectively kill cancer cells. The intermediate 13 displayed less potent cytotoxicity activities than compound (25R)-5 and intermediates 8 and 11. Therefore, compound (25R)-5 and intermediates 8 and 11 were chosen for further specific cytotoxicity studies.

Table 3. Anti-cancer activities of compounds (25R)-5, 8, 11 and 13 [a].

Cell Lines	Compds.				
	Inhibition Rate (%)				
	8 (at 20 µM)	11 (at 20 µM)	13 (at 20 µM)	(25R)-5 (at 20 µM)	Doxorubicin (at 10 µM)
K-562	7.2 ± 2.2	13.1 ± 1.8	7.8 ± 2.3	17.1 ± 2.8	67.5 ± 1.0
A549	53.0 ± 2.7	31.2 ± 3.9	3.9 ± 2.7	35.3 ± 1.3	75.9 ± 2.5
MKN-45	54.4 ± 1.9	53.8 ± 1.6	52.7 ± 2.4	61.1 ± 1.4	89.8 ± 0.5
HCT 116	61.7 ± 2.1	19.8 ± 1.4	19.3 ± 1.2	59.3 ± 3.8	88.9 ± 1.5
HeLa	49.7 ± 3.6	14.9 ± 2.2	−2.3 ± 1.7	22.7 ± 1.2	97.7 ± 0.4
786-O	69.0 ± 1.8	65.9 ± 2.4	20.5 ± 1.3	65.3 ± 0.5	86.3 ± 1.9
TE-1	34.0 ± 3.8	27.7 ± 0.6	13.5 ± 2.6	29.5 ± 2.2	83.3 ± 1.1
5637 (HTB-9)	75.1 ± 0.8	80.5 ± 2.5	52.2 ± 4.5	64.7 ± 3.4	99.3 ± 0.3
GBC-SD	26.8 ± 1.3	10.4 ± 3.3	6.0 ± 2.4	28.1 ± 1.5	76.7 ± 1.5
L-02	8.1 ± 1.3	2.8 ± 2.1	6.3 ± 3.2	−4.9 ± 3.4	99.2 ± 0.1
MCF7	31.2 ± 1.4	14.1 ± 0.5	19.0 ± 1.1	19.3 ± 2.1	55.9 ±1.7
HepG2	76.8 ± 1.3	64.2 ± 2.5	58.0 ± 1.2	66.8 ± 2.1	95.9 ±1.9
SF126	30.7 ± 2.4	11.7 ± 2.9	4.7 ± 1.3	28.1 ± 0.5	97.1 ± 1.0
DU145	26.0 ± 1.7	18.4 ± 3.7	−0.4 ± 3.9	12.2 ± 2.0	76.4 ± 1.6
CAL-62	28.0 ± 4.0	12.5 ± 3.9	7.5 ± 2.7	18.2 ± 1.9	92.6 ± 1.3
PATU8988T	62.7 ± 2.0	63.3 ± 4.2	53.6 ± 1.7	65.9 ± 4.2	98.4 ± 0.6
HOS	2.7 ± 4.0	9.3 ± 4.3	52.6 ± 1.5	22.2 ± 1.1	98.4 ± 0.9
A-375	72.3 ± 0.6	60.8 ± 1.4	54.8 ± 1.7	76.3 ± 1.7	95.3 ± 1.0
A-673	51.9 ± 2.8	26.5 ± 2.1	66.3 ± 3.2	49.4 ± 1.4	98.7 ± 0.6
293T	42.4 ± 2.1	−18.2 ± 1.3	37.3 ± 2.7	26.2 ± 1.5	88.2 ± 1.2

[a] The values are the mean ± SEM of at least three independent experiments. The inhibition rates (%) are calculated by the calculation formula as follows: inhibition rate (%) = (OD$_{Control}$ − OD$_{Compound}$)/(OD$_{Control}$ − OD$_{Blank}$) × 100%. K-562 (human myeloid leukemia cell); A549 (human lung adenocarcinoma cell); MKN-45 (human gastric cancer cell); HCT 116 (human colorectal cancer cell); HeLa (human cervical cancer cell); 786-O (human renal cancer cell); TE-1 (human esophageal cancer cell); 5637 (HTB-9) (human bladder cancer cell); GBC-SD (human gallbladder carcinoma cell); L-02 (human hepatocyte cell); MCF7 (human breast cancer cell); HepG2 (human liver carcinoma cell); SF126 (human glioblastoma cell); DU145 (human prostate carcinoma cell); CAL-62 (human thyroid anaplastic carcinoma cell); PATU8988T (human pancreatic cancer cell); HOS (human osteosarcoma cell); A-375 (human melanoma cell); A-673 (Ewing sarcoma); 293T (human embryonic kidney cell).

Then, the IC$_{50}$ values of compound (25R)-5 and intermediates 8 and 11 were investigated against 5637 (HTB-9) and HepG2 cancer cell lines, as summarized in Figure 3. As depicted in Figure 3A, all three compounds displayed similar micromolar IC$_{50}$ values (5.8 µM for 8, 3.0 µM for 11 and 4.8 µM for (25R)-5, respectively) against 5637 (HTB-9) cancer cells. Interestingly, intermediate 11 proved to be the best compound against HepG2 cancer cells, with an IC$_{50}$ value of 5.6 µM (Figure 3B). Additionally, compound (25R)-5 and intermediate 8 showed very similar anti-proliferation activities against HepG2 cancer cells, with an IC$_{50}$ value of 15.5 µM and 12.0 µM, respectively (Figure 3B). Taken together, compound (25R)-5 represented a promising drug discovery lead towards human liver cancer and is worthy of further discovery.

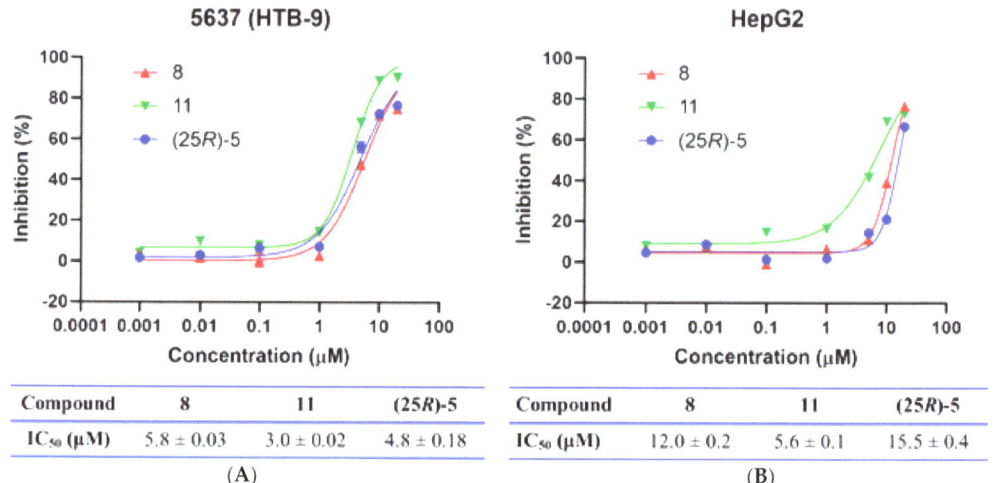

Figure 3. CCK8 assays of 5637 (HTB-9) and HepG2 cells treated with compounds **8**, **11** or (25R)-**5** at the indicated concentrations for 48 h. (**A**) Dose-dependent curves of compounds **8**, **11** or (25R)-**5** at the indicated concentrations against 5637 (HTB-9) cells. (**B**) Dose-dependent curves of compounds **8**, **11** or (25R)-**5** at the indicated concentrations against HepG2 cells. All results are presented as mean ± SEM from triplicate testing in a representative experiment, with similar results observed in at least 3 experiments.

Next, the apoptosis study of compound (25R)-**5** was investigated against 5637 (HTB-9) cells based on a standard flow cytometry technique and assessed by Annexin V-FITC/PI staining. As depicted in Figure 4, the results showed that compound (25R)-**5** induced apoptotic cell death in a dose-dependent manner of both early-stage (Annexin VFITC+/PI-) and late-stage (Annexin VFITC+/PI+). Hence, these data strongly suggested that compound (25R)-**5** was able to kill cancer cells with the mechanism of inducing cancer cell apoptosis.

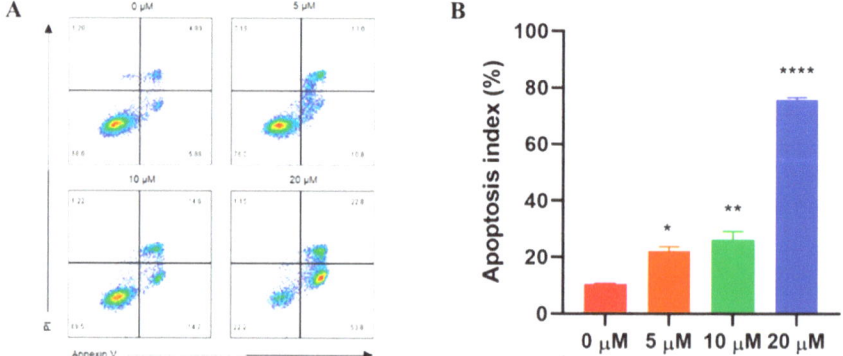

Figure 4. Compound (25R)-5 inhibited the proliferation of and induced apoptosis in 5637 (HTB-9) cells. (**A**) 5637 (HTB) cells were treated with different concentrations of compound (25R)-5 for 48 h, then stained with Annexin-V/PI and analyzed by flow cytometry. (**B**) Quantitative analysis of annexin V-FITC/PI staining after the treatment with (25R)-5 for 48 h, mean ± SEM, $n = 3$; * $p < 0.05$, ** $p < 0.01$, **** $p < 0.0001$; all data in this experiment are expressed as the mean ± SEM of at least three independent experiments.

3. Materials and Methods

3.1. Chemistry

All commercially available starting materials and solvents were reagent grade and used without further purification. The diosgenin was purchased from Shanghai Macklin Biochemical Co., Ltd., Shanghai, China, with a purity of over 95%. Column chromatography was carried out on silica gel (200–300 mesh) manufactured by Qingdao Haiyang Chemical Group Co., Ltd. Analytical TLC was performed on silica gel plates and visualized under ultraviolet light (254 nm or 365 nm). 1H and 13C NMR spectra were recorded on a BRUKER AVANCE NEO with 400 MHz for proton (1H NMR) and 100 MHz for carbon (13C NMR). Chemical shifts downfield from TMS were expressed in ppm and the signals are described as d (doublet), dd (doublet of doublet), m (multi-plet), q (quartet), s (singlet) and t (triplet). Coupling constants (J values) were given in Hz. HRMS (ESI) and LC-MS (ESI) were recorded on a SHIMADZU LCMS-IT-TOF mass spectrometer and Thermo TSQ QUANTUM LC-MS spectrometer, respectively. Purity of representative compounds (>95%) was established by 1H NMR and analytical HPLC, which was carried out on a Waters Xbridge C18 (250 mm × 4.6 mm, 5 µm), a flow rate 1.0 mL/min, UV detection at 203 nm and linear gradient from 90% MeOH in water to 100% MeOH in 20 min followed by 30 min of the last-named solvent.

3.1.1. Synthesis of (3S,8S,9S,10R,13S,14S,16S,17R)-17-((2R,6R)-7-Hydroxy-6-Methylheptan-2-yl)-10,13-Dimethyl-2,3,4,7,8,9,10,11,12,13,14,15,16,17-Tetradecahydro-1H-Cyclopenta[a]Phenanthrene-3,16-diol (**8**)

Pre-activated zinc dust (46.1 g, 708 mmol) was added to a solution of diosgenin (2.0 g, 4.8 mmol) in ethanol (100 mL) in a three-necked flask and the mixture solution was heated to reflux. Then, 80 mL of concentrated HCl was added dropwise over 30 min; after the addition of concentrated HCl, the mixture was stirred at reflux for 1 h. After the reaction was completed (detected by TLC), the solution was worked up by the addition of water (100 mL). The excess zinc dust was removed by filtration and washed with CH_2Cl_2. The filtrate was extracted with CH_2Cl_2 (50 mL × 3) and the combined CH_2Cl_2 extracts were washed with brine and dried over anhydrous Na_2SO_4. The solution was filtered and condensed by rotary evaporation. The residue was purified by silica gel column chromatography (gradient: 1 to 5% MeOH in CH_2Cl_2) to afford compound **8** (1.6 g, 78%, R_f = 0.2 in CH_2Cl_2: MeOH = 20:1) as a white solid. ^{1}H NMR (400 MHz, DMSO-d_6) δ 5.25 (d, J = 4.6 Hz, 1H), 4.59 (d, J = 4.6 Hz, 1H), 4.34 (t, J = 5.2 Hz, 1H), 4.27 (d, J = 4.9 Hz, 1H), 4.16–4.09 (m, 1H), 3.28–3.20 (m, 2H), 3.17–3.11 (m, 1H), 2.17–2.02 (m, 3H), 1.96–1.18 (m, 16H), 1.09–0.95 (m, 5H), 0.93 (s, 3H), 0.89 (d, J = 6.6 Hz, 3H), 0.82 (s, 3H), 0.81 (d, J = 6.7 Hz, 3H). ^{13}C NMR (100 MHz, DMSO-d_6) δ 141.7, 120.9, 70.5, 70.3, 66.9, 61.5, 54.5, 50.1, 42.7, 42.2, 37.7, 37.3, 36.6, 36.0, 35.9, 33.8, 31.9, 31.8, 31.6, 29.8, 23.9, 20.8, 19.6, 18.5, 17.3, 13.3.

3.1.2. Synthesis of (3S,8S,9S,10R,13S,14S,16S,17R)-16-Hydroxy-10,13-Dimethyl-17-((2R,6R)-6-Methyl-7-(Pivaloyloxy)Heptan-2-yl)-2,3,4,7,8,9,10,11,12,13,14,15,16,17-Tetradecahydro-1H-Cyclopenta[a]Phenanthren-3-yl Pivalate (**9**)

Pivaloyl chloride (0.5 mL, 4.0 mmol) was slowly added to a solution of compound **8** (513 mg, 1.2 mmol) in 10 mL of THF and 5 mL of pyridine at 0 °C with an ice bath, then the ice bath was removed and the mixture was stirred at room temperature overnight. After the reaction was completed (detected by TLC), the solution was worked up by the addition of water (10 mL) and then extracted with EtOAc (20 mL × 3). The combined EtOAc extracts were washed with brine, dried over Na_2SO_4, filtered and condensed by rotary evaporation to yield a yellow oil. The residue was purified by silica gel chromatography (gradient: 10% to 20% EtOAc in petroleum ether) and provided product **9** (355 mg, 49%, R_f = 0.3 in petroleum ether: EtOAc = 5:1) as a white solid. ^{1}H NMR (CDCl$_3$, 400 MHz) δ 5.30 (d, J = 4.5 Hz, 1H), 4.55–4.45 (m, 1H), 4.28 (m, 1H), 3.91 (dd, J = 10.7, 5.6 Hz, 1H), 3.74 (dd, J = 10.7, 6.9 Hz, 1H), 2.25–2.13 (m, 3H), 1.96–1.87 (m, 2H), 1.82–1.71 (m, 4H), 1.13 (s, 9H),

1.11 (s, 9H), 0.97 (s, 3H), 0.91 (d, J = 6.7 Hz, 3H), 0.86 (d, J = 6.8 Hz, 3H), 0.82 (s, 3H). ^{13}C NMR (CDCl$_3$, 100 MHz) δ 178.7, 178.1, 139.9, 122.2, 73.5, 72.4, 69.2, 61.4, 54.4, 50.9, 42.2, 39.8, 38.9, 38.6, 38.0, 36.9, 36.7, 36.6, 36.1, 33.7, 32.6, 31.8, 31.5, 29.8, 27.6, 27.2, 27.2, 23.6, 20.7, 19.4, 18.2, 17.0, 13.0.

3.1.3. Synthesis of (2R,6R)-6-((3S,8S,9S,10R,13S,14S,16S,17R)-10,13-Dimethyl-16-((Methylsulfonyl)oxy)-3-(Pivaloyloxy)-2,3,4,7,8,9,10,11,12,13,14,15,16,17-Tetradecahydro-1H-Yclopenta[a]Phenanthren-17-yl)-2-Methylheptyl Pivalate (10)

A solution of methanesulfonic anhydride (1.4 g, 8.2 mmol) in 15 mL dry pyridine was added to a solution of compound **9** (1.0 g, 1.6 mmol) in 6 mL dry pyridine at 0 °C with an ice bath. The mixture was stirred at 0 °C to room temperature for overnight. After the reaction was completed (detected by TLC), the solution was worked up by the addition of water (10 mL) and then extracted with EtOAc (20 mL × 3). The combined EtOAc extracts were washed with 1 N HCl, NaHCO$_3$ (aq. sat.), brine, dried over Na$_2$SO$_4$, filtered and condensed by rotary evaporation to yield a yellow oil. The residue was purified by silica gel chromatography (gradient: 10% to 20% EtOAc in petroleum ether) and provided product **10** (1.1 g, 99%, R$_f$ = 0.2 in petroleum ether: EtOAc = 5:1) as a white solid. ^{1}H NMR (CDCl$_3$, 400 MHz) δ 5.28 (d, J = 5.1 Hz, 1H), 5.17–5.09 (m, 1H), 4.55–4.44 (m, 1H), 3.89–3.83 (m, 1H), 3.82–3.74 (m, 1H), 2.90 (s, 3H), 2.32 (dt, J = 14.3, 7.5 Hz, 1H), 2.22 (d, J = 8.2 Hz, 2H), 1.98 (d, J = 12.1 Hz, 1H), 1.91 (d, J = 12.6 Hz, 1H), 1.83–1.65 (m, 5H), 1.56–1.16 (m, 14H), 1.13 (s, 9H), 1.11 (s, 9H), 1.08–1.04 (m, 2H), 0.97 (s, 3H), 0.91 (d, J = 6.7 Hz, 3H), 0.85 (d, J = 6.8 Hz, 3H), 0.81 (s, 3H). ^{13}C NMR (100 MHz, CDCl$_3$) δ 178.7, 178.0, 139.9, 121.9, 83.2, 73.4, 69.2, 60.7, 54.7, 49.8, 42.4, 39.3, 38.9, 38.9, 38.6, 37.9, 36.9, 36.6, 35.3, 34.8, 33.6, 32.6, 31.6, 31.3, 30.1, 27.6, 27.2, 27.2, 23.8, 20.6, 19.3, 18.0, 16.9, 12.6.

3.1.4. Synthesis of (3S,8S,9S,10R,13R,14S,17R)-17-((2R,6R)-7-Hydroxy-6-Methylheptan-2-yl)-10,13-Dimethyl-2,3,4,7,8,9,10,11,12,13,14,15,16,17-Tetradecahydro-1H-Cyclopenta[a]Phenanthren-3-ol (11)

Compound **10** (1.1 g, 1.6 mmol) was dissolved in 15 mL of dry ether and was added dropwise to a mixture of LiAlH$_4$ (623 mg, 16.4 mmol) in 15 mL of dry ether. The mixture was heated to reflux and stirred at reflux for 10 h. After the reaction was completed (detected by TLC), the reaction was quenched with water. The solution was worked up by the addition of 1 N NaOH (4 mL) and then extracted with EtOAc (20 mL × 3). The combined EtOAc extracts were washed with brine, dried over Na$_2$SO$_4$, filtered and condensed by rotary evaporation to yield a yellow oil. The residue was purified by silica gel chromatography (gradient: 1 to 5% MeOH in CH$_2$Cl$_2$) and provided product **11** (600 mg, 91%, R$_f$ = 0.2 in CH$_2$Cl$_2$: MeOH = 20:1) as a white solid. ^{1}H NMR (400 MHz, DMSO-d_6) δ 5.26 (d, J = 5.0 Hz, 1H), 4.60 (d, J = 4.6 Hz, 1H), 4.35 (t, J = 5.3 Hz, 1H), 3.29–3.19 (m, 2H), 3.19–3.11 (m, 1H), 2.18–2.02 (m, 2H), 2.01–1.85 (m, 2H), 1.81–1.71 (m, 2H), 1.67 (d, J = 12.2 Hz, 1H), 1.58–0.95 (m, 20H), 0.94 (s, 3H), 0.89 (d, J = 6.5 Hz, 3H), 0.80 (d, J = 6.6 Hz, 3H), 0.65 (s, 3H). ^{13}C NMR (100 MHz, DMSO-d_6) δ 141.7, 120.9, 70.5, 66.8, 56.7, 56.1, 50.1, 42.7, 42.3, 37.4, 36.5, 36.2, 35.8, 35.6, 33.7, 31.9, 31.9, 31.8, 29.5, 28.3, 24.4, 23.3, 21.1, 19.6, 19.0, 17.2, 12.2.

3.1.5. Synthesis of (2R,6R)-6-((3S,8S,9S,10R,13R,14S,17R)-3-Hydroxy-10,13-Dimethyl-2,3,4,7,8,9,10,11,12,13,14,15,16,17-Tetradecahydro-1H-Cyclopenta[a]Phenanthren-17-yl)-2-Methylheptyl Acetate (12)

Acetyl chloride (0.1 mL, 2.0 mmol) and Et$_3$N (0.4 mL, 3.0 mmol) was added dropwise to a solution of compound **11** (676 mg, 1.7 mmol) and DMAP (24.2 mg, 0.2 mmol) in 20 mL of dry CH$_2$Cl$_2$ at 0 °C with an ice bath, then the ice bath was removed and the mixture was stirred at room temperature overnight. After the reaction was completed (detected by TLC), the solution was worked up by the addition of water (10 mL) and then extracted with EtOAc (20 mL × 3). The combined EtOAc extracts were washed with 1 N HCl, NaHCO$_3$ (aq. sat.), brine, dried over Na$_2$SO$_4$, filtered and condensed by rotary evaporation to yield a yellow oil. The residue was purified by silica gel chromatography (gradient: 1 to 5% MeOH in CH$_2$Cl$_2$) and provided product **12** as a colorless oil (314.0 mg, 42% yield, R$_f$ = 0.3 in CH$_2$Cl$_2$: MeOH = 30:1). ^{1}H NMR (400 MHz, CDCl$_3$) δ 5.35 (d, J = 5.3 Hz, 1H), 3.97–3.91 (m, 1H), 3.84 (dd, J = 10.7, 6.9 Hz, 1H), 3.57–3.48 (m, 1H), 2.06 (s, 3H), 1.01 (s, 3H), 0.92 (s, 3H), 0.91 (s, 3H), 0.68 (s, 3H). ^{13}C NMR (101 MHz, CDCl$_3$) δ 171.4, 140.8, 121.7, 71.8, 69.7, 56.8, 56.1, 50.1, 42.3, 42.3, 39.8, 37.3, 36.5, 36.1, 35.7, 33.8, 32.5, 31.9, 31.7, 29.7, 28.3, 24.3, 23.2, 21.1, 21.0, 19.4, 18.7, 16.8, 11.9.

3.1.6. Synthesis of (2R,6R)-2-Methyl-6-((3S,5R,6R,8S,9S,10R,13R,14S,17R)-3,5,6-Trihydroxy-10,13-Dimethylhexadecahydro-1H-Cyclopenta[a]Phenanthren-17-yl) Heptyl Acetate (**13**)

MMPP (485.0 mg, 1.0 mmol) was added to a solution of compound **12** (291.0 mg, 0.6 mmol) in 6 mL of acetone at reflux and the reaction was stirred at reflux for 30 min. Then, the mixture solution was cooled to room temperature, the acetone was evaporated, the residue was dissolved in 20 mL of CH$_2$Cl$_2$ and the mixture solution was washed with water and brine and dried over anhydrous Na$_2$SO$_4$, filtered and condensed by rotary evaporation. The residue was dissolved in 6 mL of acetone, Bi(OTf)$_3$ (46.0 mg, 0.1 mmol) was added and the mixture was stirred at room temperature for 1 h. After the reaction was completed (detected by TLC), the solution was worked up by the addition of water (10 mL) and then extracted with EtOAc (20 mL × 3). The combined EtOAc extracts were washed with brine, dried over Na$_2$SO$_4$, filtered and condensed by rotary evaporation to yield a yellow oil. The residue was purified by silica gel chromatography (gradient: 1 to 5% MeOH in CH$_2$Cl$_2$) and provided product **13** (127.0 mg, 41%, R$_f$ = 0.2 in CH$_2$Cl$_2$: MeOH = 20:1) as a white solid. M.p. 201–202 °C. ^{1}H NMR (400 MHz, DMSO-d_6) δ 4.39 (d, J = 4.1 Hz, 1H), 4.17 (d, J = 5.5 Hz, 1H), 3.86 (dd, J = 10.7, 6.0 Hz, 1H), 3.78 (dd, J = 10.7, 6.6 Hz, 2H), 3.63 (s, 1H), 3.30 (d, J = 3.8 Hz, 1H), 2.00 (s, 3H), 1.95–1.82 (m, 2H), 1.80–1.66 m, 2H), 1.62–1.42 (m, 5H), 1.41–1.03 (m, 17H), 1.02 (s, 3H), 0.98 (m, 2H), 0.88 (d, J = 6.3 Hz, 3H), 0.86 (d, J = 6.7 Hz, 3H), 0.63 (s, 3H). ^{13}C-NMR (101 MHz, DMSO-d_6) δ 170.9, 74.8, 74.6, 69.1, 66.2, 56.3, 56.2, 45.0, 42.8, 41.4, 38.3, 36.0, 35.6, 35.0, 33.5, 32.5, 32.4, 31.6, 30.5, 28.3, 24.4, 23.1, 21.2, 21.2, 19.0, 17.0, 16.8, 12.4. HRMS (ESI) [M + NH$_4$]$^+$ m/z calcd for C$_{29}$H$_{54}$O$_5$N 496.3997, found: 476.3987.

3.1.7. Synthesis of (2R,6R)-6-((3S,5R,8S,9S,10R,13R,14S,17R)-3,5-Dihydroxy-10,13-Dimethyl-6-Oxohexadecahydro-1H-Cyclopenta[a]Phenanthren-17-yl)-2-Methylheptyl Acetate ((25R)-**5**)

N-bromosuccinimide (79.0 mg, 0.4 mmol) was added in three portions to a mixture solution of compound **13** (105.0 mg, 0.2 mmol) in acetone (4 mL), acetic acid (15.0 μL, 0.3 mmol) and H$_2$O (180.0 μL) at 0 °C with an ice bath, then the ice bath was removed and the mixture was stirred at room temperature for 1 h. After the reaction was completed (detected by TLC), the reaction solution was quenched by the addition of Na$_2$SO$_3$ (aq. sat.). The solution was extracted with EtOAc (20 mL × 3). The combined EtOAc extracts were washed with brine, dried over Na$_2$SO$_4$, filtered and condensed by rotary evaporation to yield a yellow oil. The residue was purified by silica gel chromatography (gradient: 1 to 5% MeOH in CH$_2$Cl$_2$) provided product (25R)-**5** (49.0 mg, 47%, R$_f$ = 0.2 in CH$_2$Cl$_2$: MeOH = 20:1) as a white solid. [α]$^{20}_D$ − 14.6 (c 0.83, MeOH). mp 202–203 °C. ^{1}H NMR (400 MHz, CDCl$_3$) δ 4.01–3.98 (m, 1H), 3.93 (dd, J = 10.6, 6.0 Hz, 1H), 3.83 (dd, J = 10.7, 6.9 Hz, 1H), 2.73 (t, J = 12.6 Hz, 1H), 2.10 (dd, J = 13.0, 4.6 Hz, 1H), 2.05 (s, 3H), 2.03–1.98 (m, 1H), 1.89–1.82 (m, 4H), 1.79–1.66 (m, 4H), 1.56–1.42 (m, 4H), 1.38–1.20 (m, 9H), 1.15–1.10 (m, 2H), 1.07–0.95 (m, 2H), 0.91 (d, J = 6.7 Hz, 3H), 0.90 (d, J = 6.5 Hz, 3H), 0.79 (s, 3H), 0.63 (s, 3H). ^{13}C NMR (100 MHz, CDCl$_3$) δ 213.5, 171.4, 80.5, 69.6, 67.2, 56.3, 56.1, 44.3, 43.1, 42.5, 41.8, 39.6, 37.4, 36.1, 36.0, 35.6, 33.7, 32.5, 30.2, 29.8, 28.1, 23.9, 23.3, 21.4, 21.0, 18.6, 16.8, 14.0, 12.0. ^{1}H NMR (400 MHz, DMSO-d_6) δ 5.29 (s, 1H), 4.35 (d, J = 5.6 Hz, 1H), 3.86 (dd, J = 10.7, 6.0 Hz, 1H), 3.78 (dd, J = 10.7, 6.7 Hz, 1H), 3.70 (m, 1H), 2.68 (t, J = 12.5 Hz, 1H), 2.00 (s, 3H), 1.95 (dd, J = 8.8, 2.7 Hz, 1H), 1.85 (d, J = 4.2 Hz, 1H), 1.82 (d, J = 4.3 Hz, 1H), 1.73–0.95 (m, 24H), 0.89 (d, J = 6.4 Hz, 3H), 0.86 (d, J = 6.6 Hz, 3H), 0.66 (s, 3H), 0.61 (s, 3H). ^{13}C NMR (100 MHz, DMSO-d_6) δ 212.7, 170.8, 79.6, 69.1, 65.7, 56.4, 56.0, 44.2, 43.1, 42.4, 41.9, 37.3,

36.2, 36.0, 35.6, 33.6, 32.4, 30.9, 30.0, 28.2, 24.0, 23.2, 21.5, 21.1, 18.9, 17.0, 14.0, 12.3. HRMS (ESI) [M + H]$^+$ m/z calcd for $C_{29}H_{49}O_5$ 477.3580, found: 477.3578; [M + Na]$^+$ m/z calcd for $C_{29}H_{48}O_5Na$ 499.3399, found: 499.3401.

3.2. Biological Studies

3.2.1. Anti-RSV Activity Assay

The anti-RSV activities of compounds (25R)-**5, 8, 11, 13** and **5** were determined by using a RT-qPCR method in HEp-2 cells, according to established procedures [28]. Remdesivir was selected and evaluated as a positive control.

3.2.2. Anti-Proliferation Assays

The anti-proliferation activities of compounds (25R)-**5, 8, 11** and **13** against nineteen human cancer cell lines and a normal liver cell line were explored by using a CCK-8 assay [29–33]. One concentration was set for each sample during preliminary screening, and three multiple holes were set for each concentration. Eight concentration gradients were set for each sample for IC$_{50}$ determination and three multiple holes were set for each concentration. The 96-well plates were cultured at 5% CO$_2$ and 37 °C for 48 h. The old culture medium with a drug solution of adherent cells was sucked out, then 100 µL of CCK-8 solution (diluted ten times with the basic medium) was added and the suspension cells was directly added 10 µL of CCK-8 stock solution, cultured at 37 °C with 5% CO$_2$ for 1–4 h (dark operation, real-time observation). The absorbance was measured at 450 nm with an enzyme labeling instrument and the original data and results were recorded. The IC$_{50}$ was calculated by software GraphPad prism 8 (version 8.0.2, from GraphPad Software Inc., San Diego, CA, USA) and the experimental results were expressed in ± SD. Doxorubicin was used as a positive control. All the cancer cell lines were obtained from Qingdao AC biotechnology Co., LTD, Qingdao, China.

3.2.3. Apoptosis Assays

The percent of apoptosis in cells was assayed according to the instructions (Vazyme, A211). 5637 (HTB-9) cells were seeded in 6-well plates at 2×10^5 cells/well overnight and treated with compound (25R)-**5** at various concentrations for 48 h. Trypsinization of the cells occurred without EDTA and they were collected in tubes and suspended in 100 µL ice-cold 1 × binding buffer after being washed twice with PBS. Cells were stained with PI and FITC Annexin V for 10 min at room temperature following the instructions of the Annexin V FITC/PI kit (Vazyme Biotech, Nanjing, China). Next, 200 µL ice-cold 1 × binding buffer was added. The result was measured by flow cytometry (MoFlo XDP, Beckman, Pasadena, CA, USA). For each condition, a minimum of 10,000 cells were analyzed. Triplicate experiments were performed independently.

4. Conclusions

In conclusion, we have first efficiently semi-synthesized the single isomer of steroid compound **5**, also named as (25R)-**5**, in seven steps from a commercially available nature product diosgenin (**7**), with a total yield of 2.8%. The structure and absolute configuration of compound (25R)-**5** was confirmed by HRMS, ^{1}H and ^{13}C NMR and HPLC analysis. Furthermore, compound (25R)-**5**, together with the important intermediates **8, 11** and **13**, was evaluated for the anti-viral activities against RSV, but none of them showed potent inhibition of RSV replication at the concentration of 10 µM. These compounds did not exhibit sufficient activity for further anti-RSV studies, but they could be seen as good leads for further structure optimization due to their derivates (**1–4**) having potent anti-RSV activities. Intriguingly, these four compounds displayed promising anti-proliferative activities against several cancer cell lines without affecting the normal human liver L-02 cell line. The initial SAR studies indicated that the hydroxyl group at the C-16 position and the double-bond of compound **8** had important roles for the anti-proliferation activity against these cancer cell lines. Results of cell flow cytometry indicated that compound

(25*R*)-**5** could exert the cell-mediated cytotoxicity with the mechanism of inducing cancer cell apoptosis. These studies suggested that compound **5** has great therapeutic potential as an anti-tumor agent. Further structure optimization and SAR study will be reported in due course.

Supplementary Materials: The following supporting information can be downloaded at: https://www.mdpi.com/article/10.3390/md21030191/s1, Figure S1: High-resolution electron spray ionization mass (HRMS-ESI) of compound (25*R*)-**5**; Figure S2: The copy of ^{1}H NMR spectrum (400 MHz, CDCl$_3$) of (25*R*)-**5**. Figure S3: The copy of ^{13}C NMR spectrum (100 MHz, CDCl$_3$) of (25*R*)-**5**. Figure S4: The copy of ^{1}H NMR spectrum (400 MHz, DMSO-d_6) of (25*R*)-**5**. Figure S5: The copy of ^{13}C NMR spectrum (100 MHz, DMSO-d_6) of (25*R*)-**5**. Figure S6: HPLC chromatograms of compounds (25*R*)-**5** and **5**. (A) HPLC chromatogram of compound (25*R*)-**5**. (B) HPLC chromatogram of compound **5**.

Author Contributions: Conceptualization and design, P.W. and Z.L.; methodology, M.M., L.L., X.Z., S.X., P.W. and Z.L.; acquisition of data M.M., L.L., X.Z., S.X. and X.L.; data analysis, all authors; writing—original draft preparation, P.W.; writing—review and editing, M.M., L.L., Z.L. and P.W.; supervision, P.W., Z.L. and C.-Y.W.; founding acquisition, P.W., Z.L. and C.-Y.W. All authors have read and agreed to the published version of the manuscript.

Funding: This work was supported by National Natural Science Foundation of China (Grant Nos. 41830535 and 42176109); Shandong Provincial Natural Science Foundation (Major Basic Research Projects) (Grant No. ZR2019ZD18); Fundamental Research Funds for the Central Universities (No. 202241008); Natural Science Foundation of Fujian Province (Grant No. 2022J01526); Taishan Scholars Program of Shandong Province, China. We appreciate the Program of Open Studio for Druggability Research of Marine Natural Products, Pilot National Laboratory for Marine Science and Technology (Qingdao, China) directed by Kai-Xian Chen and Yue-Wei Guo.

Institutional Review Board Statement: Not applicable.

Data Availability Statement: The data presented in this study are available in the manuscript and in the Supplementary Materials.

Acknowledgments: In this section, you can acknowledge any support given which is not covered by the author contribution or funding sections. This may include administrative and technical support, or donations in kind (e.g., materials used for experiments).

Conflicts of Interest: The authors declare no conflict of interest.

References

1. Bhatti, H.N.; Khera, R.A. Biological transformations of steroidal compounds: A review. *Steroids* **2012**, *77*, 1267–1290. [CrossRef]
2. Sharma, K.; Kumar, H.; Priyanka. Formation of nitrogen-containing six-membered heterocycles on steroidal ring system: A review. *Steroids* **2022**, *191*, 109171. [CrossRef] [PubMed]
3. Huo, H.; Li, G.; Shi, B.; Li, J. Recent advances on synthesis and biological activities of C-17 aza-heterocycle derived steroids. *Bioorg. Med. Chem.* **2022**, *69*, 116882. [CrossRef]
4. Bansal, R.; Acharya, P.C. Man-made cytotoxic steroids: Exemplary agents for cancer therapy. *Chem. Rev.* **2014**, *114*, 6986–7005. [CrossRef]
5. Dabbah-Assadi, F.; Handel, R.; Shamir, A. What we know about the role of corticosteroids in psychiatric disorders; evidence from animal and clinical studies. *J. Psychiatr. Res.* **2022**, *155*, 363–370. [CrossRef]
6. Guevara, M.A.; Lu, J.; Moore, R.E.; Chambers, S.A.; Eastman, A.J.; Francis, J.D.; Noble, K.N.; Doster, R.S.; Osteen, K.G.; Damo, S.M.; et al. Vitamin D and streptococci: The interface of nutrition, host immune response, and antimicrobial activity in response to infection. *ACS Infect. Dis.* **2020**, *6*, 3131–3140. [CrossRef]
7. Thomas, C.; Pellicciari, R.; Pruzanski, M.; Auwerx, J.; Schoonjans, K. Targeting bile-acid signalling for metabolic diseases. *Nat. Rev. Drug Discov.* **2008**, *7*, 678–693. [CrossRef] [PubMed]
8. Plum, L.A.; DeLuca, H.F. Vitamin D, disease and therapeutic opportunities. *Nat. Rev. Drug Discov.* **2010**, *9*, 941–955. [CrossRef]
9. Hurley, M.J.; Bates, R.; Macnaughton, J.; Schapira, A.H.V. Bile acids and neurological disease. *Pharmacol. Ther.* **2022**, *240*, 108311. [CrossRef]
10. Madasu, C.; Xu, Y.-M.; Wijeratne, E.M.K.; Liu, M.X.; Molnár, I.; Gunatilaka, A.A.L. Semi-synthesis and cytotoxicity evaluation of pyrimidine, thiazole, and indole analogues of argentatins A–C from guayule (*Parthenium argentatum*) resin. *Med. Chem. Res.* **2022**, *31*, 1088–1098. [CrossRef]

11. Xu, Y.-m.; Madasu, C.; Liu, M.X.; Wijeratne, E.M.K.; Dierig, D.; White, B.; Molnár, I.; Gunatilaka, A.A.L. Cycloartane- and Lanostane-Type Triterpenoids from the Resin of Parthenium argentatum AZ-2, a Byproduct of Guayule Rubber Production. *ACS Omega* **2021**, *6*, 15486–15498. [CrossRef] [PubMed]
12. Tong, W.Y.; Dong, X. Microbial biotransformation: Recent developments on steroid drugs. *Recent Pat. Biotechnol.* **2009**, *3*, 141–153 [CrossRef] [PubMed]
13. Gundamraj, S.; Hasbun, R. The Use of Adjunctive Steroids in Central Nervous Infections. *Front. Cell. Infect. Microbiol.* **2020**, *10*, 592017. [CrossRef] [PubMed]
14. Chen, B.; Gu, Y.C.; Voogd, N.J.; Wang, C.Y.; Guo, Y.W. Xidaosterols A and B, two new steroids with unusual alpha-keto-enol functionality from the south China sea sponge neopetrosia chaliniformis. *Nat. Prod. Res.* **2022**, *36*, 1941–1947. [CrossRef]
15. Chen, B.; Li, W.S.; Gu, Y.C.; Zhang, H.Y.; Luo, H.; Wang, C.Y.; Guo, Y.W. New sterols from the south China sea sponges halichondria sp. *Fitoterapia* **2021**, *152*, 104918. [CrossRef]
16. Cao, F.; Shao, C.L.; Chen, M.; Zhang, M.Q.; Xu, K.X.; Meng, H.; Wang, C.Y. Antiviral C-25 epimers of 26-acetoxy steroids from the south China sea gorgonian echinogorgia rebekka. *J. Nat. Prod.* **2014**, *77*, 1488–1493. [CrossRef]
17. Zhang, Y.H.; Zhao, Y.J.; Qi, L.; Du, H.F.; Cao, F.; Wang, C.Y. Talasteroid, a new withanolide from the marine-derived fungus talaromyces stollii. *Nat. Prod. Res.* **2022**, *36*, 1–7. [CrossRef]
18. Sun, X.P.; Cao, F.; Shao, C.L.; Chen, M.; Liu, H.J.; Zheng, C.J.; Wang, C.Y. Subergorgiaols A-L, 9,10-secosteroids from the South China Sea gorgonian Subergorgia rubra. *Steroids* **2015**, *94*, 7–14. [CrossRef]
19. Cao, F.; Shao, C.-L.; Wang, Y.; Xu, K.-X.; Qi, X.; Wang, C.-Y. Polyhydroxylated Sterols from the South China Sea Gorgonian Verrucella umbraculum. *Helv. Chim. Acta* **2014**, *97*, 900–908. [CrossRef]
20. Chen, M.; Wu, X.D.; Zhao, Q.; Wang, C.Y. Topsensterols A-C, Cytotoxic Polyhydroxylated Sterol Derivatives from a Marine Sponge Topsentia sp. *Mar. Drugs* **2016**, *14*, 146. [CrossRef]
21. Battles, M.B.; McLellan, J.S. Respiratory syncytial virus entry and how to block it. *Nat. Rev. Microbiol.* **2019**, *17*, 233–245. [CrossRef] [PubMed]
22. Atanasov, A.G.; Zotchev, S.B.; Dirsch, V.M.; Supuran, C.T. Natural products in drug discovery: Advances and opportunities. *Nat. Rev. Drug Discov.* **2021**, *20*, 200–216. [CrossRef] [PubMed]
23. Rho, J.-R.; Lee, H.-S.; Seo, Y.; Cho, K.W.; Shin, J. New bioactive steroids from the gorgonian *acalycigorgia inermis*. *Bull. Korean Chem. Soc.* **2000**, *21*, 518–520.
24. Gong, H.; Williams, J.R. Synthesis of the aglycone of the shark repellent pavoninin-4 using remote functionalization. *Org. Lett.* **2006**, *8*, 2253–2255. [CrossRef] [PubMed]
25. Martin, R.; Schmidt, A.W.; Theumer, G.; Krause, T.; Entchev, E.V.; Kurzchalia, T.V.; Knölker, H.J. Synthesis and biological activity of the (25R)-cholesten-26-oic acids–ligands for the hormonal receptor DAF-12 in Caenorhabditis elegans. *Org. Biomol. Chem.* **2009**, *7*, 909–920. [CrossRef]
26. Carvalho, J.F.S.; Silva, M.M.C.; Moreira, J.N.; Simões, S.; Sá e Melo, M.L. Sterols as anticancer agents: Synthesis of ring-B oxygenated steroids, cytotoxic profile, and comprehensive SAR analysis. *J. Med. Chem.* **2010**, *53*, 7632–7638. [CrossRef]
27. Carvalho, J.F.S.; Silva, M.M.C.; Sá e Melo, M.L. Efficient trans-diaxial hydroxylation of Δ5-steroids. *Tetrahedron* **2010**, *66*, 2455–2462. [CrossRef]
28. Joshi, S.; Chaudhari, A.A.; Dennis, V.; Kirby, D.J.; Perrie, Y.; Singh, S.R. Anti-RSV peptide-loaded liposomes for the inhibition of respiratory syncytial virus. *Bioengineering* **2018**, *5*, 37. [CrossRef]
29. Tominaga, H.; Ishiyama, M.; Ohseto, F.; Sasamoto, K.; Hamamoto, T.; Suzuki, K.; Watanabe, M. A water-soluble tetrazolium salt useful for colorimetric cell viability assay. *Anal. Commun.* **1999**, *36*, 47–50. [CrossRef]
30. Liu, X.; Wei, W.; Wang, C.; Yue, H.; Ma, D.; Zhu, C.; Ma, G.; Du, Y. Apoferritin-camouflaged Pt nanoparticles: Surface effects on cellular uptake and cytotoxicity. *J. Mater. Chem.* **2011**, *21*, 7105–7110. [CrossRef]
31. Lin, S.Z.; Wei, W.T.; Chen, H.; Chen, K.J.; Tong, H.F.; Wang, Z.H.; Ni, Z.L.; Liu, H.B.; Guo, H.C.; Liu, D.L. Antitumor activity of emodin against pancreatic cancer depends on its dual role: Promotion of apoptosis and suppression of angiogenesis. *PLoS ONE* **2012**, *7*, e42146. [CrossRef] [PubMed]
32. Li, X.; Zheng, S.L.; Li, X.; Li, J.L.; Qiang, O.; Liu, R.; He, L. Synthesis and anti-breast cancer activity of new indolylquinone derivatives. *Eur. J. Med. Chem.* **2012**, *54*, 42–48. [CrossRef] [PubMed]
33. Xu, M.Y.; Lee, S.Y.; Kang, S.S.; Kim, Y.S. Antitumor activity of jujuboside B and the underlying mechanism via induction of apoptosis and autophagy. *J. Nat. Prod.* **2014**, *77*, 370–376. [CrossRef] [PubMed]

Disclaimer/Publisher's Note: The statements, opinions and data contained in all publications are solely those of the individual author(s) and contributor(s) and not of MDPI and/or the editor(s). MDPI and/or the editor(s) disclaim responsibility for any injury to people or property resulting from any ideas, methods, instructions or products referred to in the content.

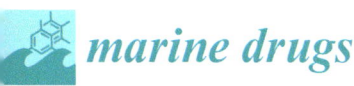

Article

Study on the Anti-*Mycobacterium marinum* Activity of a Series of Marine-Derived 14-Membered Resorcylic Acid Lactone Derivatives

Qian-Qian Jing [1,†], Jun-Na Yin [1,†], Ya-Jie Cheng [1], Qun Zhang [1], Xi-Zhen Cao [1], Wei-Feng Xu [1,2], Chang-Lun Shao [1,3,4,*] and Mei-Yan Wei [1,*]

[1] Key Laboratory of Marine Drugs, The Ministry of Education of China, School of Medicine and Pharmacy, Ocean University of China, Qingdao 266003, China; jingqianqian1231@163.com (Q.-Q.J.); yinjunna@163.com (J.-N.Y.); yajiecheng1212@163.com (Y.-J.C.); zhangqunnn@163.com (Q.Z.); caoxizhen2022@163.com (X.-Z.C.); xuweifeng_u@163.com (W.-F.X.)
[2] State Key Laboratory for Chemistry and Molecular Engineering of Medicinal Resources, College of Chemistry and Pharmaceutical Sciences, Guangxi Normal University, Guilin 541004, China
[3] Laoshan Laboratory, Qingdao 266237, China
[4] Key Laboratory of Tropical Medicinal Resource Chemistry of Ministry of Education, College of Chemistry and Chemical Engineering, Hainan Normal University, Haikou 571158, China
* Correspondence: shaochanglun@163.com (C.-L.S.); mywei95@126.com (M.-Y.W.)
† These authors contributed equally to this work.

Abstract: With the emergence of drug-resistant strains, the treatment of tuberculosis (TB) is becoming more difficult and there is an urgent need to find new anti-TB drugs. *Mycobacterium marinum*, as a model organism of *Mycobacterium tuberculosis*, can be used for the rapid and efficient screening of bioactive compounds. The 14-membered resorcylic acid lactones (RALs) have a wide range of bioactivities such as antibacterial, antifouling and antimalarial activity. In order to further study their bioactivities, we initially constructed a 14-membered RALs library, which contains 16 new derivatives. The anti-*M. marinum* activity was evaluated in vitro. Derivatives **12**, **19**, **20** and **22** exhibited promising activity with MIC_{90} values of 80, 90, 80 and 80 μM, respectively. The preliminary structure–activity relationships showed that the presence of a chlorine atom at C-5 was a key factor to improve activity. Further studies showed that **12** markedly inhibited the survival of *M. marinum* and significantly reduced the dosage of positive drugs isoniazid and rifampicin when combined with them. These results suggest that **12** is a bioactive compound capable of enhancing the potency of existing positive drugs, and its effective properties make it a very useful leads for future drug development in combating TB resistance.

Keywords: 14-membered resorcylic acid lactones; *Mycobacterium marinum*; *Mycobacterium tuberculosis*; marine natural products; anti-tuberculosis

1. Introduction

Tuberculosis (TB) is caused by *Mycobacterium tuberculosis* and is one of the deadliest infectious diseases worldwide [1,2]. By 2022, TB became the second leading cause of death globally from a single infectious source after COVID-19, with almost twice as many deaths as HIV/AIDS [3]. Multidrug-resistant tuberculosis (MDR-TB) is a public health crisis and health security threat, and cases of drug-resistant tuberculosis are increasing gradually due to the emergence of multidrug-resistant strains [4–7]. However, due to the difficulty of anti-tuberculosis drug development and other factors, only bedaquiline, delamanid and pretomanid have been approved for clinical treatment in the past decade, and the first-line drugs are still mainly isoniazid and rifampicin, which were discovered in the 1950s [8–10]. Therefore, the development of new anti-TB drugs is crucial.

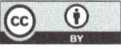

M. tuberculosis is highly infectious and pathogenic, and its culture must be carried out in biosafety level-3 (BSL-3) laboratories [11,12]. Specifically, *M. tuberculosis* grows slowly under in vitro culture conditions, taking about 15 to 20 h to proliferate one generation and 12 days to culture, resulting in a long study cycle. These factors limit the in-depth research of anti-TB drugs [13,14]. In contrast, *Mycobacterium marinum*, from the same genus as *M. tuberculosis*, which grows rapidly with a growth time of about 4 h, is less pathogenic and can be operated in BSL-2 laboratories. More importantly, *M. marinum* and *M. tuberculosis* have high genetic and protein sequence homology. The former's genome size is 6.5 Mb, which is 2.1 Mb longer than the genes of *M. tuberculosis* [15]. It shares more than 85% of its genome with *M. tuberculosis* and shares major virulence factors. Additionally, *M. marinum* infection in humans usually occurs when broken skin comes into direct contact with infected fish or water sources. After infection, patients exhibit pathological features of TB, such as granuloma. Clinically, *M. marinum* can be effectively treated with anti-TB drugs such as rifampicin, ethambutol and quinolones. Based on the advantages of its good biosafety and ease of operation, *M. marinum* is also widely used as one of the model organisms to study the pathogenesis of *M. tuberculosis* [16–18].

Natural products are an important source of new drug development, and more than two-thirds of small molecules approved by the FDA between 1981 and 2019 were related to natural products [19]. The value of natural products of marine origin cannot be ignored. The unique marine environment has created complex, novel and diverse natural products, and endow marine natural products with diversity and particularity in pharmacological activity [20,21]. In terms of anti-TB activity, marine compounds have shown important research value and are valuable resources for the development of anti-TB drugs [22].

The search for new bioactive natural products and derivatives from marine-derived fungi is an ongoing focus of our laboratory. One of our research subjects focuses on resorcylic acid lactones (RALs), polyketide natural products with a 14-membered macrocyclic ring fused to a resorcylic acid residue, which have antibacterial, antifouling, antimalarial and other activities [23,24]. In our previous research, a series of bioactive natural 14-membered RALs (Cochliomycins A–G, 5-Bromozeaenol and 3,5-Dibromozeaenol) were isolated from the marine-derived fungus *Cochliobolus lunatus* (Figure 1) [23,25–27]. Especially, cochliomycin A, at a concentration of 1.2 µg/mL, showed significant antifouling activity against the barnacle *Balanus Amphitrite* [23]. In addition, a series of 14-membered RAL derivatives with antiplasmodial and antifouling activities have been discovered [25–30].

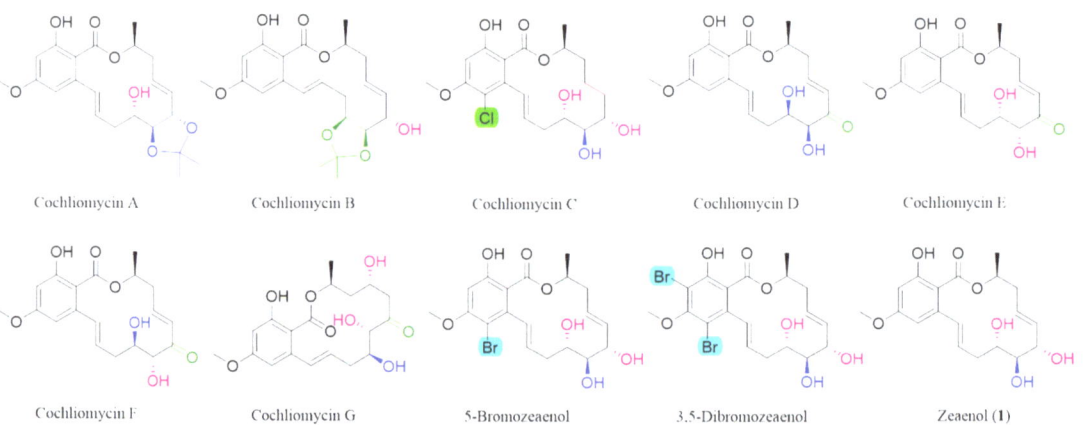

Figure 1. Fourteen-membered lactones isolated from *Cochliobolus lunatus* [23,25–27].

In this study, we constructed a library consisting of zeaenol (1) and its derivatives, **2–97**, aimed to enrich the structural diversity of 14-membered RALs and evaluate their structure–activity relationships. Among the synthesized compounds, **19** and **24–38** are new derivatives. In addition, six different bacteria and fungi were selected for the in vitro screening of activity. Derivatives **12**, **19**, **20** and **22** have selective activity against *M. marinum*. A further study showed that compound **12** significantly inhibited the survival of *M. marinum*, and the combination with positive drugs significantly reduced the dose of positive drugs isoniazid and rifampicin.

2. Results and Discussion

2.1. Chemistry

The fermentation condition of *Cochliobolus lunatus* (CHNSCLM-0009) was liquid fermentation. The crude extract obtained after fermentation was subjected to silica gel column chromatography (CC) and recrystallization, and a total of 7.54 g of zeaenol (**1**) was obtained [29,30]. 97 derivatives were semi-synthesized using zeaenol (**1**) as a starting material through one to three steps (Scheme 1). Synthetic schemes for some of the compounds (**2–18**, **20–23** and **39–97**) can be seen in reference [30].

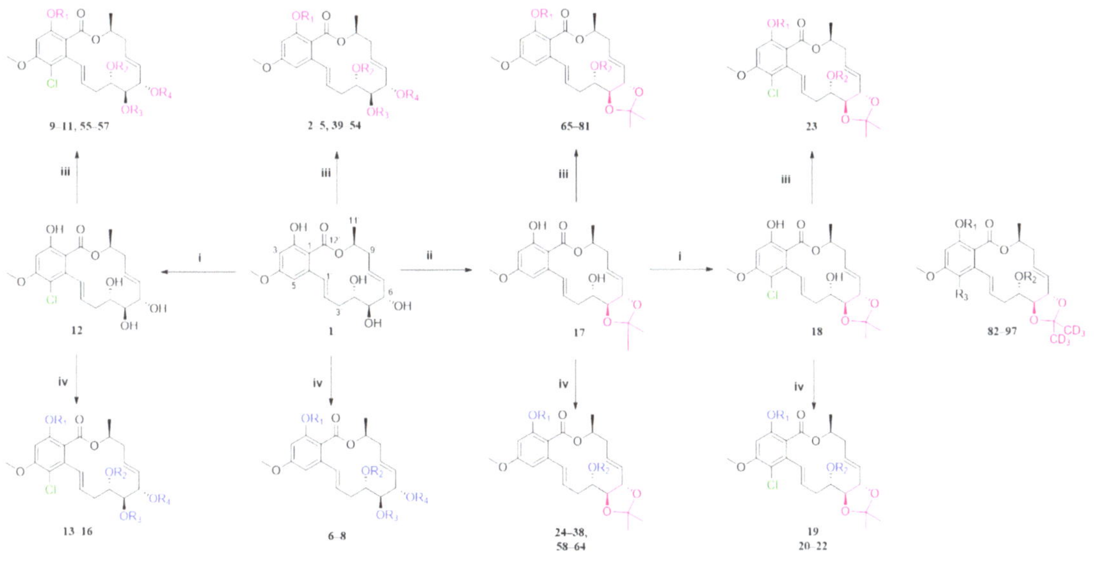

Scheme 1. The synthetic route. i SO$_2$Cl$_2$, 0 °C; ii *p*-TsOH, acetone, room temperature, 5 h; iii ArCH$_2$Br reagent, K$_2$CO$_3$, acetone, 50 °C, 24 h; iv anhydride, acyl chloride reagents or carboxylic acids, DMAP, EDCl, DCM, 45 °C, 3–4 h. Compounds **82–97** were synthesized in the same way as other compounds were, except acetone-*d*$_6$ was used for acetal formation. The specific information of compounds **2–18**, **20–23**, **39–97** was shown in Ref. [27].

Among the 97 compounds of the library, 38 representative derivatives are shown in Table 1, including the new compounds **19** and **24–38**. Compounds **39–97** are shown in Table S1.

Table 1. Zeaenol (**1**) and its derivatives **2–38**.

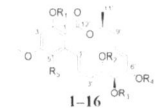

No.	R₁	R₂	R₃	R₄	R₅	No.	R₁	R₂	R₃	R₄	R₅
1	H	H	H	H	H	9	⟨aryl⟩	H	H	H	Cl
2	⟨benzyl⟩	H	H	H	H	10	⟨Cl-aryl⟩	H	H	H	Cl
3	⟨tBu-benzyl⟩	H	H	H	H	11	⟨CN-aryl⟩	H	H	H	Cl
4	⟨Me-benzyl⟩	H	H	H	H	12	H	H	H	H	Cl
5	⟨naphthyl⟩	H	H	H	H	13	Ac	Ac	Ac	Ac	Cl
6	Ac	Ac	Ac	Ac	H	14	⟨acyl⟩	⟨acyl⟩	⟨acyl⟩	⟨acyl⟩	Cl
7	⟨acyl⟩	⟨acyl⟩	⟨acyl⟩	⟨acyl⟩	H	15	Piv	Piv	H	Piv	Cl
8	Piv	Piv	H	Piv	H	16	Piv	H	H	H	Cl

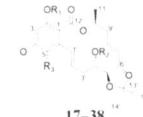

No.	R₁	R₂	R₃	No.	R₁	R₂	R₃
17	H	H	H	28	Bz	H	H
18	H	H	Cl	29	Bz	Bz	H
19	Ac	H	Cl	30	⟨F-Bz⟩	H	H
20	⟨propanoyl⟩	H	Cl	31	⟨F-Bz⟩	⟨F-Bz⟩	H
21	Piv	H	Cl	32	H	⟨F-Bz⟩	H
22	⟨MeO-acyl⟩	⟨MeO-acyl⟩	Cl	33	⟨nicotinoyl⟩	H	H
23	⟨MeO-benzoyl⟩	H	Cl	34	⟨nicotinoyl⟩	⟨nicotinoyl⟩	H
24	⟨MeO-Bz⟩	H	H	35	H	⟨nicotinoyl⟩	H
25	⟨furoyl⟩	H	H	36	Ac	H	H
26	⟨furoyl⟩	⟨furoyl⟩	H	37	⟨thienoyl⟩	H	H
27	H	⟨furoyl⟩	H	38	⟨thienoyl⟩	⟨thienoyl⟩	H

2.2. Evaluation of Biological Activity

2.2.1. Anti-*M. marinum* and Other Antimicrobial Activity

The cases of drug-resistant tuberculosis are increasing gradually due to the emergence of multidrug-resistant strains [31,32]. As a model organism of *M. tuberculosis*, *M. marinum* can quickly and efficiently screen bioactive compounds. The antibacterial and antifungal activity of the 97 RAL derivatives were evaluated. We discovered several compounds exhibiting potent antibacterial activity, as evidenced by the data presented in Table 2. The activities of the remaining derivatives (MIC$_{90}$ > 200 µM) are not shown in Table 2. Derivatives **12**, **19**, **20** and **22** exhibited promising anti-*M. marinum* activity with MIC$_{90}$ values of 80, 90, 80 and 80 µM, respectively (Figure 2). Comparatively, the MIC$_{90}$ of isoniazid was 40 µM, which indicated the presence of derivatives **12**, **19**, **20** and **22**, and these exhibit good activity. It is worth noting that they also have antibacterial activity selectivity. Compound **1** was the raw material for all derivatives and did not exhibit antimicrobial activity. Derivatives **12**, **19**, **20** and **22** showed substantially improved anti-*M. marinum* activity compared with compound **1**. In order to determine the safety of these compounds, we selected the active derivatives **12**, **19**, **20** and **22** to evaluate non-small cell lung cancer (A549), and the results showed that the IC$_{50}$ values of the above compounds were between 100 and 600 µM, which fully verified that the compounds had own antibacterial effects rather than toxicity.

Table 2. Antimicrobial activity of representative compounds in the RAL library [1].

Compound	MIC$_{90}$ (µM)					
	M. marinum	*S. aureus*	*E. coli*	*P. aeruginosa*	*C. albicans*	*A. fumigatus*
1	>200	>100	>100	>100	>100	>100
4	>200	12.5	>100	>100	>100	>100
11	100	>100	>100	>100	>100	>100
12	80	>100	>100	>100	>100	>100
18	>200	>100	>100	>100	>100	>100
19	90	>100	>100	>100	>100	>100
20	80	>100	>100	>100	>100	>100
22	80	>100	>100	>100	>100	>100
Isoniazid	40	nt	nt	nt	nt	nt
Rifampicin	10	nt	nt	nt	nt	nt
Ciprofloxacin	nt	3.13	0.10	1.56	nt	nt
Amphotericin B	nt	nt	nt	nt	0.84	0.07

[1] Results are the average of three independent experiments, each performed in duplicate. Standard deviations were less than ±10%. nt = not tested.

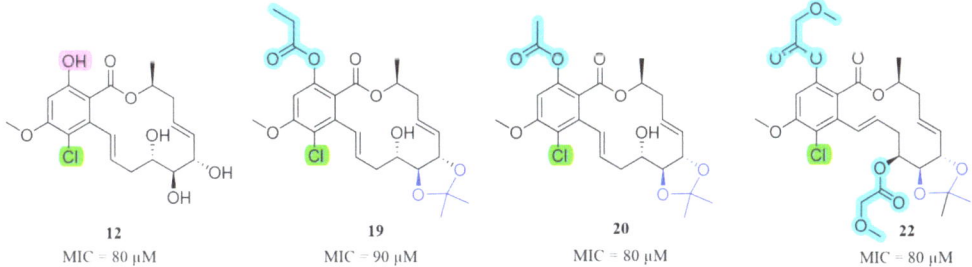

Figure 2. Chemical structures of derivatives **12**, **19**, **20** and **22**, and their anti-*M. marinum* activity.

An overview of the MICs of this 14-membered RAL library in combination with their structures gives preliminary insights of SARs: (1) the anti-*M. marinum* activity of 14-membered RALs can be significantly improved via the introduction of the chlorine atom at the C-5 position, as seen by comparing the MICs of **1/12**; (2) bearing an acetonide group at position 5'6' reduces activity, as seen by comparing the MICs of **12/18**; (3) the acetyl- and propanoyl-substituted phenolic hydroxy group enhanced activity when both the chlorine atom, and an acetonide group at 5'6' were also present (**19**, **20** and **22**); (4) a comparison of compound **12** with compounds **9–11** indicates that when the phenolic hydroxy group is transformed into an ether, the activity decreases.

2.2.2. Time–Growth Curves of *M. marinum* Strain Treated with Different Concentrations of Compound **12**

According to the above results, derivatives **12**, **19**, **20** and **22** have selective anti-*M. marinum* activity. Initially, we tested the solubility of the active compounds. In the aqueous solution of 1% DMSO, the solubility of **12** was 0.30 mg/mL, and the solubility of derivatives **19**, **20** and **22** was less than 0.10 mg/mL. Due to the high solubility and strong activity of **12**, it was selected for further study.

To investigate its effect on the survival of the *M. marinum* strain, we treated the *M. marinum* strain with different concentrations of compound **12** and plotted a time–growth curve (Figure 3). The results showed that the higher the concentration of compound **12**, the stronger its inhibitory effect on the survival of *M. marinum*, showing a certain concentration dependence. The anti-*M. marinum* effect of **12** began to play a role in 24 h. From that point onwards, the inhibition rate of **12** significantly exceeded the growth rate of the bacteria, resulting in a gradually widening gap between the number of bacteria in the treated group and the control group. By 48 h, a noticeable difference between the groups emerged, however, neither completely eradicated the bacteria.

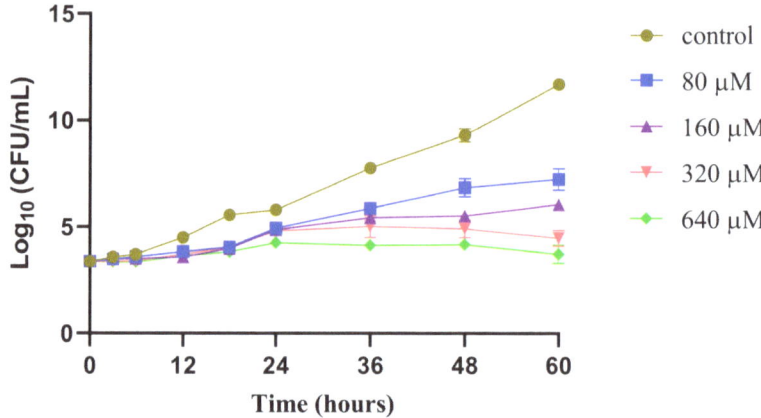

Figure 3. Time–growth curves of *M. marinum* strain treated with different concentrations of compound **12**. Results are expressed as mean ± SEM, $n = 6$.

2.2.3. Anti-*M. marinum* Effects of Compound **12** in Combination with Positive Drugs

Current TB treatment regimens are extremely challenging, with about 20% of TB deaths caused by drug-resistant *M. tuberculosis*. MDR-TB is at least resistant to isoniazid and rifampicin, the two most important first-line drugs with which to treat TB. It is necessary to reduce the use of both drugs. We used the checkerboard method [33] to combine **12** with positive drugs for a drug sensitivity test, and the MIC$_{90}$ values for combined medication are shown in Table 3. The results showed that **12** combined with isoniazid and rifampicin had an obvious additive effect. We observed that **12** can significantly reduce the dosage of the positive drugs isoniazid and rifampicin. Compound **12** at 40 μM made *M. marinum* four-fold more sensitive to isoniazid and rifampicin, while 20 μM isoniazid or 2.5 μM rifampicin did not inhibit bacterial growth on average. In particular, when the concentration of **12** was adjusted to 60 μM, *M. marinum* was eight-fold more sensitive to isoniazid and six-fold more sensitive to rifampicin. We selected **12** in combination with isoniazid for bacterial count statistics (Figure 4). It is worth mentioning that **12** did not significantly inhibit bacterial growth in the concentration range of 40–60 µM. Therefore, **12** is considered to be an active compound that can improve the sensitivity of positive drugs.

Table 3. Anti-*M. marinum* effects of compound **12** in combination with positive drugs.

	Positive Drugs MIC$_{90}$ (µM)		Compound 12 MIC$_{90}$ (µM)		FICI [1]	Mode of Action
	Alone	Combined	Alone	Combined		
Isoniazid	40	10	80	40	0.75	additive
Rifampicin	10	2.5	80	40	0.75	additive

[1] The mode of action was determined using the fractional inhibitory concentration index (FICI): (1) FICI ≤ 0.5, synergistic effect; (2) 0.5 < FICI ≤ 1, additive effect; (3) 1 < FICI ≤ 2, irrelevant; (4) FICI > 2, antagonistic effect.

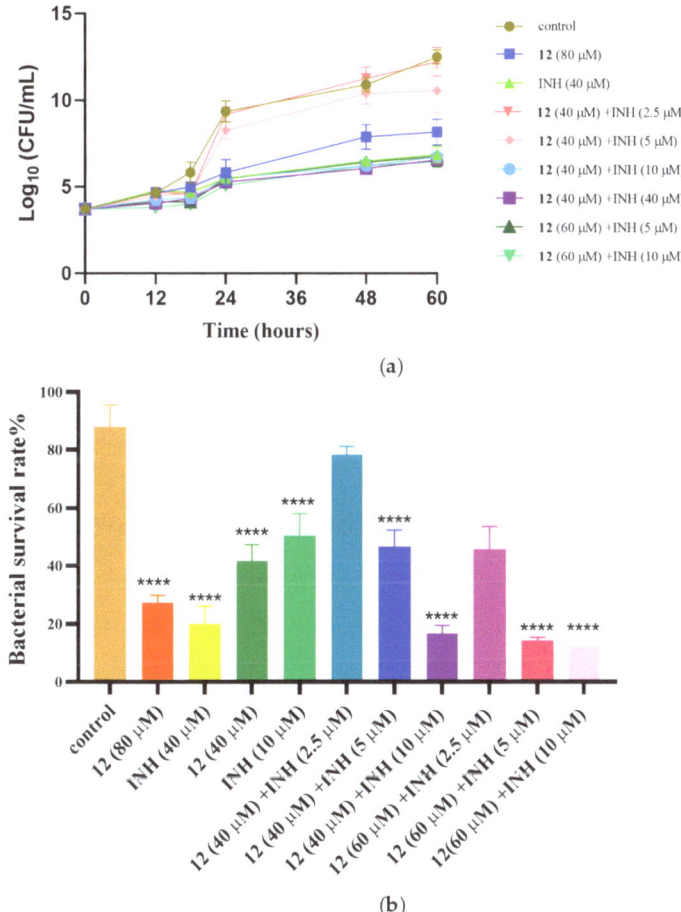

Figure 4. Compound **12** in combination with positive drugs isoniazid (INH). (**a**) Time–growth curves of *M. marinum* strain treated with different concentrations of compound **12** and INH; (**b**) different concentrations of **12** and INH inhibit the growth of *M. marinum*. The number of bacterial cells was measured at 48 h. Data are presented as the mean of three experiments ± SD. **** $p < 0.0001$ compared with the control group.

3. Materials and Methods

3.1. General Experimental Procedures

Reagents and solvents were purchased from commercial suppliers and used without further purification. Column chromatography (CC) was performed on silica gel (Qingdao Haiyang Chemical Group Co., Qingdao, China; 200–300 mesh) and Sephadex LH-20 (Amersham Biosciences, Amersham, UK). TLC silica gel plates (Yantai Zifu Chemical Group) were used for thin-layer chromatography. Semi-preparative HPLC was performed on a Waters 1525 system using a C18 column (Amsterdam, The Netherland; Kromasil, 5 µm, 10 × 250 mm) equipped with a Waters 2996 photodiode array detector, and the flow rate was 2.0 mL/min. NMR spectra were recorded on Bruker Advance NEO 400. Chemical shifts, δ, were measured in ppm, the internal standard was TMS and coupling constants (J) were measured in Hz.

3.2. Fungal Material

The fungal strain *Cochliobolus lunatus* (CHNSCLM-0009) was isolated from a piece of tissue from the inner part of the freshly collected gorgonian coral *Dichotella gemmacea* (GX-WZ-20080034), which was collected from the Weizhou coral reef in the South China Sea in September 2008. The fungus was identified as *C. lunatus* via 16*S* rRNA gene analysis, and code ZJ2008002 was obtained. The strain was stored at the Key Laboratory of Marine Drugs, the Ministry of Education of China, School of Medicine and Pharmacy, Ocean University of China, Qingdao, China.

3.3. Fermentation, Extraction and Isolation

The fermentation condition of *Cochliobolus lunatus* (CHNSCLM-0009) was liquid fermentation. This fungus was placed in a 500 mL flask with 200 mL of liquid medium (soluble starch 10 g/L, NaNO$_3$ 5 g/L, NaOAc 1 g/L, 1% salinity), and fermented on a rotating shaker at 120 r/min at 28 °C for 10 days [29,30].

The fermentation liquid was extracted with an equal volume of EtOAc 3–4 times, and concentrated to obtain 25 g of crude extract. The total crude extract was separated via silica gel column chromatography (CC). Ethyl acetate and petroleum ether were selected as eluents. Zeaenol (**1**) was obtained in a 60% ethyl acetate/petroleum ether composition. After repeated recrystallization of the crude product (ethyl acetate/petroleum ether/methanol), a total of 7.54 g of zeaenol (**1**) was obtained.

3.4. General Synthetic Methods for Compounds **2**–**97**

The synthesis of reported compounds (**2**–**18**, **20**–**23** and **39**–**97**) is not described in this article. The synthesis and detailed data of these compounds can be found in reference [30]. Here, we describe in detail the synthetic steps of compound **19** and **24**–**38**.

3.4.1. General Procedure for the Synthesis of **19**

Compound **18** (438.14 µmol, 1 equiv), acetyl chloride (77.99 µmol, 2 equiv), DMAP (753.56 µmol, 3 equiv) and EDCl (753.56 µmol, 3 equiv) in dry CH$_2$Cl$_2$ (15 mL) were stirred at 45 °C for 2 h, and the reaction process was monitored via TLC. After the reaction was completed, it was quenched with saturated NaHCO$_3$ (30 mL) aqueous solution and extracted with CH$_2$Cl$_2$ (30 mL), and the organic layer was evaporated to dryness, leaving the crude product. The crude product was purified via silica gel CC column chromatography (EtOAc/petroleum ether, 1:5, v/v) to give derivative **19**.

3.4.2. General Procedure for the Synthesis of **24**–**38**

Compounds **17** (404.18 µmol, 1 equiv), anhydride, acyl chloride or carboxylic acid reagents (5 equiv, Supplementary Table S2), DMAP (753.56 µmol, 3 equiv) and EDCl (753.56 µmol, 3 equiv) in dry CH$_2$Cl$_2$ (15 mL) were stirred at 45 °C for 4 h, and the reaction process was monitored via TLC. After the reaction was completed, it was quenched with saturated NaHCO$_3$ (30 mL) aqueous solution and extracted with CH$_2$Cl$_2$ (30 mL), and the organic layer was evaporated to dryness, leaving the crude product. Derivatives **24–38** were purified via silica gel column chromatography.

3.4.3. Characterization Data of Compounds **19**, and **24–38**

The structures of all compounds were identified using NMR data and the HR-ESI-MS spectrum. Compounds **19** and **24–38** were new derivatives, the details of which are in the Supplementary Materials. Detailed structural information on other known compounds is not indicated.

Compound **19**, white, solid; yield 70.7%; $[\alpha]_D^{20}$–14.6° (c 0.05, MeOH); ^{1}H NMR (400 MHz, CDCl$_3$): δ ppm 6.61 (1H, s), 6.50 (1H, dd, J = 16.0, 1.9 Hz), 5.95 (1H, dt, J = 16.0, 4.6 Hz), 5.78 (1H, ddd, J = 16.0, 10.0, 3.8 Hz), 5.67–5.48 (2H, overlapped), 4.51 (1H, t, J = 8.4 Hz), 4.12 (1H, m), 3.89 (3H, s), 3.80 (1H, dd, J = 8.4, 2.2 Hz), 2.77 (1H, ddd, J = 14.6, 6.5, 3.9 Hz), 2.47–2.39 (2H, overlapped), 2.32 (1H, m), 2.28 (3H, s), 1.42 (3H, s), 1.38 (3H, s), 1.30 (3H, d, J = 6.3 Hz). ^{13}C NMR (100 MHz, CDCl$_3$): δ 169.0 (C), 165.0 (C), 156.9 (C), 147.7 (C), 136.8 (C), 133.2 (CH), 131.4 (CH), 128.9 (CH), 127.1 (CH), 119.7 (C), 119.4 (CH), 108.5 (CH), 105.4 (CH), 81.2 (CH), 75.5 (CH), 69.2 (CH), 67.9 (CH), 56.5(CH$_2$), 37.0 (CH$_3$), 35.5 (CH$_2$), 26.9(CH$_3$ × 2), 26.9(CH$_3$ × 2), 20.8 (CH$_3$), 20.7 (CH$_3$). HRESIMS m/z 479.1480 [M − H]$^-$ (calcd for C$_{24}$H$_{28}$O$_8$Cl$^-$, 479.1467).

Compound **24**, White, solid; yield 83.2%; $[\alpha]_D^{20}$–23.6° (c 0.1, MeOH); ^{1}H NMR (400 MHz, CDCl$_3$) δ 8.05 (1H, dd, J = 7.8, 1.8 Hz), 7.53 (1H, ddd, J = 8.4, 7.4, 1.8 Hz), 7.10–6.99 (3H, overlapped), 6.81 (1H, d, J = 2.5 Hz), 6.70 (1H, d, J = 2.5 Hz), 5.98 (1H, dt, J = 15.8, 5.1 Hz), 5.83 (1H, ddd, J = 15.1, 10.8, 3.9 Hz), 5.57–5.37 (2H, overlapped), 4.54 (1H, t, J = 8.4 Hz), 4.16(1H, m), 3.94–3.86 (4H, overlapped), 3.83 (3H, s), 2.67 (1H, dtd, J = 14.0, 4.1, 2.2 Hz), 2.57–2.41 (3H, overlapped), 2.29 (1H, ddd, J = 13.9, 12.0, 10.6 Hz), 1.43 (3H, s), 1.34 (6H, m).^{13}C NMR (100 MHz, CDCl$_3$) δ 165.6 (C), 164.1 (C), 161.9 (C), 160.5 (C), 151.6 (C), 139.9 (C), 134.8 (CH), 133.3 (CH), 133.0 (CH), 131.8 (CH), 130.7 (CH), 128.4 (CH), 120.7 (C), 119.1 (CH), 117.9 (CH), 112.6 (CH), 110.7 (C), 108.9 (CH), 108.5 (CH), 81.5 (CH), 76.2 (CH), 69.8 (CH), 67.0 (CH), 56.5 (CH$_2$), 56.1 (CH$_3$), 37.5 (CH$_3$), 36.4 (CH$_2$), 27.4 (CH$_3$ × 2), 20.5 (CH$_3$). HRESIMS m/z 539.2273 [M + H]$^+$ (calcd for C$_{30}$H$_{35}$O$_9^+$, 539.2276).

Compound **25**, White, solid; yield 70.3%; $[\alpha]_D^{20}$–21.4° (c 0.1, MeOH); ^{1}H NMR (400 MHz, CDCl$_3$) δ 7.66 (1H, dd, J = 1.7, 0.8 Hz), 7.37 (1H, dd, J = 3.5, 0.9 Hz), 7.05 (1H, dd, J = 15.6, 2.0 Hz), 6.82 (1H, d, J = 2.5 Hz), 6.68 (1H, d, J = 2.5 Hz), 6.58 (1H, dd, J = 3.5, 1.7 Hz), 5.98 (1H, dt, J = 15.7, 5.2 Hz), 5.84 (1H, ddd, J = 15.1, 10.8, 3.9 Hz), 5.49 (1H, ddt, J = 15.7, 8.9, 1.8 Hz), 5.39 (1H, pd, J = 6.4, 3.8 Hz), 4.54 (1H, t, J = 8.4 Hz), 4.16 (1H, ddd, J = 12.2, 4.3, 2.3 Hz), 3.88 (1H, dd, J = 8.0, 2.3 Hz), 3.83 (3H, s), 2.67 (1H, dtd, J = 14.0, 4.3, 2.3 Hz), 2.59–2.46 (3H, overlapped), 2.29 (1H, ddd, J = 14.0, 12.0, 10.6 Hz), 1.42 (3H, s), 1.36–1.31 (6H, overlapped).^{13}C NMR (100 MHz, CDCl$_3$) δ 165.1 (C), 161.7 (C), 156.7 (C), 150.5 (C), 147.4 (CH), 143.9 (C), 139.9 (C), 132.8 (CH), 131.4 (CH), 130.6 (CH), 128.4 (CH), 119.9 (C), 117.3 (CH), 112.4 (C), 110.6 (CH), 108.6 (CH), 108.0 (CH), 81.2 (CH), 75.9 (CH), 69.7 (CH), 68.6 (CH), 55.8 (CH$_2$), 37.1 (CH$_3$), 36.1 (CH$_2$), 27.1 (CH$_3$), 27.0 (CH$_3$), 20.1 (CH$_3$) HRFSIMS m/z 499.1968 [M + H]$^+$ (calcd for C$_{27}$H$_{31}$O$_9^+$, 499.1963).

Compound **26**, White, solid; yield 60.6%; $[\alpha]_D^{20}$–17.2° (c 0.1, MeOH); ^{1}H NMR (400 MHz, CDCl$_3$) δ 7.67 (1H, dd, J = 1.8, 0.8 Hz), 7.60 (1H, dd, J = 1.8, 0.8 Hz), 7.38 (1H, dd, J = 3.5, 0.9 Hz), 7.23 (1H, dd, J = 3.5, 0.9 Hz), 7.12 (1H, dd, J = 15.5, 1.9 Hz), 6.84 (1H, d, J = 2.5 Hz), 6.70 (1H, d, J = 2.5 Hz), 6.59 (1H, dd, J = 3.5, 1.7 Hz), 6.53 (1H, dd, J = 3.5, 1.7 Hz), 6.06 (1H, dt, J = 15.8, 5.2 Hz), 5.93 (1H, ddd, J = 15.1, 10.7, 3.9 Hz), 5.65–5.49 (2H, overlapped), 5.41 (1H, m), 4.73 (1H, t, J = 8.2 Hz), 4.06 (1H, dd, J = 7.8, 2.3 Hz), 3.85 (3H, s), 2.77 (1H, dtd, J = 13.8, 4.3, 2.2 Hz), 2.55–2.40 (3H, overlapped), 1.34 (6H, overlapped), 1.26 (3H, s).^{13}C NMR (100 MHz, CDCl$_3$) δ 165.0 (C), 161.8 (C), 158.1 (C), 156.7 (C), 150.6 (C), 147.4 (C), 146.6 (CH), 144.7 (CH), 143.9 (CH), 139.6 (C), 133.4 (CH), 131.5 (CH), 130.6 (CH), 127.3 (CH), 119.9 (C), 118.3 (CH), 117.3 (CH), 112.4 (C), 112.0 (CH), 110.5 (CH), 109.3 (CH), 108.3 (CH), 79.8 (CH), 70.8 (CH), 69.8 (CH), 55.8 (CH), 37.3 (CH$_2$), 35.2 (CH$_3$), 29.8 (CH$_2$), 27.3 (CH$_3$), 26.7 (CH$_3$), 20.1 (CH$_3$). HRESIMS m/z 593.2027 [M + H]$^+$ (calcd for C$_{32}$H$_{33}$O$_{11}^+$, 593.2017).

Compound **27**, White, solid; yield 73.4%; $[\alpha]_D^{20}$ –19.7° (c 0.1, MeCN); ^{1}H NMR (400 MHz, CDCl$_3$) δ 11.51 (1H, s), 7.61 (1H, dd, J = 1.8, 0.8 Hz), 7.24 (1H, d, J = 2.5 Hz), 6.54 (1H, dd, J = 3.5, 1.8 Hz), 6.49 (1H, d, J = 2.6 Hz), 6.41 (1H, d, J = 2.6 Hz), 6.08 (1H, ddd, J = 15.3, 7.5, 5.5 Hz), 5.81 (1H, ddd, t, J = 15.4, 10.6, 3.1 Hz), 5.71–5.54 (2H, overlapped), 5.45 (1H, m), 4.76 (1H, t, J = 8.1 Hz), 4.06 (1H, dd, J = 7.8, 2.3 Hz), 3.83 (3H, s), 2.84 (1H, ddt, J = 14.4, 5.4, 2.9 Hz), 2.61–2.39 (3H, overlapped), 1.46 (3H, d, J = 6.3 Hz), 1.35 (3H, s), 1.26 (3H, s). ^{13}C NMR (100 MHz, CDCl$_3$) δ 170.9 (C), 164.9 (C), 164.2 (C), 158.1 (C), 146.7 (CH), 144.7 (CH), 141.9 (C), 134.7 (CH), 132.5 (CH), 129.6 (CH), 125.8 (CH), 118.4 (C), 112.0 (CH), 109.3 (CH), 107.4 (C), 104.5 (CH), 100.6 (CH), 80.3 (CH), 76.2 (CH), 71.0 (CH), 70.9 (CH), 55.6 (CH$_2$), 38.1 (CH$_3$), 35.1 (CH$_2$), 27.4 (CH$_3$), 26.7 (CH$_3$), 19.6 (CH$_3$). HRESIMS m/z 499.1962 [M + H]$^+$ (calcd for C$_{27}$H$_{31}$O$_9^+$, 499.1963).

Compound **28**, White, solid; yield 63.7%; $[\alpha]_D^{20}$ –38.1° (c 0.1, MeOH); ^{1}H NMR (400 MHz, CDCl$_3$) δ 8.20–8.13 (2H, overlapped), 7.63 (1H, m), 7.50 (2H, overlapped), 7.06 (1H, dd, J = 17.2, 2.0 Hz), 6.82 (1H, d, J = 2.5 Hz), 6.69 (1H, d, J = 2.5 Hz), 5.98 (1H, dt, J = 15.8, 5.1 Hz), 5.84 (1H, ddd, J = 15.2, 10.8, 3.9 Hz), 5.50 (1H, ddt, J = 15.7, 8.8, 1.8 Hz), 5.39 (1H, m), 4.54 (1H, t, J = 8.4 Hz), 4.17–4.09 (1H, overlapped), 3.89 (1H, dd, J = 8.0, 2.3 Hz), 3.84 (3H, s), 2.67 (1H, dtd, J = 14.0, 4.1, 2.2 Hz), 2.58–2.44 (3H, overlapped), 2.30 (1H, ddd, J = 14.0, 12.0, 10.6 Hz), 1.42 (3H, s), 1.35 (3H, s), 1.30 (3H, d, J = 6.3 Hz). ^{13}C NMR (100 MHz, CDCl$_3$) δ 165.2 (C), 165.1 (C), 161.7 (C), 151.3 (C), 139.8 (C), 133.8 (CH), 132.7 (CH), 131.4 (CH), 130.4 (CH), 129.4 (C), 128.7 (CH), 128.3 (CH), 117.4 (CH), 110.4 (CH), 108.6 (CH), 108.0 (C), 81.2 (C), 75.9 (CH), 69.5 (CH), 68.6 (CH), 60.5 (CH), 55.8 (CH$_3$), 37.1 (CH), 36.1 (CH$_2$), 27.1 (CH$_3$), 27.1 (CH$_2$), 21.2 (CH$_3$), 20.1 (CH$_3$), 14.3 (CH$_3$). HRESIMS m/z 509.2176 [M + H]$^+$ (calcd for C$_{29}$H$_{33}$O$_8^+$, 509.2170).

Compound **29**, White, solid; yield 77.8%; $[\alpha]_D^{20}$ –8.1° (c 0.1, MeCN); ^{1}H NMR (400 MHz, CDCl$_3$) δ 8.21–8.15 (2H, overlapped), 8.12–8.06 (2H, overlapped), 7.61 (2H, m), 7.49 (4H, overlapped), 7.13 (1H, dd, J = 15.5, 1.9 Hz), 6.85 (1H, d, J = 2.5 Hz), 6.72 (1H, d, J = 2.5 Hz), 6.07 (1H, dt, J = 15.7, 5.2 Hz), 5.97 (1H, ddd, J = 15.1, 10.7, 3.9 Hz), 5.66 (1H, ddd, J = 12.3, 4.6, 2.2 Hz), 5.58 (1H, dd, J = 15.8, 8.6 Hz), 5.41 (1H, q, J = 5.9 Hz), 4.78 (1H, t, J = 8.2 Hz), 4.11 (1H, dt, J = 7.8, 2.4 Hz), 3.86 (3H, s), 2.78 (1H, m), 2.56–2.43 (3H, overlapped), 1.32–1.31 (6H, overlapped), 1.23 (3H, s). ^{13}C NMR (100 MHz, CDCl$_3$) δ 165.9 (C), 165.2 (C), 161.8 (C), 151.4 (C), 139.5 (C), 133.8 (C), 133.4 (CH), 133.3 (CH), 131.2 (CH), 130.7 (C), 130.4 (C), 130.4 (CH), 129.8 (CH), 129.4 (CH), 128.8 (CH×2), 128.6 (CH×2), 127.5 (CH), 117.5 (CH), 110.4 (C), 109.3 (C), 108.3 (CH), 79.9 (CH), 70.8 (CH), 69.7 (CH), 55.8 (CH), 37.3 (CH), 35.3 (CH$_2$), 29.9 (CH$_3$), 27.2 (CH$_2$), 27.0 (CH$_3$ × 2), 20.2 (CH$_3$). HRESIMS m/z 613.2433 [M + H]$^+$ (calcd for C$_{36}$H$_{37}$O$_9^+$, 613.2433).

Compound **30**, White, solid; yield 83.5%; $[\alpha]_D^{20}$ –19.3° (c 0.1, MeOH); ^{1}H NMR (400 MHz, CDCl$_3$) δ 8.10 (1H, td, J = 7.5, 1.9 Hz), 7.59 (m, 1H), 7.28 (1H, dd, J = 7.7, 1.1Hz), 7.19 (1H, ddd, J = 10.8, 8.3, 1.1 Hz), 7.07 (1H, dd, J = 15.5, 2.0 Hz), 6.83 (1H, d, J = 2.5 Hz), 6.70 (1H, d, J = 2.5 Hz), 5.98 (1H, dt, J = 15.8, 5.1 Hz), 5.84 (1H, ddd, J = 15.2, 10.8, 3.9 Hz), 5.50 (1H, ddt, J = 15.6, 8.8, 1.8 Hz), 5.41 (1H, q, J = 5.9 Hz), 4.54 (1H, t, J = 8.4 Hz), 4.16 (1H, ddd, J = 12.3, 4.4, 2.2 Hz), 3.89 (1H, dd, J = 8.0, 2.3 Hz), 3.84 (3H, s), 2.68 (1H, dtd, J = 14.0, 4.2, 2.3 Hz), 2.56–2.46 (3H, overlapped), 2.30 (1H, ddd, J = 14.0, 12.0, 10.6 Hz), 1.42 (3H, s), 1.37–1.31 (6H, overlapped). ^{13}C NMR (100 MHz, CDCl$_3$) δ 165.2 (C), 163.8 (C), 162.6 (C), 161.8 (C), 151.1 (C), 139.9 (C), 135.4 (CH), 135.4 (CH), 132.9 (CH), 132.9 (CH), 131.5 (CH), 130.4 (CH), 128.4 (CH), 124.3 (C), 124.3 (C), 117.9 (CH), 117.2 (C), 110.7 (CH), 108.6 (CH), 108.0 (CH), 81.2 (CH), 75.9 (CH), 69.6 (CH), 68.6 (CH$_2$), 55.8 (CH$_3$), 37.2 (CH$_2$), 36.1 (CH$_3$), 27.1 (CH$_3$), 20.1 (CH$_3$). HRESIMS m/z 527.2080 [M + H]$^+$ (calcd for C$_{29}$H$_{32}$O$_8$F$^+$, 527.2076).

Compound **31**, White, solid; yield 87.2%; $[\alpha]_D^{20}$ –28.4° (c 0.1, MeOH); ^{1}H NMR (400 MHz, CDCl$_3$) δ 8.12 (1H, td, J = 7.5, 1.9 Hz), 8.03 (1H, m), 7.65–7.49 (2H, overlapped), 7.32–7.11 (5H, overlapped), 6.85 (1H, d, J = 2.6 Hz), 6.72 (1H, d, J = 2.6 Hz), 6.06 (1H, dt, J = 15.8, 5.1 Hz), 5.94 (1H, ddd, J = 15.1, 10.8, 3.8 Hz), 5.69 (1H, ddd, J = 12.4, 4.8, 2.3 Hz), 5.56 (1H, ddt, J = 15.6, 8.5, 1.8 Hz), 5.44 (1H, td, J = 6.5, 4.5 Hz), 4.76 (1H, t, J = 8.3 Hz), 4.08 (1H, dd, J = 7.9, 2.3 Hz), 3.86 (3H, s), 2.80 (1H, ddq, J = 13.8, 4.3, 2.3 Hz), 2.60–2.43 (3H, overlapped),

1.38–1.31 (6H, overlapped), 1.26 (3H, s). ^{13}C NMR (100 MHz, CDCl$_3$) δ 169.2 (C), 165.2 (C), 163.4 (C), 162.6 (C), 161.8 (C), 161.4 (C), 151.1 (C), 139.6 (C), 135.7 (CH), 135.5 (CH), 134.9 (CH), 133.5 (CH), 132.9 (CH), 132.9 (CH), 132.4 (CH), 131.3 (CH), 130.3 (CH), 127.5 (CH), 124.3 (C), 117.4 (C), 117.3 (C), 117.2 (CH), 117.1 (CH), 110.6 (C), 109.1 (CH), 108.2 (CH), 79.7 (CH), 77.0 (CH), 71.2 (CH), 69.7 (CH), 55.8 (CH$_2$), 37.3 (CH$_3$), 35.2 (CH$_2$), 27.2 (CH$_3$), 26.7 (CH$_3$), 20.2 (CH$_3$). HRESIMS m/z 649.2242 [M + H]$^+$ (calcd for C$_{36}$H$_{35}$O$_9$F$_2^+$, 649.2244).

Compound **32**, White, solid; yield 73.9%; $[α]_D^{20}$ −31.5° (c 0.1, MeOH); ^{1}H NMR (400 MHz, CDCl$_3$) δ 11.53 (1H, s), 8.01 (1H, td, J = 7.5, 1.9 Hz), 7.55 (1H, m), 7.23 (1H, m), 7.17 (1H, ddd, J = 10.9, 8.4, 1.1 Hz), 6.49 (1H, d, J = 2.6 Hz), 6.42 (1H, d, J = 2.6 Hz), 6.06 (1H, ddd, J = 15.4, 7.2, 5.6 Hz), 5.82 (1H, ddd, J = 15.4, 10.6, 3.1 Hz), 5.72 (1H, ddd, J = 12.4, 5.2, 2.2 Hz), 5.61 (1H, ddt, J = 15.5, 8.5, 1.5 Hz), 5.44 (1H, qd, J = 6.4, 3.6 Hz), 4.77 (1H, t, J = 8.1 Hz), 4.07 (1H, dd, J = 7.8, 2.2 Hz), 3.83 (3H, s), 2.87 (1H, ddt, J = 14.4, 5.4, 2.8 Hz), 2.50 (3H, m), 2.59–2.42 (4H, overlapped), 1.46 (3H, d, J = 6.3 Hz), 1.35 (3H, s), 1.27 (3H, s). ^{13}C NMR (100 MHz, CDCl$_3$) δ 171.0 (C), 165.0 (C), 164.2 (C), 142.0 (C), 134.9 (C), 134.8 (C), 134.7 (CH), 132.5 (CH), 132.4 (CH), 129.6 (CH), 126.0 (CH), 124.2 (CH), 118.7 (CH), 117.4 (C), 117.1 (CH), 109.1 (CH), 107.4 (C), 104.5 (CH), 100.5 (CH), 80.2 (CH), 76.3 (CH), 71.4 (CH), 71.0 (CH), 55.6 (CH$_2$), 38.2 (CH$_3$), 35.2 (CH$_2$), 27.3 (CH$_3$), 26.8 (CH$_3$), 19.7 (CH$_3$). HRESIMS m/z 527.2077 [M + H]$^+$ (calcd for C$_{29}$H$_{32}$O$_8$F$^+$, 527.2076).

Compound **33**, White, solid; yield 67.7%; $[α]_D^{20}$ −24.4° (c 0.1, MeOH); ^{1}H NMR (400 MHz, CDCl$_3$) δ 9.35 (1H, dd, J = 2.2, 0.9 Hz), 8.85 (1H, dd, J = 4.9, 1.8 Hz), 8.43 (1H, dt, J = 7.9, 2.0 Hz), 7.46 (1H, ddd, J = 7.9, 4.9, 0.9 Hz), 7.08 (1H, dd, J = 15.5, 2.0 Hz), 6.85 (1H, d, J = 2.5 Hz), 6.70 (1H, d, J = 2.5 Hz), 5.98 (1H, dt, J = 15.7, 5.2 Hz), 5.85 (1H, ddd, J = 15.1, 10.8, 3.8 Hz), 5.48 (1H, ddt, J = 15.7, 8.9, 1.8 Hz), 5.35 (1H, m), 4.55 (1H, t, J = 8.4 Hz), 4.17 (1H, dt, J = 12.3, 3.5 Hz), 3.91–3.84 (4H, overlapped), 2.69 (1H, dtd, J = 14.0, 4.1, 2.3 Hz), 2.56 (1H, d, J = 1.5 Hz), 2.49 (2H, overlapped), 2.30 (1H, m), 1.42 (3H, s), 1.35 (3H, s), 1.31 (3H, d, J = 6.4 Hz). ^{13}C NMR (100 MHz, CDCl$_3$) δ 165.1 (C), 164.0 (C), 161.9 (C), 154.1 (C), 151.6 (CH), 151.1 (CH), 140.2 (C), 137.8 (CH), 132.8 (CH), 131.4 (CH), 130.5 (CH), 128.5 (C), 125.6 (CH), 123.7 (CH), 117.0 (C), 110.7 (C), 108.6 (CH), 108.0 (C), 81.2 (CH), 75.9 (CH), 69.8 (CH), 68.6 (CH), 55.8 (CH$_2$), 37.1 (CH$_3$), 36.2 (CH$_2$), 27.1 (CH$_3$ × 2), 20.1 (CH$_3$). HRESIMS m/z 510.2127 [M + H]$^+$ (calcd for C$_{28}$H$_{32}$O$_8$N$^+$, 510.2122).

Compound **34**, White, solid; yield 85.6%; $[α]_D^{20}$ −10.3° (c 0.05, MeOH); ^{1}H NMR (400 MHz, CDCl$_3$) δ 9.36 (1H, dd, J = 2.2, 0.9 Hz), 9.29 (1H, dd, J = 2.2, 0.9 Hz), 8.85 (1H, dd, J = 4.9, 1.8 Hz), 8.81 (1H, dd, J = 4.9, 1.8 Hz), 8.44 (1H, dt, J = 8.0, 2.0 Hz), 8.35 (1H, dt, J = 8.0, 2.0 Hz), 7.45 (2H, dddd, J = 16.4, 8.0, 4.9, 0.9 Hz), 7.17 (1H, dd, J = 15.5, 1.9 Hz), 6.88 (1H, d, J = 2.5 Hz), 6.73 (1H, d, J = 2.5 Hz), 6.07 (1H, dt, J = 15.7, 5.2 Hz), 5.96 (1H, ddd, J = 15.1, 10.7, 3.8 Hz), 5.70 (1H, ddd, J = 12.5, 4.7, 2.3 Hz), 5.55 (1H, ddt, J = 15.7, 8.7, 1.7 Hz), 5.39 (1H, td, J = 6.5, 4.4 Hz), 4.74 (1H, t, J = 8.2 Hz), 4.10 (1H, dd, J = 7.8, 2.3 Hz), 3.87 (3H, s), 2.80 (1H, dtd, J = 13.8, 4.3, 2.3 Hz), 2.59–2.45 (3H, overlapped), 1.33 (6H, overlapped), 1.22 (3H, s). ^{13}C NMR (100 MHz, CDCl$_3$) δ 165.1 (C), 164.6 (C), 164.0 (C), 162.0 (C), 154.2 (C), 153.8 (CH), 151.6 (CH), 151.2 (CH), 151.0 (CH), 139.7 (C), 137.9 (CH), 137.3 (CH), 133.5 (CH), 131.3 (CH), 130.6 (CH), 127.3 (C), 126.2 (C), 125.6 (CH), 123.7 (CH), 123.6 (CH), 117.0 (C), 110.7 (C), 109.3 (CH), 108.4 (CH), 79.7 (CH), 71.3 (CH), 69.9 (CH), 55.9 (CH), 37.2 (CH$_2$), 35.2 (CH$_3$), 27.2 (CH$_2$), 27.0 (CH$_3$ × 2), 20.2 (CH$_3$). HRESIMS m/z 615.2318 [M + H]$^+$ (calcd for C$_{34}$H$_{35}$O$_9$N$_2^+$, 615.2337).

Compound **35**, White, solid; yield 72.4%; $[α]_D^{20}$ −17.0° (c 0.1, MeOH); ^{1}H NMR (400 MHz, CDCl$_3$) δ 11.52 (1H, s), 9.29 (1H, m), 8.81 (1H, d, J = 4.0 Hz), 8.35 (1H, dt, J = 7.9, 1.9 Hz), 7.44 (1H, dd, J = 7.9, 4.8 Hz), 7.25 (1H, d, J = 15.4, 2.2Hz), 6.50 (1H, d, J = 2.6 Hz), 6.42 (1H, d, J = 2.6 Hz), 6.09 (1H, ddd, J = 15.3, 7.6, 5.5 Hz), 5.83 (1H, ddd, J = 15.4, 10.5, 3.1 Hz), 5.74 (1H, m), 4.77 (1H, t, J = 8.0 Hz), 4.11 (1H, dd, J = 7.7, 2.3 Hz), 3.83 (3H, s), 2.86 (1H, ddt, J = 14.4, 5.5, 2.9 Hz), 2.60–2.44 (3H, overlapped), 1.47 (3H, d, J = 6.3 Hz), 1.35 (3H, s), 1.23 (3H, s). ^{13}C NMR (100 MHz, CDCl$_3$) δ 170.9 (C), 165.0 (C), 164.6 (C), 164.2 (C), 153.8 (CH), 151.0 (CH), 141.8 (C), 137.3 (CH), 134.8 (CH), 132.6 (CH), 129.7 (CH), 125.6 (CH), 123.6 (CH), 109.3 (CH), 107.5 (C), 104.5 (C), 100.6 (CH), 80.2 (CH), 77.4 (CH), 76.4 (CH), 71.5 (CH),

70.9 (CH), 55.6 (CH$_2$), 38.1 (CH$_3$), 35.2 (CH$_2$), 27.2 (CH$_3$), 27.0 (CH$_3$), 19.6 (CH$_3$). HRESIMS m/z 510.2126 [M + H]$^+$ (calcd for C$_{28}$H$_{32}$O$_8$N$^+$, 510.2122).

Compound **36**, White, solid; yield 63.7%; $[\alpha]_D^{20}$ –24.6° (c 0.1, MeOH); ^{1}H NMR (400 MHz, CDCl$_3$) δ 7.05 (1H, dd, J = 15.6, 2.1 Hz), 6.79 (1H, d, J = 2.5 Hz), 6.55 (1H, d, J = 2.5 Hz), 5.99 (1H, dt, J = 15.7, 5.3 Hz), 5.81 (1H, ddd, J = 15.5, 10.8, 3.8 Hz), 5.56–5.34 (2H, overlapped), 4.55 (1H, t, J = 8.4 Hz), 4.16 (1H, ddd, J = 12.3, 4.5, 2.4 Hz), 3.93–3.79 (4H, overlapped), 2.67 (1H, dtd, J = 14.0, 4.1, 2.3 Hz), 2.57–2.44 (3H, overlapped), 2.29 (4H, s), 1.39 (9H, m). ^{13}C NMR (100 MHz, CDCl$_3$) δ 169.7 (C), 165.2 (C), 161.8 (C), 151.4 (C), 140.0 (C), 132.9 (CH), 131.3 (CH), 130.7 (CH), 128.2 (CH), 117.0 (C), 110.4 (C), 108.6 (CH), 108.0 (CH), 81.2 (CH), 75.9 (CH), 69.7 (CH), 68.7 (CH), 55.7 (CH$_2$), 37.2 (CH$_3$), 36.1 (CH$_2$), 27.1 (CH$_3$ × 2), 21.1 (CH$_3$), 20.0 (CH$_3$). HRESIMS m/z 447.2011 [M + H]$^+$ (calcd for C$_{24}$H$_{31}$O$_8^+$, 447.2013).

Compound **37**, White, solid; yield 85.2%; $[\alpha]_D^{20}$ –28.3° (c 0.1, MeOH); ^{1}H NMR (400 MHz, CDCl$_3$) δ 7.97 (1H, dd, J = 3.8, 1.3 Hz), 7.66 (1H, dd, J = 5.0, 1.3 Hz), 7.17 (1H, dd, J = 5.0, 3.8 Hz), 7.06 (1H, dd, J = 15.5, 2.0 Hz), 6.82 (1H, d, J = 2.5 Hz), 6.71 (1H, d, J = 2.5 Hz), 5.98 (1H, dt, J = 15.7, 5.1 Hz), 5.84 (1H, ddd, J = 15.2, 10.8, 3.9 Hz), 5.55–5.36 (2H, overlapped), 4.54 (1H, t, J = 8.5 Hz), 4.15 (1H, ddd, J = 12.2, 4.3, 2.3 Hz), 3.88 (1H, dd, J = 8.0, 2.3 Hz), 3.84 (3H, s), 2.67 (1H, dtd, J = 13.9, 4.1, 2.2 Hz), 2.49 (3H, overlapped), 2.29 (1H, ddd, J = 14.1, 12.0, 10.6 Hz), 1.42 (3H, s), 1.40–1.30 (6H, overlapped). ^{13}C NMR (100 MHz, CDCl$_3$) δ 165.2 (C), 161.7 (C), 160.4 (C), 150.8 (C), 139.8 (C), 135.1 (C), 133.8 (CH), 132.9 (CH), 132.6 (CH), 131.5 (CH), 130.3 (CH), 128.4 (CH), 128.2 (CH), 117.4 (C), 110.6 (C), 108.6 (CH), 108.0 (CH), 81.2 (CH), 69.6 (CH), 68.6 (CH), 55.8 (CH), 37.2 (CH$_2$), 36.1 (CH$_3$), 29.8 (CH$_2$), 27.1 (CH$_3$), 27.1 (CH$_3$), 20.2 (CH$_3$). HRESIMS m/z 515.1730 [M + H]$^+$ (calcd for C$_{27}$H$_{31}$O$_8$S$^+$, 515.1734).

Compound **38**, White, solid; yield 87.7%; $[\alpha]_D^{20}$ –26.7° (c 0.1, MeOH); ^{1}H NMR (400 MHz, CDCl$_3$) δ 7.98 (1H, dd, J = 3.8, 1.3 Hz), 7.86 (1H, dd, J = 3.8, 1.3 Hz), 7.66 (1H, dd, J = 5.0, 1.3 Hz), 7.58 (1H, dd, J = 5.0, 1.3 Hz), 7.17 (1H, dd, J = 5.0, 3.8 Hz), 7.12 (2H, m), 6.83 (1H, d, J = 2.5 Hz), 6.72 (1H, d, J = 2.5 Hz), 6.06 (1H, dt, J = 15.8, 5.0 Hz), 5.93 (1H, ddd, J = 15.1, 10.7, 3.9 Hz), 5.63–5.51 (2H, overlapped), 5.44 (1H, td, J = 6.5, 4.7 Hz), 4.72 (1H, t, J = 8.2 Hz), 4.05 (1H, dd, J = 7.9, 2.3 Hz), 3.85 (3H, s), 2.78 (1H, dtd, J = 13.6, 4.3, 2.2 Hz), 2.55–2.41 (3H, overlapped), 1.34 (6H, overlapped), 1.27 (3H, s). ^{13}C NMR (100 MHz, CDCl$_3$) δ 165.1 (C), 161.8 (C), 161.5 (C), 160.4 (C), 150.9 (C), 139.5 (C), 135.1 (C), 133.9 (C), 133.7 (CH×2), 133.4 (CH), 132.7 (CH), 132.6 (CH), 131.4 (CH), 130.3 (CH), 128.2 (CH), 128.0 (CH), 127.5 (CH), 117.4 (C), 110.5 (C), 109.2 (CH), 108.3 (CH), 79.8 (CH), 71.0 (CH), 69.7 (CH), 55.8 (CH), 37.3 (CH$_2$), 35.2 (CH$_3$), 27.3 (CH$_2$), 27.0 (CH$_3$ × 2), 20.3 (CH$_3$). HRESIMS m/z 625.1545 [M + H]$^+$ (calcd for C$_{32}$H$_{33}$O$_9$S$_2^+$, 625.1561).

3.5. Antimicrobial Activity

The methods described by Fromtling et al. were used to evaluate the derivatives' antibacterial activity [34]. Isoniazid and rifampicin were used as a positive control anti-*M. marinum*, ciprofloxacin as a positive control anti-bacteria, and amphotericin B as a positive control anti-fungi. The strains were cultured in the corresponding medium at 32 °C for 8 h and diluted to 10^5 CFU/mL using 96-well plates with 2 μL of sample and 198 μL of bacterial solution. Incubation was carried out at 32 °C for 24 h or 48 h, and DMSO was used as a negative control.

3.6. Time–Growth Curve Assay

The time–growth curve was determined using the method of Li et al. [35]. Initially, the concentration of *M. marinum* was set at 10^5 CFU/mL, and 5 groups were chosen, each group tested on 6 times. The drug concentration of the dosing group was set at 640, 320, 160 and 80 μM. An equal amount of DMSO was added to the blank group, and the suspension of *M. marinum* was incubated at 32 °C (100 rpm) by oscillating it. The colony count was determined and counted using the OD600 at the planned time points (0, 3, 6, 12, 18, 24, 36, 48 and 60 h).

3.7. In Vitro Synergic Anti-M. marinum Activity Assay

An in vitro synergistic antibacterial assay was performed as described by Li et al., and synergistic activity was evaluated on 96-well plates [33]. Based on the MIC_{90} data of the compound and each positive drug as the design basis, the chessboard dilution method was used to combine $4 \times MIC_{90}$, $2 \times MIC_{90}$, MIC_{90}, $1/2 \times MIC_{90}$, $1/4 \times MIC_{90}$, $1/8 \times MIC_{90}$ and $1/16 \times MIC_{90}$ in the 96-well plate with bacterial solution added. The measurements were repeated three times per well. The 96-well plates were placed in a constant-temperature incubator at 32 °C, the results were observed and recorded 48 h later, and an optical density of 600 nm (OD600) was measured.

3.8. Statistical Analysis

All statistical analyses were performed using GraphPad Prism 8.3 software. Data are presented as the mean of three experiments. For two-group comparison, the *p* value was derived from a one-way Student *t* test to determine the difference between groups with normally distributed data. For all comparisons, $p < 0.05$ was considered statistically significant. * $p < 0.05$, ** $p < 0.01$, *** $p < 0.001$ and **** $p < 0.0001$.

4. Conclusions

In summary, 16 new derivatives were successfully synthesized through two to three steps, which enriched the diversity of 14-membered RALs. Through the activity evaluation of the derivative library, four derivatives showed promising anti-*M. marinum* activity. The preliminary structure–activity relationships showed that the anti-*M. marinum* activity of 14-membered RALs can be significantly improved via the introduction of a chlorine atom at the C-5 position. The substitution of positions 5'6' of dihydroxy with an acetonide group reduced the activity. The etherification modification of the phenolic hydroxy group did not significantly improve the activity. Further studies showed that compound **12** enhanced the effects of positive drugs isoniazid and rifampicin on *M. marinum*. These results suggest that **12** is an active compound capable of enhancing the potency of existing positive drugs, and its effective properties make it a very useful lead for future drug development in combating TB resistance.

Supplementary Materials: The following supporting information can be downloaded at https://www.mdpi.com/article/10.3390/md22030135/s1; Table S1: All compounds that not appear in the text in the derivative library. Table S2: Anhydride, acyl chloride or carboxylic acid reagents used to generate compounds **24–38**. Figures S1–S48: ^{1}H NMR, ^{13}C NMR and HRESIMS of compounds **19** and **24–38**.

Author Contributions: Q.-Q.J. contributed to preparation of all compounds; writing—original draft; writing—review and editing. J.-N.Y. contributed to related work on bioactivity; writing—original draft; writing—review and editing, Y.-J.C., Q.Z., X.-Z.C. and W.-F.X. contributed to providing the compounds and their derivatives. C.-L.S. and M.-Y.W. were the project leaders, organizing and guiding the experiments and manuscript writing. All authors have read and agreed to the published version of the manuscript.

Funding: This work was supported by the Special Funds of Shandong Province for Qingdao National Laboratory of Marine Science and Technology (No. 2022QNLM030003), the State Key Laboratory for Chemistry and Molecular Engineering of Medicinal Resources, Guangxi Normal University (No. CMEMR2023-B16), Shandong Province Special Fund "Frontier Technology and Free Exploration" from Laoshan Laboratory (No. 8-01), the National Key Research and Development Program of China (No. 2022YFC2601305) and the Innovation Center for Academicians of Hainan Province.

Institutional Review Board Statement: Not applicable.

Data Availability Statement: The data are contained within the article or Supplementary Materials.

Acknowledgments: We thank Syngenta for the fellowship to Qun Zhang. We also thank Xiu-Li Zhang and Cong Wang at the School of Medicine and Pharmacy, Ocean University of China, for the NMR test.

Conflicts of Interest: The authors declare no conflicts of interest.

References

1. Daniel, T.M. The History of Tuberculosis. *Respir. Med.* **2006**, *100*, 1862–1870. [CrossRef]
2. Public Health Online. Available online: https://www.publichealthonline.org/worst-global-pandemics-in-history (accessed on 13 October 2021).
3. Global Tuberculosis Report 2023. World Health Organization: Geneva, Switzerland, 2023. Licence: CC BY-NC-SA 3.0 IGOnization. Available online: https://www.who.int/publications/i/item/9789240083851 (accessed on 7 November 2023).
4. Bloom, B.R. A half-century of research on tuberculosis: Successes and challenges. *J. Exp. Med.* **2023**, *220*, e20230859. [CrossRef] [PubMed]
5. Maitre, T.; Aubry, A.; Jarlier, V.; Robert, J.; Veziris, N.; Bernard, C.; Sougakoff, W.; Brossier, F.; Cambau, E.; Mougari, F.; et al. Multidrug and Extensively Drug-Resistant Tuberculosis. *Med. Mal. Infect.* **2017**, *47*, 3–10. [CrossRef] [PubMed]
6. Lange, C.; Dheda, K.; Chesov, D.; Mandalakas, A.M.; Udwadia, Z.; Horsburgh, C.R., Jr. Management of drug-resistant tuberculosis. *Lancet* **2019**, *394*, 953–966. [CrossRef] [PubMed]
7. Elsevier. Patient safety: Too little, but not too late. *Lancet* **2019**, *394*, 895. [CrossRef]
8. Kakkar, A.K.; Dahiya, N. Bedaquiline for the treatment of resistant tuberculosis: Promises and pitfalls. *Tuberculosis* **2014**, *94*, 357–362. [CrossRef] [PubMed]
9. Ryan, N.J.; Lo, J.H. Delamanid: First global approval. *Drugs* **2014**, *74*, 1041–1045. [CrossRef]
10. Keam, S.J. Pretomanid: First Approval. *Drugs* **2019**, *79*, 1797–1803. [CrossRef]
11. Xu, Y.; Wang, G.Z.; Xu, M. Biohazard levels and biosafety protection for *Mycobacterium tuberculosis* strains with different virulence. *Biosaf. Health* **2020**, *2*, 135–141. [CrossRef]
12. van Soolingen, D.; Wisselink, H.J.; Lumb, R.; Anthony, R.; van der Zanden, A.; Gilpin, C. Practical biosafety in the tuberculosis laboratory: Containment at the source is what truly counts. *Int. J. Tuberc. Lung Dis.* **2014**, *18*, 885–889. [CrossRef]
13. Lambrecht, R.S.; Carriere, J.F.; Collins, M.T. A model for analyzing growth kinetics of a slowly growing *Mycobacterium* sp. *Appl. Environ. Microbiol.* **1988**, *54*, 910–916. [CrossRef]
14. Gao, L.Y.; Groger, R.; Cox, J.S.; Beverley, S.M.; Lawson, E.H.; Brown, E.J. Transposon mutagenesis of *Mycobacterium marinum* identifies a locus linking pigmentation and intracellular survival. *Infect. Immun.* **2003**, *71*, 922–929. [CrossRef]
15. Cronin, R.M.; Ferrell, M.J.; Cahir, C.W.; Champion, M.M.; Champion, P.A. Proteo-genetic analysis reveals clear hierarchy of ESX-1 secretion in *Mycobacterium marinum*. *Proc. Natl. Acad. Sci. USA* **2022**, *119*, e2123100119. [CrossRef] [PubMed]
16. Van Seymortier, P.; Verellen, K.; De Jonge, I. *Mycobacterium marinum* causing tenosynovitis. 'Fish tank finger'. *Acta. Orthop. Belg.* **2004**, *70*, 279–282. [PubMed]
17. Stinear, T.P.; Seemann, T.; Harrison, P.F.; Jenkin, G.A.; Davies, J.K.; Johnson, P.D.; Abdellah, Z.; Arrowsmith, C.; Chillingworth, T.; Churcher, C.; et al. Insights from the complete genome sequence of *Mycobacterium marinum* on the evolution of *Mycobacterium tuberculosis*. *Genome Res.* **2008**, *18*, 729–741. [CrossRef] [PubMed]
18. Habjan, E.; Ho, V.Q.T.; Gallant, J.; van Stempvoort, G.; Jim, K.K.; Kuijl, C.; Geerke, D.P.; Bitter, W.; Speer, A. An anti-tuberculosis compound screen using a zebrafish infection model identifies an aspartyl-tRNA synthetase inhibitor. *Dis. Model. Mech.* **2021**, *14*, dmm049145. [CrossRef] [PubMed]
19. Newman, D.J.; Cragg, G.M. Natural Products as Sources of New Drugs over the Nearly Four Decades from 01/1981 to 09/2019. *J. Nat. Prod.* **2020**, *83*, 770–803. [CrossRef] [PubMed]
20. Hai, Y.; Cai, Z.M.; Li, P.J.; Wei, M.Y.; Wang, C.Y.; Gu, Y.C.; Shao, C.L. Trends of antimalarial marine natural products: Progresses, challenges and opportunities. *Nat. Prod. Rep.* **2022**, *39*, 969–990. [CrossRef] [PubMed]
21. Carroll, A.R.; Copp, B.R.; Davis, R.A.; Keyzers, R.A.; Prinsep, M.R. Marine natural products. *Nat. Prod. Rep.* **2022**, *39*, 1122–1171. [CrossRef] [PubMed]
22. Han, J.; Liu, X.; Zhang, L.; Quinn, R.J.; Feng, Y. Anti-mycobacterial natural products and mechanisms of action. *Nat. Prod. Rep.* **2022**, *39*, 77–89. [CrossRef]
23. Shao, C.L.; Wu, H.X.; Wang, C.Y.; Liu, Q.A.; Xu, Y.; Wei, M.Y.; Qian, P.Y.; Gu, Y.C.; Zheng, C.J.; She, Z.G.; et al. Potent antifouling resorcylic acid lactones from the gorgonian-derived fungus *Cochliobolus lunatus*. *J. Nat. Prod.* **2011**, *74*, 629–633. [CrossRef] [PubMed]
24. Jana, N.; Nanda, S. Resorcylic acid lactones (RALs) and their structural congeners: Recent advances in their biosynthesis, chemical synthesis and biology. *New J. Chem.* **2018**, *42*, 17803–17873. [CrossRef]
25. Liu, Q.A.; Shao, C.L.; Gu, Y.C.; Blum, M.; Gan, L.S.; Wang, K.L.; Chen, M.; Wang, C.Y. Antifouling and Fungicidal Resorcylic Acid Lactones from the Sea Anemone-Derived Fungus *Cochliobolus lunatus*. *J. Agric. Food. Chem.* **2014**, *62*, 3183–3191. [CrossRef]
26. Xu, W.F.; Xue, X.J.; Qi, Y.X.; Wu, N.N.; Wang, C.Y.; Shao, C.L. Cochliomycin G, a 14-membered resorcylic acid lactone from a marine-derived fungus *Cochliobolus lunatus*. *Nat. Prod. Res.* **2021**, *35*, 490–493. [CrossRef] [PubMed]
27. Zhang, W.; Shao, C.L.; Chen, M.; Liu, Q.A.; Wang, C.Y. Brominated resorcylic acid lactones from the marine-derived fungus *Cochliobolus lunatus* induced by histone deacetylase inhibitors. *Tetrahedron Lett.* **2014**, *55*, 4888–4891. [CrossRef]
28. Wang, K.L.; Zhang, G.; Sun, J.; Xu, Y.; Han, Z.; Liu, L.L.; Shao, C.L.; Liu, Q.A.; Wang, C.Y.; Qian, P.Y. Cochliomycin A inhibits the larval settlement of *Amphibalanus amphitrite* by activating the NO/cGMP pathway. *Biofouling* **2016**, *32*, 35–44. [CrossRef]

29. Zhang, X.Q.; Spadafora, C.; Pineda, L.M.; Ng, M.G.; Sun, J.H.; Wang, W.; Wang, C.Y.; Gu, Y.C.; Shao, C.L. Discovery, Semisynthesis, Antiparasitic and Cytotoxic Evaluation of 14-Membered Resorcylic Acid Lactones and Their Derivatives. *Sci. Rep.* **2017**, *7*, 11822. [CrossRef]
30. Xu, W.F.; Wu, N.N.; Wu, Y.W.; Qi, Y.X.; Wei, M.Y.; Pineda, L.M.; Ng, M.G.; Spadafora, C.; Zheng, J.Y.; Lu, L.; et al. Structure modification, antialgal, antiplasmodial, and toxic evaluations of a series of new marine-derived 14-membered resorcylic acid lactone derivatives. *Mar. Life Sci. Technol.* **2022**, *4*, 88–97. [CrossRef]
31. Koul, A.; Arnoult, E.; Lounis, N.; Guillemont, J.; Andries, K. The challenge of new drug discovery for tuberculosis. *Nature* **2011**, *469*, 483–490. [CrossRef]
32. Smith, T.C., 2nd; Aldridge, B.B. Targeting drugs for tuberculosis. *Science* **2019**, *364*, 1234–1235. [CrossRef]
33. Li, Z.; Huang, Y.; Tu, J.; Yang, W.; Liu, N.; Wang, W.; Sheng, C. Discovery of BRD4-HDAC Dual Inhibitors with Improved Fungal Selectivity and Potent Synergistic Antifungal Activity against Fluconazole-Resistant *Candida albicans*. *J. Med. Chem.* **2023**, *66*, 5950–5964. [CrossRef] [PubMed]
34. Fromtling, R.A.; Galgiani, J.N.; Pfaller, M.A.; Espinel-Ingroff, A.; Bartizal, K.F.; Bartlett, M.S.; Body, B.A.; Frey, C.; Hall, G.; Roberts, G.D. Multicenter evaluation of a broth macrodilution antifungal susceptibility test for yeasts. *Antimicrob. Agents Chemother.* **1993**, *37*, 39–45. [CrossRef] [PubMed]
35. Li, Z.; Liu, N.; Tu, J.; Ji, C.; Han, G.; Sheng, C. Discovery of simplified sampangine derivatives with potent antifungal activities against cryptococcal meningitis. *ACS Infect. Dis.* **2019**, *5*, 1376–1384. [CrossRef] [PubMed]

Disclaimer/Publisher's Note: The statements, opinions and data contained in all publications are solely those of the individual author(s) and contributor(s) and not of MDPI and/or the editor(s). MDPI and/or the editor(s) disclaim responsibility for any injury to people or property resulting from any ideas, methods, instructions or products referred to in the content.

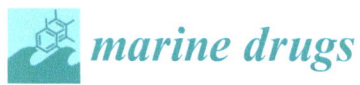 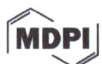

Article

Avellanin A Has an Antiproliferative Effect on TP-Induced RWPE-1 Cells via the PI3K-Akt Signalling Pathway

Chang Xu [1], Guangping Cao [1,2], Hong Zhang [1], Meng Bai [1,2,*], Xiangxi Yi [1,2,*] and Xinjian Qu [1,2,*]

1. Faculty of Pharmacy/Institute of Marine Drugs, Guangxi University of Chinese Medicine, Nanning 530200, China; xuchang2022@stu.gxtcmu.edu.cn (C.X.); cao15765981927@163.com (G.C.); zhanghong2023@stu.gxtcmu.edu.cn (H.Z.)
2. Guangxi Key Laboratory of Marine Drugs, Guangxi University of Chinese Medicine, Nanning 530200, China
* Correspondence: xxbai2014@163.com (M.B.); yixiangxi2017@163.com (X.Y.); quxj2022@gxtcmu.edu.cn (X.Q.)

Abstract: Cyclic pentapeptide compounds have garnered much attention as a drug discovery resource. This study focused on the characterization and anti-benign prostatic hyperplasia (BPH) properties of avellanin A from *Aspergillus fumigatus* fungus in marine sediment samples collected in the Beibu Gulf of Guangxi Province in China. The antiproliferative effect and molecular mechanism of avellanin A were explored in testosterone propionate (TP)-induced RWPE-1 cells. The transcriptome results showed that avellanin A significantly blocked the ECM–receptor interaction and suppressed the downstream PI3K-Akt signalling pathway. Molecular docking revealed that avellanin A has a good affinity for the cathepsin L protein, which is involved in the terminal degradation of extracellular matrix components. Subsequently, qRT-PCR analysis revealed that the expression of the genes *COL1A1*, *COL1A2*, *COL5A2*, *COL6A3*, *MMP2*, *MMP9*, *ITGA2*, and *ITGB3* was significantly downregulated after avellanin A intervention. The Western blot results also confirmed that it not only reduced ITGB3 and FAK/p-FAK protein expression but also inhibited PI3K/p-PI3K and Akt/p-Akt protein expression in the PI3K-Akt signalling pathway. Furthermore, avellanin A downregulated Cyclin D1 protein expression and upregulated Bax, p21$^{WAF1/Cip1}$, and p53 proapoptotic protein expression in TP-induced RWPE-1 cells, leading to cell cycle arrest and inhibition of cell proliferation. The results of this study support the use of avellanin A as a potential new drug for the treatment of BPH.

Keywords: marine organisms; *Aspergillus fumigatus*; benign prostatic hyperplasia; avellanin A

Citation: Xu, C.; Cao, G.; Zhang, H.; Bai, M.; Yi, X.; Qu, X. Avellanin A Has an Antiproliferative Effect on TP-Induced RWPE-1 Cells via the PI3K-Akt Signalling Pathway. *Mar. Drugs* 2024, 22, 275. https://doi.org/10.3390/md22060275

Academic Editor: Chang-Lun Shao

Received: 15 May 2024
Revised: 10 June 2024
Accepted: 10 June 2024
Published: 13 June 2024

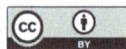

Copyright: © 2024 by the authors. Licensee MDPI, Basel, Switzerland. This article is an open access article distributed under the terms and conditions of the Creative Commons Attribution (CC BY) license (https://creativecommons.org/licenses/by/4.0/).

1. Introduction

Benign prostatic hyperplasia (BPH), which refers to the prostate transition zone and periurethral hyperplasia of epithelial and fibromuscular tissue growth, is one of the most common urological diseases in middle-aged and older men worldwide, and its incidence gradually increases with age [1]. At present, BPH is mainly treated with drugs such as 5α-reductase inhibitors and α blockers. Although both antagonists are effective in the treatment of BPH, these drugs have many adverse side effects, such as abnormal ejaculation, erectile dysfunction, and gynaecomastia [2]. Therefore, to more effectively prevent and treat BPH, improve the quality of life of patients, and reduce the adverse reactions caused by drugs, finding new targets and developing effective drug candidates with fewer adverse reactions are hot research directions [3].

The growth of marine microorganisms in a special environment produces a variety of secondary metabolites with special chemical structures [4]. Many secondary metabolites have a variety of pharmacological effects, such as antibacterial, anti-inflammatory, anti-tumour, or antiviral effects, so they have received extensive attention and application [5–7]. As a result, marine microbial secondary metabolites have become a very promising source of drug candidates [8]. Mangrove plants mainly grow in tropical and subtropical intertidal zones and are an important part of coastal wetland ecosystems, which are of great significance in terms of their ecological and economic value [9]. As endophytic fungi in mangrove plants have become a new hotspot for drug research and development, in recent years, many scientific research groups around the world have carried out research on the secondary metabolites of mangrove endophytic fungi and obtained a series of compounds with novel biological activities such as anti-inflammatory, anti-tumour, antibacterial, or antiviral effects [10].

Naturally occurring cyclic peptides have garnered much attention as a drug discovery resource [11,12]. This is because cyclic peptides are composed of amino acid residues, including nonproteinogenic residues, which are arranged in a three-dimensional structure and have high affinity for their target biomolecules [12]. In addition, cyclic peptides are reported to be more stable and membrane-permeable than general linear peptides [13].

Avellanin A ($C_{31}H_{39}N_5O_5$, m/z: 561.2951) is a cyclic pentapeptide compound, which was first found in *Hamigers avellanea* [14]. We report here the re-isolation of this compound from *Aspergillus fumigatus* fungus in marine sediment samples collected in the Beibu Gulf of Guangxi Province in China. Avellanin A was obtained as a white powder, and HRESIMS analysis gave a pseudomolecular ion $[M + H]^+$ at m/z 562.3024, corresponding to the molecular formula of $C_{31}H_{39}N_5O_5$ (Δ −0.05 mmu for $C_{31}H_{40}N_5O_5$; Figure S1). To date, the biological activity associated with avellanin A has only inhibited apoB in HepG2 cells without exhibiting cytotoxicity, and other biological activities need to be further explored [15]. Avellanin A is a cyclic pentapeptide compound linked in the order Ant-L-Pro-D-Ala- N-Me-D-Phe-L-Ile (Figures 1, S2 and S3 and Table S1). The present study was designed to further explore the antiproliferative effects of avellanin A on RWPE-1 cells, ultimately revealing that this novel candidate therapeutic agent may inhibit PI3K-Akt pathway activity, suggesting that it may be useful as a new option for treating BPH patients.

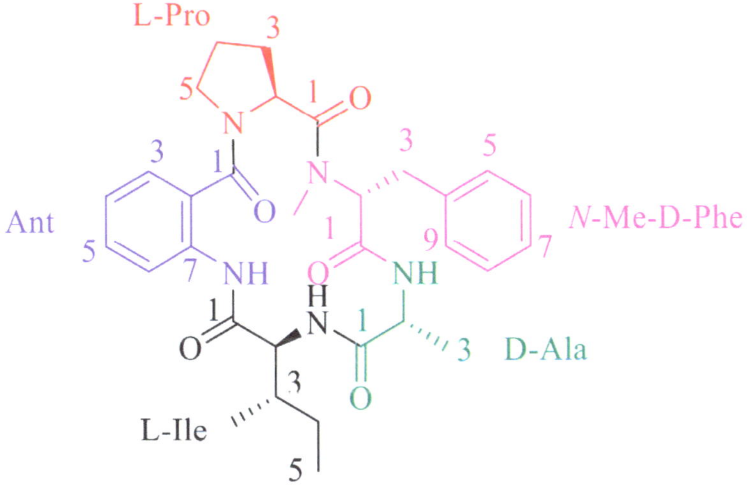

Figure 1. Avellanin A structure.

2. Results

2.1. Antiproliferative Efficacy of Avellanin A on RWPE-1 Cells

Initially, the antiproliferative efficacy of avellanin A was investigated by treating it with testosterone propionate (TP)-induced RWPE-1 cells and performing a CCK-8 analysis.

This approach revealed that avellanin A strongly inhibited RWPE-1 cell proliferation after treatment for 48 h in a dose-dependent manner. The avellanin A IC_{50} values for the RWPE-1 cell lines were calculated to be 0.72 µM (Figure 2A).

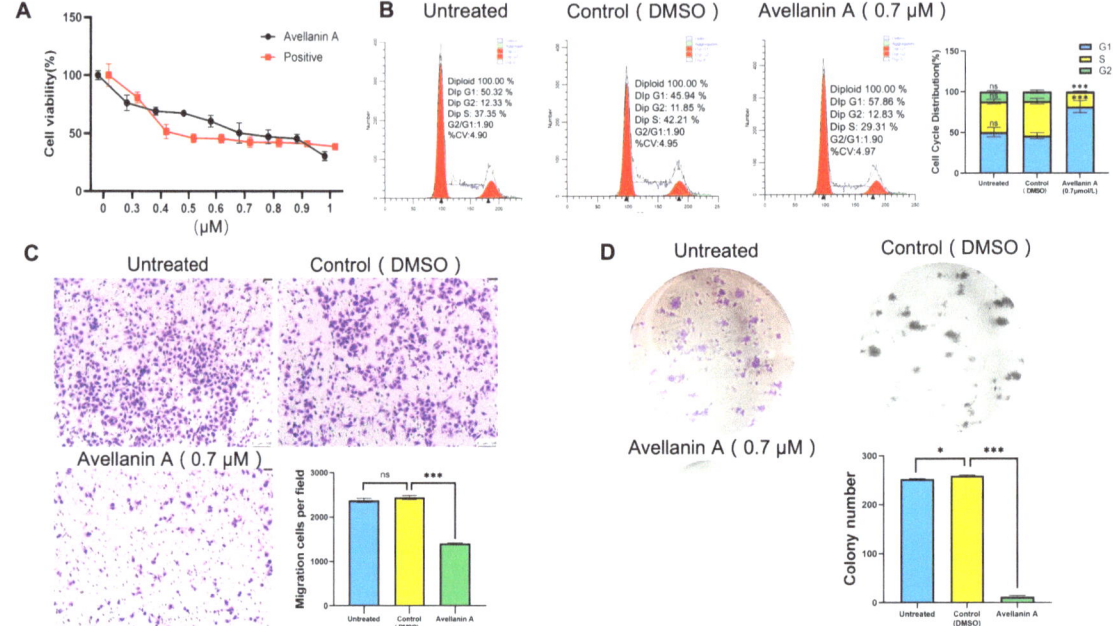

Figure 2. Antiproliferative efficacy of compound avellanin A on RWPE-1 cells: (**A**) RWPE-1 cells were treated with the indicated concentrations of compound avellanin A for 48 h, and the cell viability was determined by a CCK-8 assay. (**B**) The RWPE-1 cells were treated with indicated concentrations of compound avellanin A for 48 h, and the cell cycle distribution was assessed by flow cytometric analysis; ns, not significant, *** $p < 0.001$, compared to the control group. (**C**) Transwell assay evaluating the migration abilities of RWPE-1 cells treated with the indicated concentrations of compound avellanin A for 7 days. ns, not significant, *** $p < 0.001$, compared to the control group. (**D**) RWPE-1 cells were treated with the indicated concentrations of compound avellanin A for 7 days, after which colony formation was assessed; * $p < 0.05$ and *** $p < 0.001$, compared to the control group.

The proliferation of normal cells is dependent on the cell growth cycle. To detect the impact of avellanin A on the cell cycle, the RWPE-1 cells were treated with avellanin A (0.7 µM) for 48 h. This process clearly showed that most of the RWPE-1 cells treated with avellanin A were arrested in the G1 phase, which inhibited the cell cycle progression (Figure 2B). Furthermore, Transwell assays were used to examine the effect of the drugs on cell migration ability. Compared with the control group, the number of transmembrane cells in RWPE-1 cells treated with avellanin A was significantly reduced, which confirmed that avellanin A significantly inhibited RWPE-1 cell migration (Figure 2C). In addition, the observations of colony formation assays demonstrated that avellanin A had the most potent inhibitory effect on RWPE-1 cell growth in a concentration-dependent manner (Figure 2D).

2.2. Transcriptome Analysis of RWPE-1 Cells Treated with Avellanin A

To investigate the mechanism of action of compound avellanin A on RWPE-1 cells, we conducted RNA-seq. After RWPE-1 cells were treated with the compound avellanin A at a concentration of 0.7 µM for 48 h, transcriptome analysis revealed that the heatmap showed a clear trend in the clustering of genes expressed in RWPE-1 cells between the compound avellanin A group and the control group (Figure 3A). A total of 1183 differentially expressed genes (DEGs) were identified, 633 of which were significantly upregulated and 550 of which were significantly downregulated.

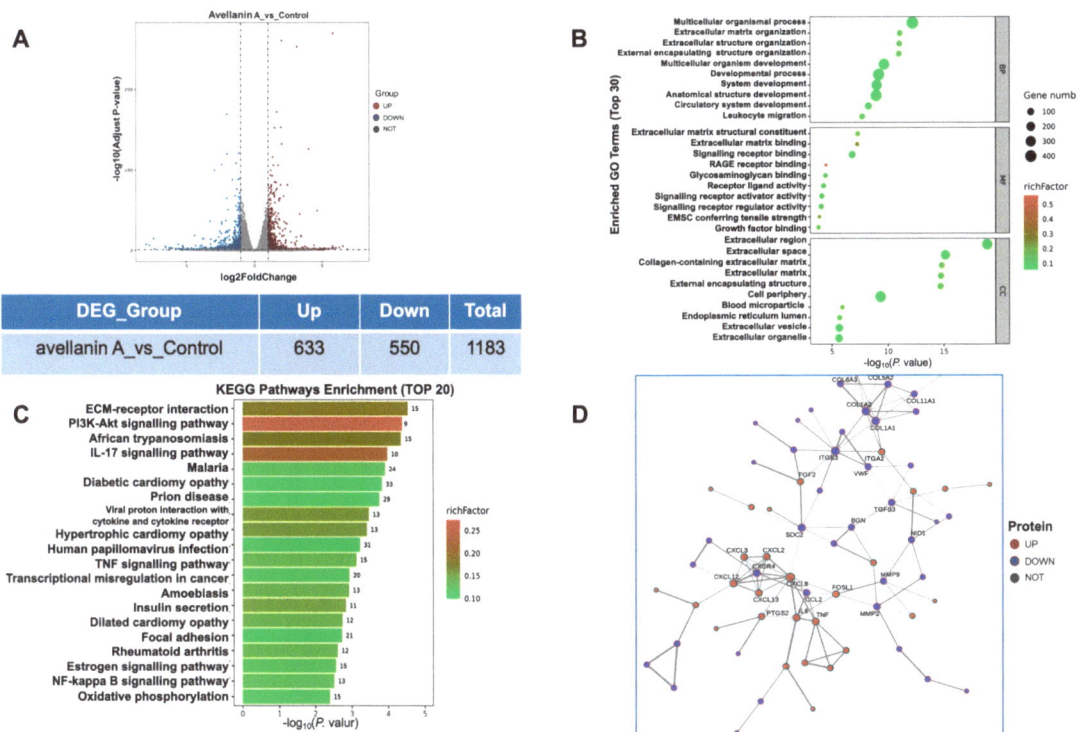

Figure 3. Transcriptome analysis of RWPE-1 cells treated with compound avellanin A vs. the control: (**A**) Volcanic map showing the differential gene expression distribution. The scattered dots in the figure represent individual genes, with grey dots indicating genes with no significant differences, red dots representing upregulated genes with significant differences, and blue dots representing downregulated genes with significant differences. Statistics of differentially expressed genes. A total of 1183 differentially expressed genes were identified, including 633 upregulated genes and 550 downregulated genes. (**B**) GO functional enrichment analysis of the DEGs. (**C**) KEGG pathway enrichment of differentially expressed genes. (**D**) PPI network construction for the identification of hub genes.

Gene Ontology (GO) is a standardised functional classification system that describes the properties of genes and gene products in organisms in three aspects: biogenesis-involved biological process (BP), molecular function (MF), and cellular component (CC). The results of GO analysis can visually show the overall functional enrichment characteristics of all differentially expressed genes, and these significantly enriched genes are related to core biological functions. The enrichment of GO results indicated that avellanin A had a significant effect on cellular components (Figure 3B), including the extracellular space, collagen-containing extracellular matrix, extracellular matrix, and external encapsulating structure.

Moreover, KEGG pathway analysis was conducted to identify the pathways involved. The enrichment results for the differentially expressed genes related to metabolic pathways indicated that the compound avellanin A had a significant effect on cellular life processes, substance transport, and metabolic pathways (Figure 3C). The analysis revealed that the differentially expressed genes were primarily enriched in several pathways, notably ECM–receptor interaction, the PI3K-Akt signalling pathway, the IL-17 signalling pathway, malaria, and diabetic cardiomyopathy. Through KEGG analysis, the top 20 pathways were identified, among which many of the enriched genes were associated with the ECM-related signalling pathway (Figure 3D).

Subsequently, PPI network analysis (Figure 3D) revealed that avellanin A significantly affected the expression of genes associated with the extracellular matrix (ECM), such as genes in the collagen subfamily (*COL1A1, COL1A2, COL5A2, COL6A3*), integrin subfamily (*ITGB3, ITGA2*), and MMP subfamily (*MMP2, MMP9*), as well as genes encoding FGF2 and VWF, which were significantly downregulated after avellanin A intervention. Therefore, bioinformatics results from transcriptome sequencing suggest that avellanin A may inhibit the expression of extracellular matrix integrins, collagen, and matrix metalloproteinases, thereby inhibiting the expression of the downstream PI3K-Akt signalling pathway and thereby inhibiting the progression of TP-induced BPH.

2.3. Interaction of Avellanin A with the Cathepsin L

To evaluate the affinity of avellanin A for its targets, we performed molecular docking analysis. According to the docking results with the cathepsin L, avellanin A interacts with the basic amino acids Gly68 and Asp162 of the cathepsin L protein through hydrogen bonding and has a low binding energy of −6.2 kcal/mol, indicating highly stable binding (Figure 4A).

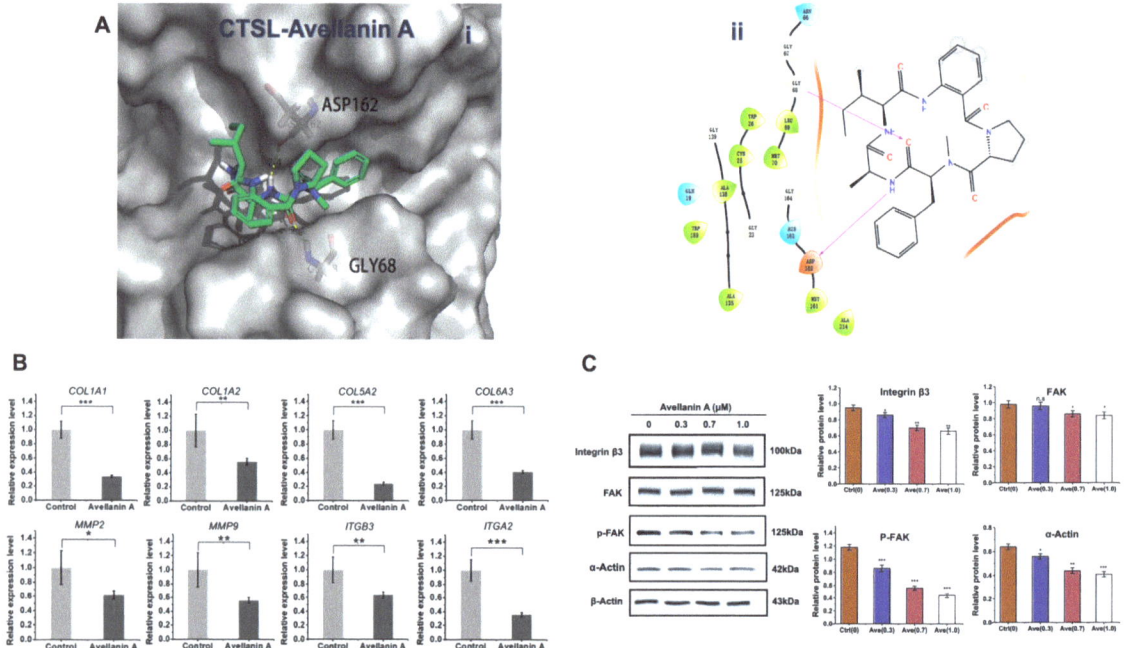

Figure 4. The binding mode of avellanin A to its targets, determined by molecular docking: (**A**) Binding mode of avellanin A to cathepsin L: (**i**) three-dimensional structures of the binding pockets were constructed with PyMOL 3.0 software; (**ii**) 2D interactions of compounds and their targets. (**B**) Relative mRNA expression of *COL1A1, COL1A2, COL5A2, COL6A3, MMP2, MMP9, ITGA2,* and *ITGB3*; * $p < 0.05$, ** $p < 0.01$, and *** $p < 0.001$, compared to the control group. (**C**) The expression of ITGB3, FAK/p-FAK, and α-Actin was analysed by Western blotting. The analysis utilized β-Actin as a reference for quantifying relative gene expression levels. * $p < 0.05$, ** $p < 0.01$, and *** $p < 0.001$, compared to the control group.

The protein cathepsin L encoded by this gene is a lysosomal cysteine proteinase that plays a major role in intracellular protein catabolism. Its substrates include collagen and integrin. Next, using fluorescence quantitative PCR analysis, it was revealed that the expression of the genes *COL1A1*, *COL1A2*, *COL5A2*, *COL6A3*, *MMP2*, *MMP9*, *ITGA2*, and *ITGB3* was significantly downregulated after avellanin A intervention ($p < 0.05$, $p < 0.01$; Figure 4B). Furthermore, Western blot experiments confirmed that the protein expression of ITGB3 and FAK/p-FAK was reduced after avellanin A intervention in TP-treated RWPE-1 cells (Figures 4C and S4). Thus, we hypothesised that avellanin A may inhibit the activity of the lysosomal cysteine proteinase cathepsin L, decrease the expression of extracellular matrix components, and decrease FAK/p-FAK expression via the downstream PI3K-Akt signalling pathway, leading to cell cycle arrest and inhibition of cell proliferation.

2.4. Avellanin A Suppressed the PI3K-Akt Pathway in RWPE-1 Cells

The PI3K/Akt pathway is significantly associated with increased proliferation and survival. To verify whether PI3K-Akt signalling might mediate avellanin A function in RWPE-1 cells, Western blotting was used to analyse changes in the expression of proteins involved in the PI3K-Akt signalling pathway.

As shown, the PI3K protein expression levels decreased in RWPE-1 cells with increasing avellanin A concentrations; the PI3K and phosphorylated PI3K protein levels were decreased. Moreover, the total Akt protein and phosphorylated Akt protein levels were decreased significantly in control and treated RWPE-1 cells, which confirmed the inhibition of the PI3K-Akt pathway by avellanin A (Figures 5A and S5). To further understand the function of avellanin A in cell proliferation and apoptosis, we assessed the expression of several proteins involved in the Akt pathway by Western blotting. The results showed that avellanin A significantly decreased the expression of cyclin D1 compared with that in the control group ($p < 0.01$). Conversely, there was a significant increase in the protein expression of the apoptosis markers Bax, p21$^{Waf1/Cip1}$, and P53 ($p < 0.01$) in RWPE-1 cells as the avellanin A concentration increased (Figure 5B). These findings suggest that avellanin A may modulate the progression of BPH by affecting the cell cycle and blocking the division and replication of RWPE-1 cells through the PI3K-Akt pathway.

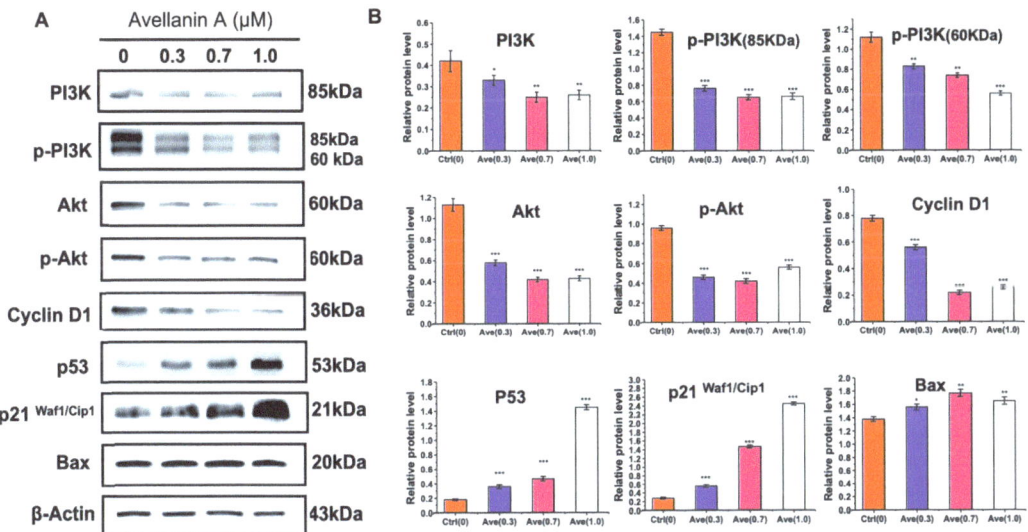

Figure 5. Effect of avellanin A on PI3K-Akt pathway-related protein expression in RWPE-1 cells. (**A**) The p-PI3K/PI3K, p-Akt/Akt, p53, Cyclin D1, P21$^{Waf1/Cip1}$, and Bax proteins were analysed by Western blotting. The analysis utilized actin as a reference for quantifying relative protein expression levels. (**B**) Relative quantitative detection of protein expression compared with control. * $p < 0.05$, ** $p < 0.01$, and *** $p < 0.001$, compared to the control group.

3. Discussion

Mangrove plants mainly include plants such as Red Sea olive plants, autumn eggplant plants [16], and so on. There is a long history of research on mangroves, and a variety of drugs for the treatment of human diseases have been extracted from mangrove plants [15] By the end of 2023, 1565 compounds with new structures had been isolated from mangrove endophytic fungi, of which 613 compounds had broad-spectrum biological activity, providing guidance for new drug development [17].

In this project, we studied the molecular mechanism of the inhibitory activity of avellanin A from *Aspergillus fumigatus* GXIMD 03099, which is an endophytic fungus in mangrove plants, to provide ideas for the development of new drugs for the treatment of BPH. Avellanin A was originally isolated from *Hamigera avellanea*. The total synthesis of this compound was subsequently completed in 1989 and 2021 [14]. Previous reports have demonstrated that it inhibits apolipoprotein B production in HepG2 cells without exhibiting cytotoxicity. To date, no other biological activities of avellanin A have been reported.

To investigate the effect of avellanin A on RWPE-1 cells, we conducted RNA-seq, and subsequent KEGG analysis found that avellanin A significantly affected ECM–receptor interactions and their downstream signalling pathways. Furthermore, molecular docking revealed that avellanin A has a good affinity for the cathepsin L protein. Cathepsin L is widely distributed in the lysosomes of mammals [18]. Cathepsin L is a lysosomal cysteine proteinase that is secreted to dissolve intracellular and endocytic proteins. Under normal circumstances, cathepsin L performs biological functions in lysosomes [19]. However, changes in the expression levels and lysosomal state cause a portion of cathepsin L to be secreted into the extracellular environment, which is involved in the terminal degradation of extracellular matrix components such as collagen and elastin [20]. Studies have shown that the downregulation of cathepsin L inhibits the proliferation, invasion, and migration of glioma cells [21]. Moreover, in vitro experiments revealed that cathepsin L overexpression promoted proliferation, migration, and invasion in MCF-7 and MDA-MB-231 cells, while cathepsin L knockdown decreased proliferation, migration, and invasion in MDA-MB-231 cells [22]. Moreover, previous studies reported that cathepsin L can promote tumour cell proliferation by activating CCAAT-displacement protein/cut homeobox (CDP/Cux) transcription factors and accelerating entry into the S phase of the cell cycle [23]. In this study, avellanin A was shown to inhibit TP-induced prostate cell proliferation by halting the G1 phase of the cell cycle. It is speculated that the reason may be that avellanin A binds to cathepsin L and inhibits its activity, resulting in a decrease in the expression of ECM components such as collagen and integrin proteins, reducing the transduction of downstream signalling pathways, and ultimately inhibiting cell proliferation, survival, and migration.

The adhesion pathway kinase FAK plays a central role in intracellular communication. Activation of the focal adhesion kinase FAK and overexpression of focal adhesion proteins lead to abnormal adhesion of the extracellular matrix to epithelial cells [24], which is essential for the development of BPH [25]. A study showed that the PI3K/Akt signalling pathway is activated by interactions with the ECM, which participates in the cell proliferation process [26,27]. The activation of the PI3K signalling pathway phosphorylates AKT, increasing cell survival and decreasing apoptosis [28]. Significantly elevated levels of phosphorylated AKT and PI3K gene expression were observed in prostate tissue from BPH patients [29]. Our results revealed that FAK and the PI3K/Akt signalling pathway were downregulated in RWPE-1 cells after avellanin A intervention, significantly reducing cell survival.

Furthermore, these interferences are most likely achieved downstream of the PI3K-AKT signalling pathway. $p21^{Waf/Cip1}$ functions as a cell cycle inhibitor and antiproliferative effector and plays an important role in controlling the cell cycle by binding to multiple Cyclin/CDK complexes of multiple phases [30,31]. Here, the protein level of $p21^{Waf/Cip1}$ increased markedly. Consistent with the above results, the protein levels of cyclin D1 decreased significantly. Cyclin D1 is recognized as a crucial indicator of cell proliferation and serves as a pivotal regulator of cell cycle checkpoints governing G2/M and G1/S transitions [32,33]. Upon cell cycle initiation, cyclin D1 is rapidly upregulated, facilitating the division and replication of prostate stromal and epithelial cells [34,35]. Cyclin D1 functions as a vital sensor and integrator of extracellular signals in normal physiological processes, modulating cellular activities by binding to cyclin-dependent kinases [36]. p53 plays an important role in many parts of the cell cycle, and when the chromosomal DNA of a cell is damaged in the G1 phase, p53 transcriptional activity is enhanced, which induces the activation of the $p21^{Waf/Cip1}$ gene, which in turn causes $p21^{Waf/Cip1}$ to inhibit the activity of cell cycle-dependent kinases (CDKs), preventing the further proliferation of cells [37,38]. When the damage signal enters the S phase, $p21^{Waf/Cip1}$ induced by p53 can bind to the DNA polymerase complex at the replication fork and prevent its activity, inducing cell repair [39]. Additionally, the expression of the well-known universal proapoptotic protein Bax increased significantly in RWPE-1 cells as the avellanin A concentration increased. Direct pharmacological modulation of BAX has long been an attractive target due to the prominent role of BAX in human diseases. Cancer cells often evade apoptosis by overexpressing the antiapoptotic inhibitor BAX [40]; however, small-molecule activators of BAX have been shown to overcome this effect and inhibit cancer growth in animal models [41,42]. These findings suggested that the compound avellanin A affects the cell cycle and blocks cell division and replication through the PI3K-AKT pathway in RWPE-1 cells.

4. Materials and Methods

4.1. Fungal Material

The fungus *Aspergillus fumigatus* GXIMD 03099 was isolated from the mangrove plant *Acanthus ilicifolius* L., which was collected from the Beibu Gulf of Guangxi Province in China in July 2020. The strain was deposited at the Institute of Marine Drug Medicine, Guangxi University of Traditional Chinese Medicine, Nanning, China. The fungus was identified according to its morphological characteristics and a molecular biological protocol involving 18S rRNA amplification and sequencing of the ITS region. The sequence data were submitted to GenBank with the accession number ON668102, and the fungal strain was identified as *Aspergillus fumigatus*.

4.2. Isolation and Purification

The mycelia and solid rice media were extracted with EtOAc. The organic extract was concentrated in vacuo to yield an oily residue (75.0 g), which was subjected to silica gel column chromatography (CC) (petroleum ether−EtOAc v/v, gradient 100:0–0:100) to generate ten fractions (Fr. 1–Fr. 10). Fr. 8 (30.1 g) was separated by silica gel CC and eluted with petroleum ether−EtOAc (from 3:1 to 1:1) to afford twelve subfractions (8-1–8-12). Subfractions 8-6 were further purified by using ODS eluted with MeOH−H$_2$O v/v to obtain avellanin A (6.82 mg, t_R = 22.5 min). The stock material was analysed using ^{1}H and ^{13}C NMR and high-resolution mass spectrometry prior to use in the studies reported here, and it was found that the material was >98% pure (Supporting Figures S2 and S3 and Table S1).

4.3. Cell Culture and Reagents

The RWPE-1 human prostate epithelial cell line was obtained from the Chinese Academy of Sciences (Shanghai, China). The cells were cultured with keratinocyte-SFM (K-SFM, Gibco, Norristown, PA, USA) supplemented with 100 mg/mL penicillin/streptomycin (HyClone, Logan, UT, USA) in an incubator at 37 °C with humidified 5% CO$_2$. After 24 h of incubation, the culture media were replaced with fresh media containing 0.5 µM TP (Wako Pure Chemical Industries, Osaka, Japan) in order to induce cell proliferation. Avellanin A was supplemented together within TP-containing media.

4.4. Cell Viability Assays

The CCK-8 assay and colony formation assays were used to assess cell viability. The cells were digested by trypsinisation and then seeded in 96-well plates at 5×10^3 cells per well. In the CCK-8 experiment, nine groups were treated with avellanin A separately at concentrations of 0, 0.1, 0.2, 0.3, 0.4, 0.5, 0.6, 0.7, 0.8, 0.9, and 1.0 µM at 37 °C for 24 h, each with eight replicates. Forty-eight hours later, 10 µL of CCK-8 reagent (KeyGEN, Nanjing, China) was added, and the absorbance was measured at 450 nm after incubation for 2–4 h. The absorbance at a wavelength of 450 nm was determined by a microplate reader (Bio Tek Instruments, Bad Friedrichshall, Germany). The CCK-8 assay was performed following the manufacturer's protocol.

4.5. Cell Cycle Assay

To detect the impact of avellanin A on the cell cycle, the RWPE-1 cells were seeded on the 6-well plates treated with avellanin A (0.7 µM) at 37 °C for 24 h. At the end of incubation, cells were trypsinised. The cells (1×10^6) were collected by centrifugation at $1000 \times g$ for 5 min, washed twice with ice-cold PBS, fixed with cold 70% ethanol, and stored at -20 °C for 24 h. The cells were subsequently centrifuged again, washed twice with cold PBS, incubated with RNase A (0.1 mg/mL) for 1 h at 37 °C, and stained with PI (0.1 mg/mL) for 30 min in the dark. The DNA content was measured by flow cytometry (LSRFortessa, BD, Canton, MA, USA), and the percentage of cells in each phase of the cell cycle was evaluated using ModFit LT version 4.0 software.

4.6. Cell Migration Assays

Cell migration assays were performed as follows: The RWPE-1 cells were digested and suspended in serum-free medium. Cells (6×10^4) were seeded in 24-well plates treated with avellanin A (0.7 µM) coated without Matrigel in the upper layer of a migration chamber (Labselect, Hangzhou, China) with 8 µm pore polycarbonate membranes containing 200 µL of FBS-free RPMI-1640 medium (Gibco, Norristown, PA, USA), and the lower layer was supplemented with 500 µL of K-SFM. After 24 h of incubation, unmigrated cells across the membranes were carefully removed with cotton swabs, while cells across the membrane were fixed with 4% paraformaldehyde (Biosharp, Shanghai, China) and then stained with crystal violet dye. Finally, the cells were photographed and counted under an optical microscope.

4.7. Colony Formation Assay

For the colony formation assay, cells (500/well) were cultured in 6-well plates treated with avellanin A (0.7 µM) for 7 days. When the colonies were clearly observed under the microscope, the cells were washed twice with PBS and fixed with 4% paraformaldehyde for 15 min, followed by staining with crystal violet dye (Yunaye, China) for 10 min. The number of cell clones was photographed and statistically analysed.

4.8. Transcriptomic Expression Profiling and Bioinformatics Analysis

RWPE-1 cells were treated with avellanin A (0.7 µM) at 37 °C for 48 h in TP-containing media and subsequently collected for transcriptomic analysis. Total RNA was extracted from the RWPE-1 cells using the TRIzol reagent kit (Invitrogen, Carlsbad, CA, USA) and assessed for quality using an Agilent 2100 Bioanalyzer system (Agilent Technologies, Palo Alto, CA, USA). Subsequently, library preparation for sequencing was conducted using the NEBNext Ultra RNA Library Prep Kit for Illumina, following the manufacturer's instructions. Clustering was carried out on the cBot Cluster Generation System (Illumina, San Diego, CA, USA) using the TruSeq PE Cluster Kit v3-cBot-HS, and sequencing was performed on the Illumina NovaSeq 6000 platform (Gene Denovo Biotechnology, Guangzhou, China).

The obtained clean data were processed by eliminating reads containing adapters and low-quality sequences from the raw data. Alignments of the clean reads with the assembled genome of GRCh38.p13 were performed using HISAT2. The FPKM value of each gene in each sample was determined using featureCounts 2.0.2 software. Genes with a p-value < 0.05 and a fold change > 2 were considered to be significantly differentially expressed. All differentially expressed genes (DEGs) were associated with Gene Ontology (GO) terms in the GO database, and the number of genes per term was calculated. The significantly enriched GO terms in DEGs were identified using the hypergeometric test. Additionally, Kyoto Encyclopedia of Genes and Genomes (KEGGs) pathway enrichment analysis was conducted to pinpoint metabolic pathways or signal transduction pathways that were significantly enriched in DEGs compared to the genome-wide background. The calculated p-value was adjusted for the false discovery rate (FDR) with a threshold of FDR $\leq$ 0.05. GO terms and KEGG pathways meeting these criteria were deemed significantly enriched in the DEGs. Then, the genes were searched in the STRING database (25 August 2023) to determine the protein–protein interaction (PPI) relationships. Cytoscape 3.7.2 software was used to construct the PPI network to visualize the relationships between avellanin A and its targets.

4.9. Molecular Docking

Molecular docking was performed to evaluate the binding affinity of avellanin A for the cathepsin L protein. The Maestro program in Glide software version 8.1 was used for docking. Human cathepsin L (UniProt ID: P07711) was obtained from the PDB protein database (7 April 2024), while the structures of the avellanin A compounds were downloaded from the PubChem database (7 April 2024). Prior to the docking process, water molecules were removed from the conformation, and the proteins were subjected to hydrogenation. Furthermore, the 3D structure of the target compound was optimised by calculating its 3D conformation at the minimum energy. The interaction between the ligand and the acceptor was analysed, and potential active substances were evaluated based on the score.

4.10. Fluorescence-Based Quantitative PCR

Total RNA from the RWPE-1 cell samples was extracted using TRIzol reagent (Invitrogen, Carlsbad, CA, USA) and then transcribed into cDNA using a reverse transcriptome kit (Applied Biosystems, Foster City, CA, USA). Quantitative PCR was performed on a real-time PCR system. Primers were designed and synthesised by Huiyuan Technology Co., Ltd. (Jinan, China). The primer sequences are shown in Table S2.

4.11. Western Blotting

The Western blot analysis was conducted as follows: Briefly, RWPE-1 cells were treated with avellanin A (0.7 µM) at 37 °C for 48 h in TP-containing media. The cells were washed twice with PBS supplemented with an appropriate amount of RIPA lysis buffer, lysed at 4 °C for 30 min, and centrifuged at 12,000 r/min for 10 min at 4 °C, after which the supernatant contained the total extracted protein. Electrophoresis was performed with a 10% concentration of polyacrylamide gel (SDS-PAGE), and the proteins were transferred to PVDF membranes. The membranes were blocked in 5% milk and incubated with the primary antibodies at 4 °C overnight. Primary antibodies against p-Akt (1:2000, No. 4060), anti-Akt (1:1000, No. 4691), anti-p-PI3K (1:1000, No. 4228), anti-PI3K (1:1000, No. 4257), anti-p53 (1:1000, No. 2527), anti-cyclin D1 (1:1000, No. 55506), anti-p21 Waf1/Cip1 (1:1000, No. 2947), and anti-Bax (1:1000, No. 5023) were purchased from Cell Signaling Technology. Then, the membranes were washed with TBST and incubated with secondary antibodies at 37 °C for two hours. Finally, the bands were visualised by using an Omni-ECL Femto Light Chemiluminescence Kit (Epizyme, Shanghai, China) and imaged by using an Amersham Imager 680 blot gel imager (Cytiva, Marlborough, MA, USA). β-Actin was used as a control, and the test was repeated at least three times.

4.12. Statistical Analysis

The data are expressed as the means ± SDs from at least three independent experiments. The unpaired *t* test was used for comparisons between groups. Statistical analyses were carried out by one-way analysis of variance with Bonferroni's multiple-comparison correction for comparisons among three or more groups. The following labels were used: ns, not significant; *, $p < 0.05$; **, $p < 0.01$; ***, $p < 0.001$; and ****, $p < 0.0001$. GraphPad Prism 10.0 software was used for statistical analysis and graphing.

5. Conclusions

In this project, the cyclic pentapeptide compound avellanin A from the *Aspergillus fumigatus fungus* was studied to explore its ability to inhibit RWPE-1 cell proliferation and its molecular mechanism. Avellanin A has a good affinity for cathepsin L, which is involved in the terminal degradation of extracellular matrix components. Avellanin A significantly blocked the ECM–receptor interaction and suppressed the downstream PI3K-Akt signalling pathway. The expression of the genes *COL1A1*, *COL1A2*, *COL5A2*, *COL6A3*, *MMP2*, *MMP9*, *ITGA2*, and *ITGB3* was significantly downregulated after avellanin A intervention. The results confirmed that it not only reduced ITGA2 and FAK/p-FAK protein expression but also inhibited PI3K/p-PI3K and Akt/p-Akt protein expression in the PI3K-Akt signalling pathway. Furthermore, avellanin A upregulated Bax, p21$^{WAF1/Cip1}$, and p53 protein expression and downregulated Cyclin D1 protein expression in TP-induced RWPE-1 cells, leading to cell cycle arrest and inhibition of cell proliferation. This study supports the use of avellanin A as a potential new drug for the treatment of BPH.

Supplementary Materials: The following supporting information can be downloaded at: https://www.mdpi.com/article/10.3390/md22060275/s1, Figure S1: HR-ESI-MS spectrum of avellanin A. Figure S2: ^{1}H NMR (d 4-methanol, 600 MHz) spectrum of avellanin A; Figure S3: ^{13}C NMR (d 4-methanol, 150 MHz) spectrum of avellanin A. Figure S4: The original Western blot image of Figure 4C. Figure S5: The original Western blot image of Figure 5. Table S1: ^{1}H and ^{13}C NMR assignments for avellanin A in DMSO-d_6. Table S2: Sequences of qPCR primers.

Author Contributions: Conceptualisation, X.Q. and M.B.; methodology, C.X. and G.C.; software, C.X.; validation, M.B.; formal analysis, C.X., G.C. and H.Z.; investigation, C.X., G.C. and H.Z.; resources, M.B., X.Y. and X.Q.; data curation, C.X., G.C. and H.Z.; writing—review and editing, C.X., G.C., M.B. and X.Q.; visualisation, C.X., M.B. and X.Q.; supervision, M.B., X.Y. and X.Q.; project administration, X.Y. and X.Q.; funding acquisition, M.B., X.Y. and X.Q.; All authors have read and agreed to the published version of the manuscript.

Funding: This study was supported by the Development Program of High-level Talent Team under the Qihuang Project of Guangxi University of Chinese Medicine (No. 202404), the Natural Science Foundation of Guangxi (No. 2021GXNSFBA220072), the Guangxi University of Chinese Medicine-Guipai Xinglin Top Talent Funding Project (2022C008), the Research Launching Fund Project from Guangxi University of Chinese Medicine Introduced Doctoral (2022BS021), and the Natural Science Foundation of Guangxi (No. 2024GXNSFAA010459).

Informed Consent Statement: Not applicable.

Data Availability Statement: The data presented in this study are available upon request from the corresponding author.

Acknowledgments: The graphical abstract was created with BioRender.com. The authors thank Bio-Render (BioRender.com) for helping with the graphical abstract preparation and the confirmation of publication and licensing rights.

Conflicts of Interest: The authors declare no conflicts of interest.

References

1. Lee, S.W.H.; Chan, E.M.C.; Lai, Y.K. The global burden of lower urinary tract symptoms suggestive of benign prostatic hyperplasia: A systematic review and meta-analysis. *Sci. Rep.* **2017**, *7*, 7984. [CrossRef]
2. Shah, A.; Shah, A.A.; Nandakumar, K.; Lobo, R. Mechanistic targets for BPH and prostate cancer-a review. *Rev. Environ. Health* **2021**, *36*, 261–270. [CrossRef]
3. Lokeshwar, S.D.; Harper, B.T.; Webb, E.; Jordan, A.; Dykes, T.A.; Neal, D.E.; Terris, M.K.; Klaassen, Z. Epidemiology and treatment modalities for the management of benign prostatic hyperplasia. *Transl. Androl. Urol.* **2019**, *8*, 529–539. [CrossRef]
4. Dhanabalan, A.K.; Kumar, P.; Vasudevan, S.; Chworos, A.; Velmurugan, D. Identification of a novel drug molecule for neurodegenerative disease from marine algae through *in-silico* analysis. *J. Biomol. Struct. Dyn.* **2024**, 1–10. [CrossRef]
5. Xu, M.W.; Bai, Z.F.; Xie, B.C.; Peng, R.; Du, Z.W.; Liu, Y.; Zhang, G.S.; Yan, S.; Xiao, X.H.; Qin, S.L. Marine-Derived Bisindoles for Potent Selective Cancer Drug Discovery and Development. *Molecules* **2024**, *29*, 933. [CrossRef]
6. Kallifidas, D.; Dhakal, D.; Chen, M.Y.; Chen, Q.Y.; Kokkaliari, S.; Rosa, N.A.C.; Ratnayake, R.; Bruner, S.D.; Paul, V.J.; Ding, Y.S.; et al. Biosynthesis of Dolastatin 10 in Marine Cyanobacteria, a Prototype for Multiple Approved Cancer Drugs. *Org. Lett.* **2024**, *26*, 1321–1325. [CrossRef]
7. Marunganathan, V.; Kumar, M.S.K.; Kari, Z.A.; Giri, J.; Shaik, M.R.; Shaik, B.; Guru, A. Marine-derived κ-carrageenan-coated zinc oxide nanoparticles for targeted drug delivery and apoptosis induction in oral cancer. *Mol. Biol. Rep.* **2024**, *51*, 89. [CrossRef]
8. Akram, W.; Rihan, M.; Ahmed, S.; Arora, S.; Ahmad, S.; Vashishth, R. Marine-Derived Compounds Applied in Cardiovascular Diseases: Submerged Medicinal Industry. *Mar. Drugs* **2023**, *21*, 193. [CrossRef]
9. Wang, J.M.; Qin, Y.N.; Lin, M.P.; Song, Y.Y.; Lu, H.M.; Xu, X.Y.; Liu, Y.H.; Zhou, X.F.; Gao, C.H.; Luo, X.W. Marine Natural Products from the Beibu Gulf: Sources, Chemistry, and Bioactivities. *Mar. Drugs* **2023**, *21*, 63. [CrossRef]
10. Wang, Z.M.; Qader, M.; Wang, Y.F.; Kong, F.D.; Wang, Q.; Wang, C. Progress in the discovery of new bioactive substances from deep-sea associated fungi during 2020–2022. *Front. Mar. Sci.* **2023**, *10*, 1232891. [CrossRef]
11. Wang, S.C.; Fan, L.M.; Pan, H.Y.; Li, Y.Y.; Qiu, Y.; Lu, Y.M. Antimicrobial peptides from marine animals: Sources, structures, mechanisms and the potential for drug development. *Front. Mar. Sci.* **2023**, *9*, 1112595. [CrossRef]
12. Ghoran, S.H.; Taktaz, F.; Sousa, E.; Fernandes, C.; Kijjoa, A. Peptides from Marine-Derived Fungi: Chemistry and Biological Activities. *Mar. Drugs* **2023**, *21*, 510. [CrossRef]
13. Yan, J.X.; Wu, Q.H.; Maity, M.; Braun, D.R.; Alas, I.; Wang, X.; Yin, X.; Zhu, Y.L.; Bell, B.A.; Rajski, S.R.; et al. Rapid Unambiguous Structure Elucidation of Streptnatamide A, a New Cyclic Peptide Isolated from A Marine-derived *Streptomyces* sp. *Chem.—A Eur. J.* **2023**, *29*, e202301813. [CrossRef]
14. Yamazaki, M.; Horie, Y.; Bae, K.; Maebayashi, Y.; Jisai, Y.; Fujimoto, H. New fungal metabolites avellanins a and B from *Hamigers avellanea* with pressor effect. *Chem. Pharm. Bull.* **1987**, *35*, 2122–2124. [CrossRef]
15. Honda, M.; Inagaki, M.; Masuda, Y. Total synthesis of the cyclic pentapeptides PF1171B, D, E, and avellanins A, B, C with inhibitory activity against apolipoprotein B production. *Tetrahedron Lett.* **2021**, *81*, 153340. [CrossRef]
16. Ismail, E.T.; El-Son, M.A.M.; El-Gohary, F.A.; Zahran, E. Prevalence, genetic diversity, and antimicrobial susceptibility of *Vibrio* spp. infected gilthead sea breams from coastal farms at Damietta, Egypt. *BMC Vet. Res.* **2024**, *20*, 129. [CrossRef]
17. Carroll, A.R.; Copp, B.R.; Grkovic, T.; Keyzers, R.A.; Prinsep, M.R. Marine natural products. *Nat. Prod. Rep.* **2024**, *41*, 162–207. [CrossRef]
18. Poreba, M.; Rut, W.; Vizovisek, M.; Groborz, K.; Kasperkiewicz, P.; Finlay, D.; Vuori, K.; Turk, D.; Turk, B.; Salvesen, G.S.; et al. Selective imaging of cathepsin L in breast cancer by fluorescent activity-based probes. *Chem. Sci.* **2018**, *9*, 2113–2129. [CrossRef]
19. Ueki, N.; Wang, W.; Swenson, C.; McNaughton, C.; Sampson, N.S.; Hayman, M.J. Synthesis and Preclinical Evaluation of a Highly Improved Anticancer Prodrug Activated by Histone Deacetylases and Cathepsin L. *Theranostics* **2016**, *6*, 808–816. [CrossRef]
20. Sudhan, D.R.; Siemann, D.W. Cathepsin L targeting in cancer treatment. *Pharmacol. Therapeut* **2015**, *155*, 105–116. [CrossRef]
21. Qian, F.; Xu, H.Y.; Zhang, Y.K.; Li, L.F.; Yu, R.T. Methionine deprivation inhibits glioma growth through downregulation of CTSL. *Am. J. Cancer Res.* **2022**, *12*, 5004–5018. [PubMed]
22. Zhang, L.M.; Zhao, Y.; Yang, J.; Zhu, Y.N.; Li, T.; Liu, X.Y.; Zhang, P.F.; Cheng, J.L.; Sun, S.; Wei, C.L.; et al. CTSL, a prognostic marker of breast cancer, that promotes proliferation, migration, and invasion in cells in triple-negative breast cancer. *Front. Oncol.* **2023**, *13*, 1158087. [CrossRef]
23. Goulet, B.; Sansregret, L.; Leduy, L.; Bogyo, M.; Weber, E.; Chauhan, S.S.; Nepveu, A. Increased expression and activity of nuclear cathepsin L in cancer cells suggests a novel mechanism of cell transformation. *Mol. Cancer Res.* **2007**, *5*, 899–907. [CrossRef]
24. Zhang, C.P.; Yu, Z.Y.; Yang, S.S.; Liu, Y.T.; Song, J.N.; Mao, J.; Li, M.H.; Zhao, Y. ZNF460-mediated circRPPH1 promotes TNBC progression through ITGA5-induced FAK/PI3K/AKT activation in a ceRNA manner. *Mol. Cancer* **2024**, *23*, 33. [CrossRef] [PubMed]
25. Ke, Z.B.; Cai, H.; Wu, Y.P.; Lin, Y.Z.; Li, X.D.; Huang, J.B.; Sun, X.L.; Zheng, Q.S.; Xue, X.Y.; Wei, Y.; et al. Identification of key genes and pathways in benign prostatic hyperplasia. *J. Cell Physiol.* **2019**, *234*, 19942–19950. [CrossRef]
26. El-Shafei, N.H.; Zaafan, M.A.; Kandil, E.A.; Sayed, R.H. Simvastatin ameliorates testosterone-induced prostatic hyperplasia in rats via modulating IGF-1/PI3K/AKT/FOXO signaling. *Eur. J. Pharmacol.* **2023**, *950*, 175762. [CrossRef] [PubMed]
27. Ding, Y.J.; Zhang, M.Y.; Hu, S.; Zhang, C.Y.; Zhou, Y.; Han, M.; Li, J.J.; Li, F.L.; Ni, H.M.; Fang, S.Q.; et al. MiRNA-766-3p inhibits gastric cancer via targeting COL1A1 and regulating PI3K/AKT signaling pathway. *J. Cancer* **2024**, *15*, 990–998. [CrossRef]

28. Li, A.A.; Wang, S.J.; Nie, J.B.; Xiao, S.N.; Xie, X.S.; Zhang, Y.; Tong, W.L.; Yao, G.L.; Liu, N.; Dan, F.; et al. USP3 promotes osteosarcoma progression via deubiquitinating EPHA2 and activating the PI3K/AKT signaling pathway. *Cell Death Dis.* **2024**, *15*, 235. [CrossRef]
29. Choi, Y.J.; Fan, M.; Wedamulla, N.E.; Tang, Y.J.; Kim, E.K. Alleviatory effect of isoquercetin on benign prostatic hyperplasia via IGF-1/PI3K/Akt/mTOR pathway. *Food Sci. Hum. Well* **2024**, *13*, 1698–1710. [CrossRef]
30. Yu, H.C.; Jeon, Y.G.; Na, A.Y.; Han, C.Y.; Lee, M.R.; Yang, J.D.; Yu, H.C.; Son, J.B.; Kim, N.D.; Kim, J.B.; et al. p21-activated kinase 4 counteracts PKA-dependent lipolysis by phosphorylating FABP4 and HSL. *Nat. Metab.* **2024**, *6*, 94–112. [CrossRef]
31. Ben-Oz, B.M.; Machour, F.E.; Nicola, M.; Argoetti, A.; Polyak, G.; Hanna, R.; Kleifeld, O.; Mandel-Gutfreund, Y.; Ayoub, N. A dual role of RBM42 in modulating splicing and translation of CDKN1A/p21 during DNA damage response. *Nat. Commun.* **2023**, *14*, 7628. [CrossRef]
32. Ma, C.Y.; Wang, D.D.; Tian, Z.F.; Gao, W.R.; Zang, Y.C.; Qian, L.L.; Xu, X.; Jia, J.H.; Liu, Z.F. USP13 deubiquitinates and stabilizes cyclin D1 to promote gastric cancer cell cycle progression and cell proliferation. *Oncogene* **2023**, *42*, 2249–2262. [CrossRef]
33. Wang, J.; Su, W.; Zhang, T.T.; Zhang, S.S.; Lei, H.W.; Ma, F.D.; Shi, M.N.; Shi, W.J.; Xie, X.D.; Di, C.X. Aberrant Cyclin D1 splicing in cancer: From molecular mechanism to therapeutic modulation. *Cell Death Dis.* **2023**, *14*, 244. [CrossRef]
34. Chen, J.; Wei, J.Q.; Hong, M.N.; Zhang, Z.; Zhou, H.D.; Lu, Y.Y.; Zhang, J.; Guo, Y.T.; Chen, X.; Wang, J.G.; et al. Mitogen-Activated Protein Kinases Mediate Adventitial Fibroblast Activation and Neointima Formation via GATA4/Cyclin D1 Axis. *Cardiovasc. Drug Ther.* **2024**, *38*, 215–222. [CrossRef]
35. Zhao, J.L.; Wu, Y.; Xiao, T.; Cheng, C.; Zhang, T.; Gao, Z.Y.; Hu, S.Y.; Ren, Z.; Yu, X.Z.; Yang, F.; et al. A specific anti-cyclin D1 intrabody represses breast cancer cell proliferation by interrupting the cyclin D1-CDK4 interaction. *Breast Cancer Res. Tr.* **2023**, *198*, 555–568. [CrossRef]
36. Fang, M.; Wu, H.K.; Pei, Y.M.; Zhang, Y.; Gao, X.Y.; He, Y.Y.; Chen, G.J.; Lv, F.X.; Jiang, P.; Li, Y.M.; et al. E3 ligase MG53 suppresses tumor growth by degrading cyclin D1. *Signal Transduct. Tar.* **2023**, *8*, 263. [CrossRef]
37. Rahimi, E.; Asefi, F.; Afzalinia, A.; Khezri, S.; Zare-Zardini, H.; Ghorani-Azam, A.; Es-haghi, A.; Yazdi, M.E.T. Chitosan coated copper/silver oxide nanoparticles as carriers of breast anticancer drug: Cyclin D1/P53 expressions and cytotoxicity studies. *Inorg. Chem. Commun.* **2023**, *158*, 111581. [CrossRef]
38. Li, S.Z.; Xue, J.C.; Zhang, H.; Shang, G.N. ARHGAP44-mediated regulation of the p53/C-myc/Cyclin D1 pathway in modulating the malignant biological behavior of osteosarcoma cells. *J. Orthop. Surg. Res.* **2023**, *18*, 972. [CrossRef]
39. Gutu, N.; Binish, N.; Keilholz, U.; Herzel, H.; Granada, A.E. p53 and p21 dynamics encode single-cell DNA damage levels, fine-tuning proliferation and shaping population heterogeneity. *Commun. Biol.* **2023**, *6*, 1196. [CrossRef]
40. Mchenry, M.W.; Shi, P.W.; Camara, C.M.; Cohen, D.T.; Rettenmaier, T.J.; Adhikary, U.; Gygi, M.A.; Yang, K.; Gygi, S.P.; Wales, T.E.; et al. Covalent inhibition of pro-apoptotic BAX. *Nat. Chem. Biol.* **2024**, 1–11. [CrossRef]
41. Shen, L.H.; Fan, L.; Luo, H.; Li, W.Y.; Cao, S.Z.; Yu, S.M. Cow placenta extract ameliorates d-galactose-induced liver damage by regulating BAX/CASP3 and p53/p21/p16 pathways. *J. Ethnopharmacol.* **2024**, *323*, 117685. [CrossRef] [PubMed]
42. Chauhan, M.; Osbron, C.A.; Koehler, H.S.; Goodman, A.G. STING dependent BAX-IRF3 signaling results in apoptosis during late-stage infection. *Cell Death Dis.* **2024**, *15*, 195. [CrossRef] [PubMed]

Disclaimer/Publisher's Note: The statements, opinions and data contained in all publications are solely those of the individual author(s) and contributor(s) and not of MDPI and/or the editor(s). MDPI and/or the editor(s) disclaim responsibility for any injury to people or property resulting from any ideas, methods, instructions or products referred to in the content.

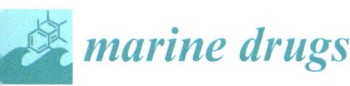

Article

A Terphenyllin Derivative CHNQD-00824 from the Marine Compound Library Induced DNA Damage as a Potential Anticancer Agent

Xi-Zhen Cao [1,2,†], Bo-Qi Zhang [1,2,†], Cui-Fang Wang [1,2], Jun-Na Yin [1,2], Waqas Haider [1,2], Gulab Said [1,3], Mei-Yan Wei [1,2] and Ling Lu [1,2,*]

[1] Key Laboratory of Marine Drugs, The Ministry of Education of China, School of Medicine and Pharmacy, Ocean University of China, Qingdao 266003, China; caoxizhen2022@163.com (X.-Z.C.); zbq2867653686@163.com (B.-Q.Z.); wangcuifang0115@163.com (C.-F.W.); yinjunna@163.com (J.-N.Y.); waqashaider07@yahoo.com (W.H.); gulabouc@gmail.com (G.S.); mywei95@126.com (M.-Y.W.)
[2] Laboratory for Marine Drugs and Biological Products, Laoshan Laboratory, Qingdao 266003, China
[3] Department of Chemistry, Women University Swabi, Swabi 23430, Pakistan
* Correspondence: linglu@ouc.edu.cn
† These authors contributed equally to this work.

Abstract: With the emergence of drug resistance and the consequential high morbidity and mortality rates, there is an urgent need to screen and identify new agents for the effective treatment of cancer. Terphenyls—a group of aromatic hydrocarbons consisting of a linear 1,4-diaryl-substituted benzene core—has exhibited a wide range of biological activities. In this study, we discovered a terphenyllin derivative—CHNQD-00824—derived from the marine compound library as a potential anticancer agent. The cytotoxic activities of the CHNQD-00824 compound were evaluated against 13 different cell lines with IC_{50} values from 0.16 to 7.64 µM. Further study showed that CHNQD-00824 inhibited the proliferation and migration of cancer cells, possibly by inducing DNA damage. Acridine orange staining demonstrated that CHNQD-00824 promoted apoptosis in zebrafish embryos. Notably, the anti-cancer effectiveness was verified in a doxycin hydrochloride (DOX)-induced liver-specific enlargement model in zebrafish. With Solafinib as a positive control, CHNQD-00824 markedly suppressed tumor growth at concentrations of 2.5 and 5 µM, further highlighting its potential as an effective anticancer agent.

Keywords: terphenyllin derivatives; marine compound library; cell cycle; apoptosis; anti-cancer

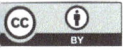

1. Introduction

Cancer is a prominent global public health issue and remains one of the primary causes of death worldwide. It is predicted that the incidence of all cancers combined will double by 2070 relative to 2020 [1]. In recent years, the COVID-19 pandemic has placed a significant burden on medical resources, impacting the diagnosis and treatment of cancer. This has led to an increase in advanced cancer cases and mortality rates [2,3]. Due to the emergence of drug resistance and high morbidity and mortality, there is an urgent need to discover new anticancer drugs. Natural products are important resources for drug development. Over the past 40 years, approximately 1400 small molecule drugs have been approved, with over two-thirds of them being related to natural products [4]. Therefore, natural products and their derivatives play important roles in drug development. The unique environment of the ocean has created complex, novel, and diverse marine natural products, making them an important component of natural products [5,6]. Marine secondary metabolites with novel structures and diverse biological activities have been demonstrated to be rich sources of chemical entities for drug discovery [7–12]. At present, among the more than 36,000 reported marine natural products, 17 have been approved for therapeutic use worldwide, especially in the field of anticancer drug research [13].

Figure 1 shows the marine natural products that have been approved as anticancer drugs Trabectedin, derived from *Ecteinascidia turbinate*, is a marine natural product that is clinically used for the treatment of advanced soft tissue sarcoma [14]. Eribulin, on the other hand, originated from the marine natural product halichondrin B [15]. Cytarabine is another marine drug developed from a marine natural product [16]. In addition, the current widely used strategies and emerging technologies, such as natural product-based antibody drug conjugates (ADCs) like brentuximab vedotin and brentuximab mafodotin, also originated from the marine natural product dolastatin 10 [17,18]. Therefore, marine natural products have consistently proved to be valuable resources for developing anticancer leads.

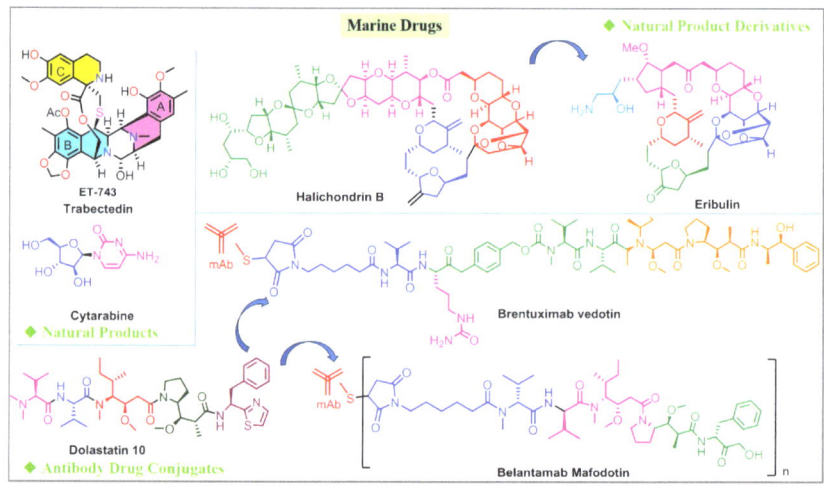

Figure 1. Marine natural products approved as the anticancer drugs.

Investigating new bioactive natural products and their derivatives from marine fungi is a significant and ongoing research focus in our laboratory [19–23]. As part of our continuous efforts to search for biologically active secondary metabolites from marine-derived fungi, terphenyllin was obtained from *Aspergillus* sp. [24]. Terphenyls—a group of aromatic hydrocarbons consisting of a linear 1,4-diaryl-substituted benzene core—exhibited a wide range of biological activities, including cytotoxicity, α-glucosidase inhibitory activity, and AMPK activator activity [23–26]. Interestingly, some of them showed strong cytotoxic activity against hepatocellular liver carcinoma cell lines (HepG2 and SMMC-7721), which were equivalent or stronger than the positive controls, Adriamycin and fluorouracil [24,27]. To date, more than 230 *p*-terphenyls have been isolated from microorganisms such as lichen endophytes, actinomycetes, and mosses [28]. The earliest chemical studies of *p*-terphenyls as one class of the pigments of mushrooms were carried out in 1877 [28]. In particular, one *p*-terphenyl derivative—MK-8722, designed by Merck—was developed as a hypoglycemic drug lead [29]. This further confirmed the significance and utility of *p*-terphenyl derivatives. Based on previous research, approximately 120 terphenyllin derivatives were designed and synthesized, which created a marine terphenyl derivatives library. Among them, two compounds—Terphenyllin and 3'-(isopentyloxy)-2',5'-dimethoxy-[1',1':4',1'-terphenyl]-4,4''-diol—not only showed strong α-glucosidase inhibitory activity, but also had relatively higher therapeutic indices, with the potential to be promising leads [24]. Additionally, eight compounds were also found to have cytotoxic potency [24,25]. Therefore, these compounds have shown value for further in-depth research.

In the present study, we scanned and identified a terphenyllin derivative—CHNQD-00824—derived from the marine-derived compound library as a potential anticancer agent. Furthermore, thirteen different cancer cells were selected for activity screening. Further study showed that this compound can inhibit the proliferation and migration of cancer cells by inducing DNA damage. CHNQD-00824 could inhibit DOX-induced liver-specific enlargement. The present results provided evidence that CHNQD-00824 exhibited great potential to be developed as an anticancer agent (Figure 2).

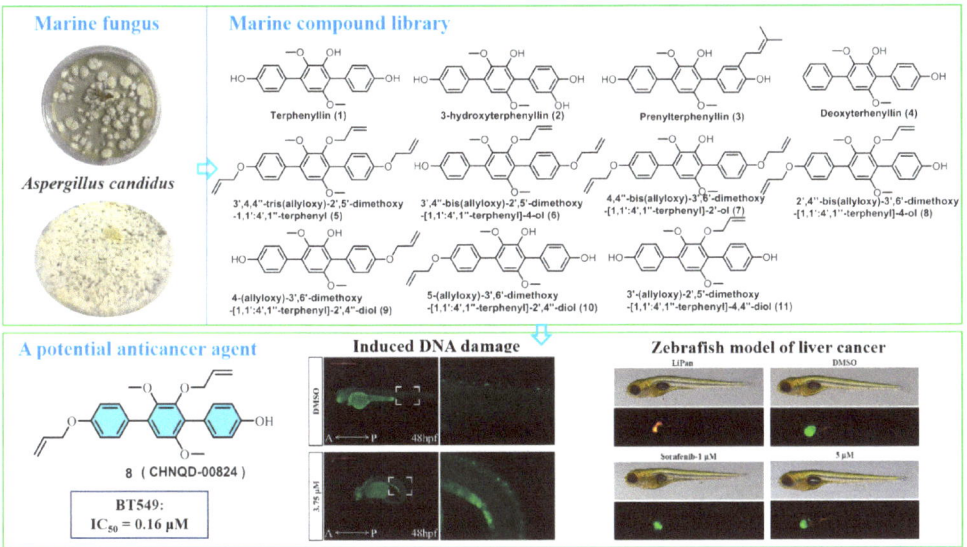

Figure 2. The discovery and biological activity research of compound CHNQD-00824.

2. Results and Discussion

2.1. Chemistry

Four terphenylated natural products, **1–4**, and seven terphenyllin derivatives, **5–11**, were scanned for their activity against BT549 cell lines from the marine-derived compound library. The four terphenylated natural products were identified from the marine fungus *Aspergillus candidus* (CHNSCLM-0393). Compound **1**, which contained three phenolic hydroxyl groups, was identified as terphenyllin [30]. Compounds **2–4** were identified as 3-hydroxyterphenyllin, prenylterphenyllin, and deoxyterphenyllin, respectively [31–34]. Seven terphenyllin derivatives, **5–11**, were obtained through the etherification reaction (Scheme 1). The etherification reaction was carried out at 45 °C for 2~3 h with dry K_2CO_3 as a catalyst and acetone as a solvent. Compound **5** was the terphenyllin trisubstituted derivative with all three phenolic hydroxyl groups alkylated, whereas compound **6** was the di-substituted derivative with allyl substituents at the R_2 and R_3 positions. Their structures were determined through nuclear magnetic resonance (NMR) analysis and ESIMS (Figures S1–S33). Their structures are shown in Figure 3.

In view of the potential biological activity of terphenyllin derivatives, we investigated the fermentation conditions of this fungus, including the effects of solid and liquid media, as well as the salinity, to increase the production of compound **1**. The liquid medium was PDB medium, which consisted of 200 g potato, 50 g glucose plus water to 1 L, adding sea salt according to the salinity, and the solid medium was rice with 4% artificial seawater. We set the salinity of the fermentation conditions as 1%, 2%, 4%, and 8%. The results showed that the yield of compound **1** was much better under solid fermentation conditions than under liquid fermentation conditions and that solid fermentation conditions are much better than liquid fermentation conditions. Among the currently set culture media, the solid culture medium with a salinity of 4% was the condition that obtained the highest yield of compound **1** (Figure S34). Accordingly, the fermentation conditions were solid rice media in 1 L Erlenmeyer flasks. Each flask contained 65 g of rice and 70 mL of PDB medium at 4% salinity for 35 days at room temperature.

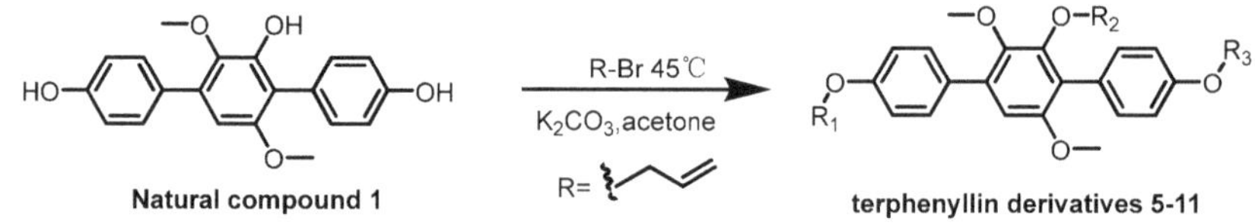

Scheme 1. Strategy for the semi-synthesis of terphenyllin derivatives **5–11**.

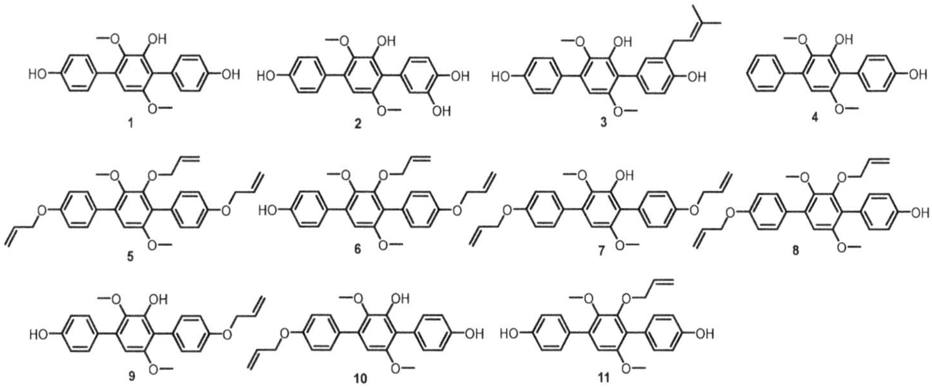

Figure 3. Natural product compounds **1–4** and terphenyllin derivatives **5–11**.

2.2. Biological Evaluation

2.2.1. Cytotoxic Activity

In this study, we first screened cytotoxic active compounds from the marine compound library using 2-(2-methoxy-4-nitrophenyl)-3-(4-nitrophenyl)-5-(2,4-disulfobenzene)-2H-tetrazolium monosodium salt CCK8 assays. Four terphenylated natural products, **1–4**, and seven terphenyllin derivatives, **5–11**, were further scanned for their activity against BT549 cell lines from the marine-derived compound library (Figure 4A). Terphenyllin derivative **8** (CHNQD-00824) was discovered as a potential anticancer agent. Furthermore, this compound was evaluated against a panel of thirteen different cancer cells, including human pancreatic cancer (Panc-1), colon cancer (HCT116), non-small cell lung cancer (A549), renal cancer (RCC4), cervical cancer (HeLa), liver cancer (HepG2), osteosarcoma (U2OS), glioma (U251), prostate cancer (DU145), esophageal cancer (TE-1), breast cancer (BT549, MCF7), and caecal adenocarcinoma (HCT8) cell lines using the CCK8 assay. As shown in Figure 4, CHNQD-00824 exhibited broad-spectrum cytotoxic activities against various cell lines, with IC_{50} values ranging between 0.16 and 7.64 µM (Table 1). Notably, it showed potent inhibitory activity against BT549, U2OS, HCT8, HCT116, and DU145 cells, with IC_{50} values in the sub-micromolar range. These findings suggest that CHNQD-00824 has significant potential for development as an anticancer agent. The above studies showed that, compared with the natural product terphenyllin **1**, only two derivatives—CHNQD-00824 and **9**—exhibited stronger cytotoxic activity. The introduction of allyl groups through alkylation reactions could affect the cytotoxic activity. In particular, when both the R_1 and R_2 positions were replaced by allyl groups, or when the allyl group was introduced only at the R_3 position, the cytotoxic activity was significantly enhanced.

Table 1. Cytotoxic activity of CHNQD-00824 against cancer cell lines.

Cell Lines	RCC4	HeLa	Hep G2	U2OS	U251	DU145	TE-1	BT549	HCT8	MCF7
IC_{50} (µM)	2.65 ± 0.04	0.45 ± 0.03	7.64 ± 0.21	0.44 ± 0.07	5.43 ± 0.05	0.91 ± 0.04	4.35 ± 0.12	0.16 ± 0.02	0.61 ± 0.06	3.66 ± 0.37

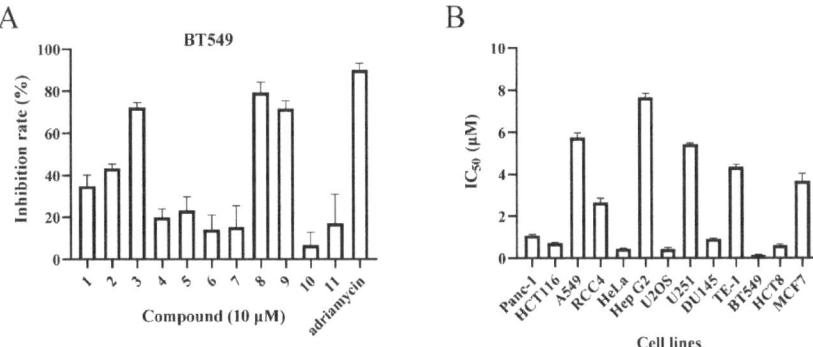

Figure 4. The cytotoxicity data of compounds **1–11**. (**A**) The inhibitory activity of compounds **1–11** against BT549 cell line. Adriamycin as a positive control. (**B**) CHNQD-00824 evaluated in thirteen different tumor cells. n = 3 biological replicate samples.

2.2.2. CHNQD-00824 Inhibited the Proliferation and Migration of Breast Cancer Cells

This CHNQD-00824 compound was found to have strong inhibitory activity on BT549 cells, with an IC$_{50}$ value of 0.16 μM. To further investigate its effect on the cell viability and proliferative capacity, single-cell clone formation and cell counting assays were performed [35]. Treatment of BT549 cells with CHNQD-00824 for 13 days dose-dependently reduced the formation of colonies, indicating its anticancer activity. Meanwhile, the cell counting assay showed that CHNQD-00824 at a concentration of 5 μM almost completely inhibited cell proliferation. Increased invasion and cell motility play a critical role in cancer progression [36,37]. Taking this fact into consideration, the anti-migratory activity of CHNQD-00824 against BT549 cells was evaluated using the scratch wound healing assay [38]. The results indicate that after 12 h treatment, there was no significant effect on the cell viability. However, a significant inhibition of cell migration was observed at concentrations of 5 μM and 10 μM. Additionally, CHNQD-00824 exhibited a notable inhibitory effect on cell migration after 24 h of treatment at concentrations of 1, 5, and 10 μM (Figure 5). Collectively, these results indicate that CHNQD-00824 inhibited the proliferation and migration of breast cancer cells in vitro.

2.2.3. CHNQD-00824 Induced G2 Phase Cell Cycle Arrest in BT549 Cells

Dysregulation of the cell cycle can lead to uncontrolled cell proliferation and cancer development. In order to further explore the mechanism of CHNQD-00824 inhibiting BT549 proliferation and migration, the cell content was analyzed to identify its impact on the BT549 cell cycle distribution. As shown in Figure 6A,C, the percentage of cells in the G2 phase decreased significantly, from 31.78% to 10.44%, in a dose-dependent manner after treatment with CHNQD-00824. The G2 phase is an important checkpoint in the cell cycle, where DNA damage is repaired before cells proceed to mitosis. Inhibiting the transition of cells from the G2 phase to mitosis can effectively halt cell division and proliferation. The observed G2 phase cell cycle arrest induced by CHNQD-00824 suggests that the compound may interfere with the normal cell cycle progression in BT549 cells. Further studies are needed to elucidate the exact molecular mechanism by which CHNQD-00824 induces G2 phase cell cycle arrest.

2.2.4. CHNQD-00824 Induced Caspase-Dependent Apoptosis in BT549 Cells

Then, we investigated whether CHNQD-00824 could induce the apoptosis of BT549 cells. According to Figure 6B, the percentage of apoptosis cells in the control group was 8.37%. However, the treatment with increasing concentrations of CHNQD-00824 (0.25, 0.5, and 1 μM) resulted in a dose-dependent increase in the percentage of apoptotic cells, reaching 10.66%, 14.67%, and 23.50%, respectively. The percentage of the cell apoptosis distribution is shown in Figure 5D. The result revealed that CHNQD-00824 could significantly induce apoptosis in a concentration-dependent manner. To gain insights into the underlying molecular mechanisms of the apoptosis induction by CHNQD-00824, the expression levels of apoptosis-related proteins were examined using western blotting analysis [39–42]. Compared to the control group, the treatment with CHNQD-00824 (0.5, 2, 8 µM) led to an increase in the levels of cleaved-PARP1 (C-PARP1) and Cytochrome C (Cyto C). Additionally, CHNQD-00824 was found to increase the level of cleaved-caspase 3 (C-Cas3) at the concentrations of 2 and 8 µM,. Furthermore, the pre-apoptotic protein, BAD, was observed to increase upon treatment with 8 µM of CHNQD-00824. Taken together, the findings indicated that CHNQD-00824 facilitated apoptosis in the BT549 cells (Figure 6E,F).

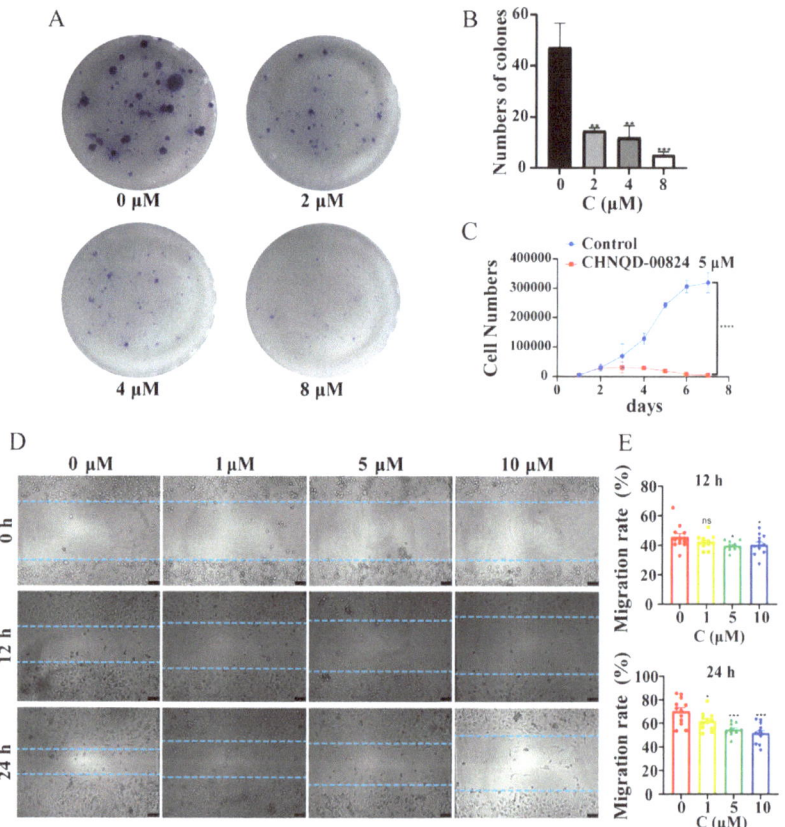

Figure 5. CHNQD-00824 inhibited the proliferation and migration of BT549 cells. (**A**,**B**) CHNQD-00824 inhibited the colony formation of BT549 cells. The BT549 cells were treated with CHNQD-00824 for 13 d, then the clones were photographed and counted. (**C**) Growth curves of BT549 cells treated with CHNQD-00824 (5 µM) and DMSO. (**D**,**E**) The scratch assay of BT549 cells after treatment with CHNQD-00824 for 12 h and 24 h. Scale bar, 100 µm. The data shown are the mean ± SD (* $p < 0.05$, ** $p < 0.01$, *** $p < 0.001$, **** $p < 0.0001$ and ns, nonsignificant). $n = 3$ biological replicate samples.

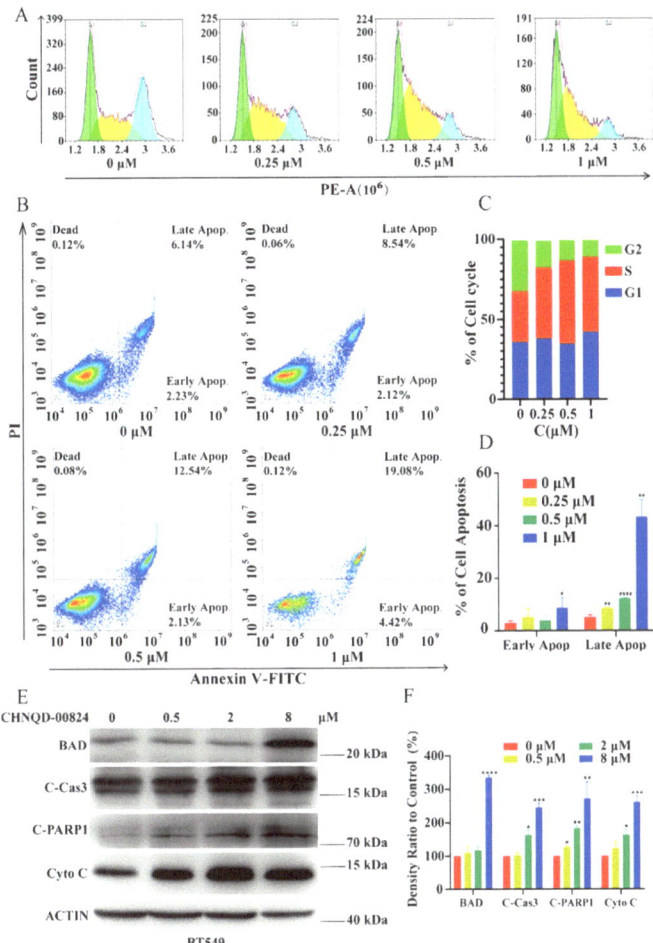

Figure 6. CHNQD-00824-induced apoptosis and cell cycle arrest in BT549 cells. (**A,C**) Flow cytometry analysis of cell cycle analysis on BT549 cells after treatment with CHNQD-00824 for 24 h. (**B,D**) Flow cytometry analysis of BT549 cells stained with the Annexin V/FITC-PI double staining solution after treatment with CHNQD-00824 for 24 h. (**E**) Effect of CHNQD-00824 on apoptosis-related proteins. BT549 cells were treated with CHNQD-00824 (0–8 µM) for 24 h, then cells were harvested and proteins were separated by electrophoresis on SDS-PAGE. Western blotting analysis were performed to detect the expression of cleaved-PARP, cleaved-caspase-3, Cyto-c and BAD. (**F**) Histogram shows the relative abundance of apoptosis-related proteins compared with the control group. The data shown are the mean ± SD (* $p < 0.05$, ** $p < 0.01$, *** $p < 0.001$, **** $p < 0.0001$, and ns, nonsignificant). $n = 3$ biological replicate samples.

2.2.5. CHNQD-00824 Caused DNA Damage in Both BT549 Cells and Zebrafish

Considering that the stability of DNA is closely related to cell apoptosis and the cell cycle, the change in the protein level of phospho-histone H2AX-S139, a marker of DNA damage, was detected [43]. After treatment with CHNQD-00824, the protein level of phospho-histone H2AX-S139 was significantly upregulated (Figure 7A,B). The accumulation of DNA damage might lead to cell death via apoptosis; therefore, we assessed the level of apoptosis using acridine orange (AO) staining in zebrafish in vivo. Fluorescent AO dye staining is an effective method for investigating cell death in zebrafish embryos [44]. The zebrafish embryos at 24 h post-fertilization (hpf) were exposed to CHNQD-00824.

Although no significant mortality was observed, developmental toxicity did occur, primarily characterized by a bent spine. The analysis of the AO-stained embryos clearly demonstrated upregulated apoptosis after the CHNQD-00824 treatment (Figure 7C,D). These results implied that CHNQD-00824 induced cell death via DNA damage.

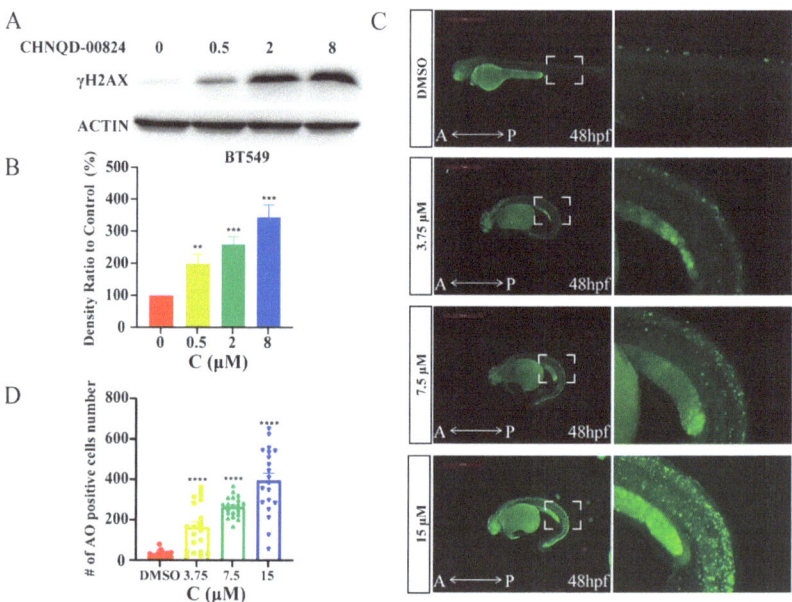

Figure 7. CHNQD-00824-induced DNA damage. (**A**) Effect of CHNQD-00824 on DNA damage marker proteins. BT549 cells were treated with CHNQD-00824 (0–8 μM) for 24 h, then cells were harvested and proteins were separated by electrophoresis on SDS-PAGE. Western blotting analysis were performed to detect the expression of γH2AX. (**B**) Histogram shows the relative abundance of γH2AX compared with the control group. (**C,D**) AO staining of zebrafish embryos at 48 hpf. When development reached 24 hpf, zebrafish embryos were treated with CHNQD-00824 (0–15 μM) to 48 hpf. AO staining was then performed. Scale bar, 1 mm. The data shown are the mean ± SD (** $p < 0.01$, *** $p < 0.001$, **** $p < 0.0001$). $n = 3$ biological replicate samples.

2.2.6. CHNQD-00824 Inhibited DOX-Induced Liver-Specific Enlargement

Traditionally, the murine model has been used in research as an in vivo model organism. Zebrafish, owing to their small size and rapid maturation time, have emerged as an important new cancer model that complements what can traditionally be achieved in mice and cell culture systems. Furthermore, the genetic pathways driving cancer are highly conserved between zebrafish and humans, and the ability to easily manipulate the zebrafish genome to rapidly generate transgenic animals makes zebrafish an excellent model organism [45–47]. In recent years, several inducible liver tumor models have been generated through the transgenic expression of oncogene in hepatocytes in zebrafish. In this report, the transgenic line—*Tg (fabp10:rtTA2s-M2; TRE2:EGFP kras^{G12V})*, named *To(kras^{G12V})*—was employed to investigate the effect of CHNQD-00824 on hepatocellular carcinoma (HCC). Under the induction of doxycin hydrochloride (DOX), *To(kras^{G12V})* exhibited the hepatocyte-specific expression of oncogenic krasV12, and eventually led to abnormal liver enlargement and even liver cancer in zebrafish [2,3,48]. In addition, a two-color transgenic zebrafish line—*Tg (fabp10:DsRed; elaA:GFP)*—with DsRed-labeled liver and GFP-labeled pancreas, was used as a normal control for the liver morphology, and was referred to as LiPan.

Therefore, the *To(kras^{G12V})* transgenic zebrafish model was used to test the effect of CHNQD-00824 on the growth of HCC in vivo. When developed to 3 dpf, the zebrafish were treated with different doses of CHNQD-00824, and DOX was added to induce abnormal liver enlargement. Following the exposure to CHNQD-00824 at this stage, no significant abnormalities or deformities were observed in the treated zebrafish. At 7 dpf, the fluorescence area of the zebrafish liver was observed and analyzed. LiPan zebrafish treated with the same concentration of DMSO were used as a control. The results showed that CHNQD-00824 could dose-dependently inhibit DOX-induced liver-specific enlargement at the concentrations of 1.25 µM, 2.5 µM, and 5 µM (Figure 8), suggesting that CHNQD-00824 has potential as a therapeutic agent for liver cancer.

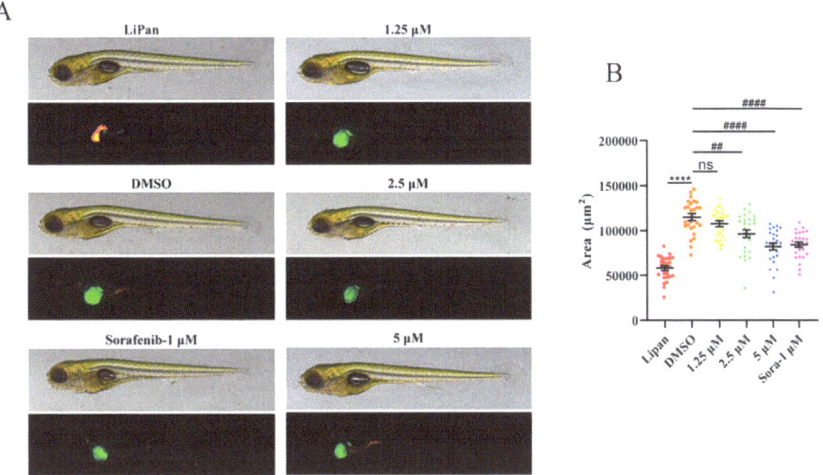

Figure 8. CHNQD-00824 inhibited tumor growth in zebrafish. (**A**) Zebrafish model of liver cancer. When development reached 3 dpf, zebrafish were treated with DOX (60 mg/L) and CHNQD-00824 (1.25–5 µM) to 7 dpf. Sorafenib as positive control. (**B**) Tumor size in zebrafish was measured by photography at 7 dpf. The data shown are the mean ± SD (**** $p < 0.0001$, ## $p < 0.01$, #### $p < 0.0001$, and ns, nonsignificant). $n = 3$ biological replicate samples.

3. Materials and Methods

3.1. General Experimental Procedures

NMR spectra were recorded on a Bruker Advance NEO 400; chemical shifts δ are reported in ppm, using TMS as internal standard, and coupling constants (*J*) are in Hz. The HRESIMS and ESIMS spectra were obtained using a Micromass Q-TOF mass spectrometer. UPLC-MS was performed on a Waters UPLC® system (Waters Ltd., Milford, MA, USA) using a C18 column [(Waters Ltd.) ACQUITY UPLC® BEH C18, 2.1 × 50 mm, 1.7 µm; 0.5 mL/min] and ACQUITY QDa ESIMS scan from 150 to 1000 Da. Column chromatography (CC) was performed on silica gel (Qingdao Haiyang Chemical Group Co., Qingdao, China; 200 to 300 mesh) and Sephadex LH-20 (Amersham Biosciences, Amersham, UK). TLC silica gel plates (Yan Tai Zi Fu Chemical Group Co., Yantai, China; G60, F-254) were used for thin layer chromatography. Semi-preparative HPLC was performed on a Waters 1525 system using a semi-preparative C18 column (Amsterdam, Netherlandish; Kromasil, 5 µm, 10 × 250 mm) equipped with a Waters 2996 photodiode array detector, and the flow rate was 2.0 mL/min.

3.2. Fungal Material

The fungal strain *A. candidus* (CHNSCLM-0393) was isolated from a piece of fresh internal tissue of the gorgonian coral *Juncella fragilis* collected from the Spratly Islands. The strain was identified through DNA amplification and sequencing of the ITS region according to the molecular biology methods described in the literature [49]. The fungus was identified as *A. candidus* with the GeneBank (NCBI) accession number MF681708.

3.3. Fermentation, Extraction, and Isolation

The fungal strain *A. candida* (CHNSCLM-0393) was grown in 60 1 L Erlenmeyer flasks in solid rice medium. Each flask contained 65 g of rice and 70 mL of 4% artificial seawater. The fungal was fermented for 35 days at room temperature. Each flask was extracted three times with 400 mL EtOAc from the fermented solid medium and then concentrated to dryness under vacuum to give an EtOAc extract (50 g). This was separated through column chromatography (CC) on silica gel, Sephadex LH-20 CC, and then recrystallized to give the two main compounds: **1** (5.6 g) and **2** (1.5 g). Further separation through semi-preparative HPLC gave compound **3** (5.0 mg) and compound **4** (8.5 mg). The structures of **1–4** were determined by analyzing the NMR data and comparing it with the literature data. The NMR data for natural products **1–4** are presented in the supplementary data.

3.4. General Synthetic Methods for Compounds 5–11

The etherification of natural product **1** was performed by alkylating the three hydroxyl groups by introducing allyl bromide to give seven derivatives, **5–11**. To an acetone solution (10 mL) of **1** (150 mg, 0.44 mM), 2.5 equivalents of allyl bromide (134.1 mg, 1.11 mM) and 3 dry equivalents of K_2CO_3 (183.8 mg, 1.33 mM) were added. The reaction was stirred at 45 °C for 3 h and monitored through TLC. The reaction solution was extracted with EtOAc and the solvent was removed from the organic layer under reduced pressure. The extracts were then separated on silica gel CC (200–300 mesh) using a gradient of petroleum ether-EtOAc from 9:1 to 4:1 (v/v). Compound **5** (16.2 mg) was obtained through the elution of 500 mL petroleum ether-EtOAc eluent at a 9:1 (v/v) eluent ratio, and compound **7** (12.8 mg) was obtained through subsequent elution. When the ratio of the petroleum ether-EtOAc eluent was 85:15 (v/v), compounds **8** and **6** could be obtained, of which compound **6** had a low content, and compounds **8** (18.9 mg) and **6** (4.5 mg) were then obtained using the semipreparative HPLC (80% MeOH-H_2O). Subsequently, semipreparative HPLC (70% MeOH-H_2O) was used to obtain compounds **10** (23.5 mg), **9** (5.2 mg), and **11** (7.9 mg), wherein compound **10** was the main reaction product. The unreacted starting compound **1** was finally eluted with a petroleum ether-EtOAc eluent ratio of 4:1 (v/v).

Their structures were all identified using the NMR data and HRESIMS spectroscopy Compounds **5** and **6** were new terphenyllin derivatives, and named 3′,4,4″-tris(allyloxy)-2′,5′-dimethoxy-1,1′:4′,1″-terphenyl (**5**) and 3′,4″-bis(allyloxy)-2′,5′-dimethoxy-[1,1′:4′,1″-terphenyl]-4-ol (**6**), respectively. Compounds **7–11** were identified using the NMR and ESIMS data, the details of which are added in the supplementary data.

3′,4,4″-tris(allyloxy)-2′,5′-dimethoxy-1,1′:4′,1″-terphenyl (**5**), White, amorphous powder; ^{1}H NMR (400 MHz, acetone-d_6) δ 7.57 (2H, d, J = 8.8 Hz), 7.30 (2H, d, J = 8.6 Hz), 7.03 (2H, d, J = 8.8 Hz), 6.98 (2H, d, J = 8.6 Hz), 6.77 (1H, s), 6.12 (2H, m), 5.78 (1H, m), 5.46 (1H, dd, J = 17.2 Hz, 1.8 Hz), 5.27 (1H, dd, J = 10.6, 1.8 Hz), 5.13 (1H, dd, J = 17.2, 1.8 Hz), 5.01 (1H, dd, J = 10.6, 1.8 Hz), 4.64 (2H, d, J = 5.2 Hz), 4.62 (2H, d, J = 5.2 Hz), 4.28 (2H, d, J = 5.2 Hz), 3.74 (3H, s), 3.56 (3H, s); ^{13}C NMR (100 MHz, acetone-d_6) δ 159.0 (C), 158.6 (C), 154.2 (C), 151.7 (C), 145.8 (C), 135.5 (C), 135.1 (CH), 134.9 (CH), 134.8 (CH), 132.8 (CH × 2), 131.7(C), 131.1 (CH × 2), 127.3(C), 125.2(C), 117.4 (CH_2), 117.3 (CH_2), 116.8 (CH_2), 115.2 (CH × 2), 114.6 (CH × 2), 108.8 (CH), 74.5 (CH_2), 69.3 (CH_2), 69.2 (CH_2), 60.9 (CH_3), 56.3 (CH_3). (+)-HR-ESI-MS m/z 459.2149 [M + H]$^+$, (calcd for $C_{29}H_{31}O_5$, 459.2166).

3′,4″-bis(allyloxy)-2′,5′-dimethoxy-[1,1′:4′,1″-terphenyl]-4-ol (**6**); White, amorphous powder; ^{1}H NMR (400 MHz, acetone-d_6) δ 8.49 (1H, s), 7.48 (2H, d, J = 8.8 Hz), 7.30 (2H, d, J = 8.8 Hz), 6.98 (2H, d, J = 8.8 Hz), 6.93 (2H, d, J = 8.8 Hz), 6.75 (1H, s), 6.12 (1H, ddt, J = 17.2, 10.5, 5.2 Hz), 5.78 (1H, ddd, J = 22.7, 10.7, 5.5 Hz), 5.45 (1H, dd, J = 17.2, 1.8 Hz), 5.27 (1H, dd, J = 10.6, 1.5 Hz), 5.13 (1H, dd, J = 17.2, 1.8 Hz), 5.01 (1H, dd, J = 10.6, 1.5 Hz), 4.62 (2H, dt, J = 5.1, 1.4 Hz), 4.28 (2H, dt, J = 5.4, 1.3 Hz), 3.73 (3H, s), 3.56 (3H, s); ^{13}C NMR (100 MHz, acetone-d_6) δ 158.5 (C), 157.8 (C), 154.1 (C), 151.7 (C), 145.8 (C), 135.6 (C), 135.4 (CH), 134.9 (CH), 132.9 (CH × 2), 131.2 (CH × 2), 130.5 (C), 127.4 (C), 125.0 (C), 117.3(CH_2), 116.8(CH_2), 115.9 (CH × 2), 114.6 (CH × 2), 108.8 (CH), 74.5 (CH_2), 69.3 (CH_2), 60.9 (CH_3), 56.3 (CH_3). (+)-HR-ESI-MS m/z 419.1841 [M + H]$^+$, (calcd for $C_{26}H_{27}O_5$, 419.1853).

3.5. Biology

3.5.1. Animals

Zerafish (Danio rerio) were maintained on a 14/10 h light/dark cycle at 28 °C and fed twice daily. *To(kras^{G12V})* and LiPan mutants were gifts from the laboratory of Zhi-yuan Gong (National University of Singapore). Zebrafish embryos were obtained through natural hybridization. To prevent melanin from affecting the liver cancer, the embryo medium was supplemented with 0.003% (w/v) 2-phenylthiourea. All experimental protocols were approved by and conducted in accordance with the Ethical Committee of Experimental Animal Care, Ocean University of China.

3.5.2. Cell Lines

Panc-1, HCT116, A549, HeLa, Hep G2, U2OS, U251, DU145, TE-1, BT549, MCF7, and HCT8 were from ATCC; RCC4 cell was gifted from Wuhan Xiao (Institute of Hydrobiology, Chinese Academy of Sciences) and cultured in high-glucose DMEM (Hyclone, Logan, UT, USA) with 10% FBS (PAN, Germany) and antibiotics (100 units/mL penicillin and 100 mg/mL streptomycin sulfate) at 37 °C in 5% CO_2. The cell lines were analyzed with short tandem repeat profiling by ShCellBank (Shanghai, China). The contamination by mycoplasmas in culture cells was tested using the EZ-PCR Mycoplasmas Detection Kit (BI, Kibbutz Beit-Haemek, Israel) every three months.

3.5.3. Antibody and Regent

The antibodies against Actin (abs137975) and Tubulin (abs137976) were obtained from Absin Bioscience. The antibodies against cleaved-PARP1 (13371-1-AP), cleaved-caspase-3 (40924), Cytochrome C (10993-1-AP), and BAD (10435-1-AP) were purchased from Proteintech. CCK8 and DMSO were purchased from Sigma (St. Louis, MO, USA). Enhanced chemiluminescence liquid (ECL) was from Sparkjade (Jinan, China). PVDF membranes were obtained from Millipore (Boston, MA, USA). Secondary antibodies against primary antibodies were provided from Millipore (Darmstadt, Germany). Chemical reagents were from Sinopharm (Shanghai, China).

3.5.4. Cytotoxic Activity of Triphenol Derivatives

The cytotoxic activity of all the compounds, **1–11**, was detected using the CCK8 assay. Cells were seeded in 96-well plates at a density of approximately 4000 cells per well. After allowing the cells to adhere, they were treated with different concentrations of the derivatives for 72 h. Following the treatment period, a CCK8 solution (10%) was added to each well and incubated for an additional 2 h. The absorbance of the samples was then measured at 450 nm using a plate reader. Based on the absorbance readings, the cell viability and IC_{50} (half-maximal inhibitory concentration) values were calculated to assess the cytotoxicity of the derivatives.

3.5.5. Plate Clone Formation Assay

BT549 cells were seeded in 3.5 cm dishes at a density of 200 cells per well. The cells were then treated with CHNQD-00824 at concentrations ranging between 0 and 8 µM for a period of 13 days. During this time, the growth medium was replaced every 3 days to maintain cell viability. After the treatment period, the cells were washed three times with pre-cooled phosphate-buffered saline (PBS) for 5 min each time. Subsequently, the cells were incubated with a 0.4% paraformaldehyde (Sigma, St. Louis, MO, USA) solution for 30 min. Following another three washes with pre-cooled PBS, the cells were stained with a 0.5% crystal violet solution for 30 min. The excess crystal violet (Sangon, Shanghai, China) solution was then rinsed off to remove any unbound dye. The samples were photographed and observed under an inverted microscope. Clonal populations consisting of more than 50 cells were considered as individual clones and were counted.

3.5.6. Cell Proliferation Assay

BT549 cells were divided into 24-well plates with 1000 cells per well. After allowing the cells to adhere, cells were treated with CHNQD-00824 at a concentration of 5 µM. The DMSO-treated group was used as a negative control. Three wells of each treatment group were digested every 24 h and counted separately using an Automated Cell Counter (LUNA-II, logos biosystems). Counts were performed for 7 consecutive days. A cell proliferation curve was drawn to compare the cell proliferation rate.

3.5.7. The Scratch Assay

Cells were seeded into 12-well plates at a density of approximately 5×10^5 cells per well. Once the cells reached confluency and formed a monolayer, a 200 µL tip was used to create a scratch across the surface of the cells, ensuring an even and consistent scratch. The suspended cells were then removed by gently washing the wells with PBS solution. Next, serum-free medium containing different concentrations of CHNQD-00824 (ranging between 0 and 10 µM) was added to each well. The plates were then incubated for a specified time period, such as 0 h, 12 h, and 24 h. At each time point, the scratches were imaged using an inverted microscope. The Image-J software (version 10.0.5, Media Cybernetics Inc., Rockville, Maryland) was used to measure the area of the scratch, allowing for a quantification of cell migration. By comparing the scratch area at different time points, the rate of cell migration can be assessed.

3.5.8. Cell Cycle Analysis

BT549 cells were plated in a 6 cm dish at a density of 2×10^6 per well. After adherence, the cells were treated with CHNQD-00824 (0–1 µM) for 24 h. The cells were digested with pancreatic enzymes and rehung in 1.5 mL medium. Then, the cells were washed twice with pre-cooled PBS. The cells were then suspended with 70% ethanol and frozen at $-20\ °C$ overnight. After centrifugation to remove 70% ethanol, they were washed twice with pre-cooling PBS. Then, the cells were stained with a propidium iodide solution (Yeasen, Shanghai, China). The results were detected through flow cytometry and analyzed using Flowjo.

3.5.9. Cell Apoptosis Assay

Approximately 2×10^6 cells per well were seeded in a 6 cm dish and incubated until the cell adhered to the well. Then, the cells were treated with CHNQD-00824 (0–1 µM) for 24 h. The cells were digested with EDTA-free pancreatic enzymes and then suspended, then washed twice with pre-cooled PBS. The PBS was removed through centrifugation and the staining solution (Yeasen, Shanghai, China) containing Annexin V/FITC-PI was added. Reaction at room temperature and away from light for 10–15 min. The apoptosis was evaluated through flow cytometry and analyzed using Flowjo.

3.5.10. Western Blotting Assay

BT549 cells were seeded in 6-well plates and treated with CHNQD-00824 for 24 h. Then, the cells were collected and lysed with loading buffer. The protein lysates were then separated using SDS-PAGE (Sangon, Shanghai, China) and transferred into nitrocellulose membranes (Millipore, Billerica, MA, USA). To prevent non-specific binding, the membranes were blocked with skim milk powder for 2 h. Then, membranes were incubated overnight with specific primary antibodies at 4 °C and secondary antibodies at room temperature for 2 h. The enhanced chemiluminescence kit was then prepared and added to the membranes in drops, and photographed and analyzed using a protein imager (Universal Hood II, BIO-RAD, Milan, Italy).

3.5.11. AO Staining Assay

Zebrafish embryos were obtained by mating wild-type female and male zebrafish. The embryos were then cultured in embryo medium containing PTU until they reached

24 h post-fertilization (hpf). After the 24 h culture period, the embryos were treated with varying concentrations of CHNQD-00824, ranging from 0 to 15 μM, for an additional 24 h. Following the treatment, the embryos were stained with acridine orange (AO) at a concentration of 2 μg/mL for 30 min. The stained embryos were then washed three times with embryo culture medium to remove any excess dye. The results were visualized and photographed using a fluorescence microscope (SMZ645, Nikon, Tokyo, Japan). The Image-pro-plus software (version 10.0.5, Media Cybernetics Inc., Rockville, Maryland) was used to analyze the images and quantify the results obtained from the stained embryos.

3.5.12. In Vivo Anticancer Assay of Zebrafish

$To(kras^{G12V})$ genotype female and male zebrafish were mated to obtain embryos. Embryos were cultured to 3 dpf in embryo medium containing PTU and then embryos were treated with CHNQD-00824 (0–5 μM) and DOX (60 mg/L, Sangon, China) for 4 days in embryo medium containing PTU. The embryo culture medium was changed once at 5 dpf. At 7 dpf, zebrafish were anesthetized with tracaine (0.08%, w/v) and transferred to methyl-cellulose (2%, w/v) for photo observation. The results were photographed using a fluorescence microscope and analyzed using image-pro-plus.

3.5.13. Statistics

The Prism 8 software was used for statistical analysis. The results were shown as the mean ± SD. For all data, p-value < 0.05 was considered statistically significant.

4. Conclusions

The findings of this study highlight the discovery of a terphenyllin derivative called CHNQD-00824 from the marine compound library. CHNQD-00824 has shown potential as an anticancer agent. Moreover, further investigations revealed that CHNQD-00824 has the ability to induce DNA damage. DNA damage is a crucial mechanism in cancer treatment as it can lead to cell death or inhibit cell proliferation. This finding suggests that CHNQD-00824 may be acting through a mechanism that disrupts the integrity of cancer cell DNA. In addition to its activity against multiple cell lines in vitro, CHNQD-00824 was evaluated in a DOX-induced liver-specific enlargement model in zebrafish. In this model, CHNQD-00824 significantly suppressed tumor growth when administered at a concentration of 5 μM. Zebrafish have emerged as a valuable model organism in cancer research, complementing the insights gained from murine models and cell culture systems. Their small size, rapid development, genetic conservation, and ease of genome manipulation make them an excellent tool for studying tumor initiation, progression, and response to treatment. This observation suggests that CHNQD-00824 may have potential in inhibiting tumor growth in vivo, making it a promising candidate for further development as a cancer drug agent. Further research is needed to explore the mechanisms, pharmacokinetics, and safety profile of CHNQD-00824 in order to assess its clinical potential.

Supplementary Materials: The following supporting information can be downloaded at: https://www.mdpi.com/article/10.3390/md21100512/s1, Figure S1–S33: 1H NMR, 13C NMR. Figure S34: Fermentation yield comparison chart. Figure S35: UPLC analysis of the reaction process of terphenyllin **1** treated with allyl bromide (2.5 equivalent).

Author Contributions: X.-Z.C. contributed to preparation of all compounds and writing—original draft, writing—review and editing; B.-Q.Z. contributed to related work of cytotoxic activity, writing—original draft, writing—review and editing; C.-F.W. contributed to providing the active compound and investigation; J.-N.Y., W.H. and G.S. contributed to the compounds and their derivatives; M.-Y.W. and L.L. were the project leaders, organizing and guiding the experiments and manuscript writing. All authors have read and agreed to the published version of the manuscript.

Funding: This work was supported by the Qingdao Marine Science and Technology Center (No 2022QNLM030003-2), the National Natural Science Foundation of China (Nos. 42006092, U1706210 and 41322037), the National Key Research and Development Program of China (No. 2022YFC2601305), the Shandong Province Special Fund "Frontier Technology and Free Exploration" from Laoshan Laboratory (No. 8-01), and the Fundamental Research Funds for the Central Universities (No. 202264001)

Data Availability Statement: The data are contained within the article or Supplementary Material.

Acknowledgments: We thank Xiu-Li Zhang and Cong Wang at the School of Medicine and Pharmacy, Ocean University of China, for the NMR analysis. We are also grateful to Tong-Yi Xu, Department of Cardiovascular and Thoracic Surgery, No. 971 Hospital of PLA Navy, for the helpful discussions of the work. We are thankful to Professor Zhi-yuan Gong, National University of Singapore, for providing the transgenic zebrafish lines.

Conflicts of Interest: The authors declare no conflict of interest.

References

1. Siegel, R.L.; Miller, K.D.; Jemal, A. Cancer statistics, 2020. *CA Cancer J. Clin.* **2020**, *70*, 7–30. [CrossRef] [PubMed]
2. Liang, W.H.; Guan, W.J.; Chen, R.C.; Wang, W.; Li, J.F.; Xu, K.; Li, C.C.; Ai, Q.; Lu, W.X.; Liang, H.R.; et al. Cancer patients in SARS-CoV-2 infection: A nationwide analysis in China. *Lancet Oncol.* **2020**, *21*, 335–337. [CrossRef] [PubMed]
3. Siegel, R.L.; Miller, K.D.; Wagle, N.S.; Jemal, A. Cancer statistics, 2023. *CA Cancer J. Clin.* **2023**, *73*, 17–48. [CrossRef]
4. Newman, D.J.; Cragg, G.M. Natural Products as Sources of New Drugs over the Nearly Four Decades from 01/1981 to 09/2019. *J. Nat. Prod.* **2020**, *83*, 770–803. [CrossRef] [PubMed]
5. Carroll, A.R.; Copp, B.R.; Davis, R.A.; Keyzers, R.A.; Prinsep, M.R. Marine natural products. *Nat. Prod. Rep.* **2022**, *39*, 1122–1171. [CrossRef]
6. Carroll, A.R.; Copp, B.R.; Davis, R.A.; Keyzers, R.A.; Prinsep, M.R. Marine natural products. *Nat. Prod. Rep.* **2023**, *40*, 275–325. [CrossRef]
7. Haque, N.; Parveen, S.; Tang, T.T.; Wei, J.E.; Huang, Z.N. Marine Natural Products in Clinical Use. *Mar. Drugs* **2022**, *20*, 528. [CrossRef]
8. Wang, C.F.; Ma, J.; Jing, Q.Q.; Cao, X.Z.; Chen, L.; Chao, R.; Zheng, J.Y.; Shao, C.L.; He, X.X.; Wei, M.Y. Integrating Activity-Guided Strategy and Fingerprint Analysis to Target Potent Cytotoxic Brefeldin A from a Fungal Library of the Medicinal Mangrove *Acanthus ilicifolius*. *Mar. Drugs* **2022**, *20*, 432. [CrossRef]
9. Lu, X.X.; Jiang, Y.Y.; Wu, Y.W.; Chen, G.Y.; Shao, C.L.; Gu, Y.C.; Liu, M.; Wei, M.Y. Semi-Synthesis, Cytotoxic Evaluation, and Structure—Activity Relationships of Brefeldin A Derivatives with Antileukemia Activity. *Mar. Drugs* **2022**, *20*, 26. [CrossRef]
10. Ren, X.H.; Xie, X.Y.; Chen, B.X.; Liu, L.; Jiang, C.Q.; Qian, Q. Marine Natural Products: A Potential Source of Anti-hepatocellular Carcinoma Drugs. *J. Med. Chem.* **2021**, *64*, 7879–7899. [CrossRef]
11. Lu, W.Y.; Li, H.J.; Li, Q.Y.; Wu, Y.C. Application of marine natural products in drug research. *Bioorgan. Med. Chem.* **2021**, *35*, 116058. [CrossRef] [PubMed]
12. Guo, F.W.; Zhang, Q.; Gu, Y.C.; Shao, C.L. Sulfur-containing marine natural products as leads for drug discovery and development. *Curr. Opin. Chem. Biol.* **2023**, *75*, 102330. [CrossRef] [PubMed]
13. Holland, D.C.; Carroll, A.R. Marine indole alkaloid diversity and bioactivity. What do we know and what are we missing? *Nat. Prod. Rep.* 2023; *advance article*. [CrossRef]
14. Maha, Z.F.; Hurley, L.H. Ecteinascidin 743: A minor groove alkylator that bends DNA toward the major groove. *J. Med. Chem.* **1999**, *42*, 1493–1497.
15. Uemura, D.; Takahashi, K.; Yamamoto, T. Norhalichondrin A: An antitumor polyether macrolide from a marine sponge. *J. Am. Chem. Soc.* **1985**, *107*, 4796–4798. [CrossRef]
16. Mayer, A.M.S.; Glaser, K.B.; Cuevas, C.; Jacobs, R.S.; Kem, W.; Little, R.D.; McIntosh, J.M.; Newman, D.J.; Potts, B.C.; Shuster, D.E. The odyssey of marine pharmaceuticals: A current pipeline perspective. *Trends Pharmacol. Sci.* **2010**, *31*, 255–265. [CrossRef]
17. Francisco, J.A.; Cerveny, C.G.; Meyer, D.L.; Mixan, B.J.; Klussman, K.; Chace, D.F.; Rejniak, S.X.; Gordon, K.A.; DeBlanc, R.; Toki, B.E. cAC10-vcMMAE, an anti-CD30-monomethyl auristatin E conjugate with potent and selective antitumor activity. *Blood* **2003**, *102*, 1458–1465. [CrossRef]
18. Tai, Y.T.; Mayes, P.A.; Acharya, C.; Zhong, M.Y.; Cea, M.; Cagnetta, A.; Craigen, J.; Yates, J.; Gliddon, L.; Fieles, W. Novel anti-B-cell maturation antigen antibody-drug conjugate (GSK2857916) selectively induces killing of multiple myeloma. *Blood* **2014**, *123*, 3128–3138. [CrossRef]
19. Hai, Y.; Wei, M.Y.; Wang, C.Y.; Gu, Y.C.; Shao, C.L. The intriguing chemistry and biology of sulfur-containing natural products from marine microorganisms (1987–2020). *Mar. Life Sci. Technol.* **2021**, *3*, 488–518. [CrossRef]
20. Hai, Y.; Cai, Z.M.; Li, P.D.; Wei, M.Y.; Wang, C.Y.; Gu, Y.C.; Shao, C.L. Trends of antimalarial marine natural products: Progresses, challenges and opportunities. *Nat. Prod. Rep.* **2022**, *39*, 969–990. [CrossRef]

21. Xu, W.F.; Wu, N.N.; Wu, Y.W.; Qi, Y.X.; Wei, M.Y.; Pineda, L.M.; Ng, M.G.; Spadafora, C.; Zheng, J.Y.; Lu, L. Structure modification, antialgal, antiplasmodial, and toxic evaluations of a series of new marine-derived 14-membered resorcylic acid lactone derivatives. *Mar. Life Sci. Technol.* **2022**, *4*, 88–97. [CrossRef]
22. Jiang, Y.Y.; Gao, Y.; Liu, J.Y.; Xu, Y.; Wei, M.Y.; Wang, C.Y.; Gu, Y.C.; Shao, C.L. Design and Characterization of a Natural Arf-GEFs Inhibitor Prodrug CHNQD-01255 with Potent Anti-Hepatocellular Carcinoma Efficacy in Vivo. *J. Med. Chem.* **2022**, *65*, 11970–11984. [CrossRef] [PubMed]
23. Chen, J.; Xu, L.; Zhang, X.Q.; Liu, X.; Zhang, Z.X.; Zhu, Q.M.; Liu, J.Y.; Iqbal, M.O.; Ding, N.; Shao, C.L.; et al. Discovery of a natural small-molecule AMP-activated kinase activator that alleviates nonalcoholic steatohepatitis. *Mar. Life Sci. Technol.* **2023**, *5*, 196–210. [CrossRef] [PubMed]
24. Zhang, X.Q.; Mou, X.F.; Mao, N.; Hao, J.J.; Liu, M.; Zheng, J.Y.; Wang, C.Y.; Gu, Y.C.; Shao, C.L. Design, semisynthesis, α-glucosidase inhibitory, cytotoxic, and antibacterial activities of p-terphenyl derivatives. *Eur. J. Med. Chem.* **2018**, *146*, 232–244. [CrossRef]
25. Haider, W.; Xu, W.F.; Liu, M.; Wu, Y.W.; Tang, Y.F.; Wei, M.Y.; Wang, C.Y.; Lu, L.; Shao, C.L. Structure-Activity Relationships and Potent Cytotoxic Activities of Terphenyllin Derivatives from a Small Compound Library. *Chem. Biodivers.* **2020**, *17*, e2000207. [CrossRef] [PubMed]
26. Bailly, C. Anti-inflammatory and anticancer p-terphenyl derivatives from fungi of the genus *Thelephora*. *Bioorgan. Med. Chem.* **2022**, *70*, 116935. [CrossRef] [PubMed]
27. Song, Y.J.; Zheng, H.B.; Peng, A.H.; Ma, J.H.; Lu, D.D.; Li, X.; Zhang, H.Y.; Xie, W.D. Strepantibins A–C: Hexokinase II inhibitors from a mud dauber wasp associated *Streptomyces* sp. *J. Nat. Prod.* **2019**, *82*, 1114–1119. [CrossRef]
28. Liu, J.K. Natural terphenyls: Developments since 1877. *Chem. Rev.* **2006**, *106*, 2209–2223.
29. Feng, D.Q.; Biftu, T.; Romero, F.A.; Kekec, A.; Dropinski, J.; Kassick, A.; Xu, S.Y.; Kurtz, M.M.; Gollapudi, A.; Shao, Q.; et al. Discovery of MK-8722: A systemic, direct pan-activator of AMP-activated protein kinase. *Med. Chem. Lett.* **2018**, *9*, 39–44. [CrossRef]
30. Marchelli, R.; Vining, L.C. Terphenyllin, a novel p-terphenyl metabolite from *Aspergillus candidus*. *J. Antibiot.* **1975**, *28*, 328–331. [CrossRef]
31. Kurobane, I.; Vining, L.C.; Mcinnes, A.G.; Smith, D.G. 3-Hydroxyterphenyllin, a new metabolite of *Aspergillus candidus*. *J. Antibio.* **1979**, *32*, 559–564. [CrossRef]
32. Wei, H.; Inada, H.; Hayashi, A.; Higashimoto, K.; Pruksakorn, P.; Kamada, S.; Arai, M.; Ishida, S.; Kobayashi, M. Prenylterphenyllin and its dehydroxyl analogs, new cytotoxic substances from a marine-derived fungus *Aspergillus candidus* IF10. *J. Antibiot.* **2007**, *60*, 586–590. [CrossRef] [PubMed]
33. Takahashi, C.; Yoshihira, K.; Natori, S.; Umeda, M.; Ohtsubo, K.; Saito, M. Toxic metabolites of *Aspergillus candidus*. *Cell. Mol. Life Sci.* **1974**, *30*, 529–530. [CrossRef] [PubMed]
34. Takahashi, C.; Yoshihira, K.; Natori, S.; Umeda, M. The structures of toxic metabolites of *Aspergillus candidus*. I. The compounds A and E, cytotoxic p-terphenyls. *Chem. Pharm. Bull.* **1976**, *24*, 613–620. [CrossRef] [PubMed]
35. Brix, N.; Samaga, D.; Belka, C.; Zitzelsberger, H.; Lauber, K. Analysis of clonogenic growth in vitro. *Nat. Protoc.* **2021**, *16*, 4963–4991. [CrossRef]
36. Lambert, A.W.; Pattabiraman, D.R.; Weinberg, R.A. Emerging Biological Principles of Metastasis. *Cell* **2017**, *168*, 670–691. [CrossRef]
37. Welch, D.R.; Hurst, D.R. Defining the Hallmarks of Metastasis. *Cancer Res.* **2019**, *79*, 3011–3027. [CrossRef]
38. Martinotti, S.; Ranzato, E. Scratch Wound Healing Assay. *Methods Mol. Biol.* **2020**, *2109*, 225–229.
39. Nagata, S. Apoptosis and Clearance of Apoptotic Cells. *Annu. Rev. Immunol.* **2018**, *36*, 489–517. [CrossRef]
40. Brown, J.S.; O'Carrigan, B.; Jackson, S.P.; Yap, T.A. Targeting DNA Repair in Cancer: Beyond PARP Inhibitors. *Cancer Discov.* **2017**, *7*, 20–37. [CrossRef]
41. Bui, N.L.; Pandey, V.; Zhu, T.; Ma, L.; Basappa, P.E.L. Bad phosphorylation as a target of inhibition in oncology. *Cancer Lett.* **2018**, *415*, 177–186. [CrossRef]
42. Kalpage, H.A.; Bazylianska, V.; Recanati, M.A.; Fite, A.; Liu, J.; Wan, J.; Mantena, N.; Malek, M.H.; Podgorski, I.; Heath, E.I.; et al. Tissue-specific regulation of cytochrome c by post-translational modifications: Respiration, the mitochondrial membrane potential, ROS, and apoptosis. *FASEB J.* **2019**, *33*, 1540–1553. [CrossRef] [PubMed]
43. Sharma, A.; Singh, K.; Almasan, A. Histone H2AX phosphorylation: A marker for DNA damage. *Methods Mol. Biol.* **2012**, *920*, 613–626. [PubMed]
44. Eimon, P.M.; Ashkenazi, A. The zebrafish as a model organism for the study of apoptosis. *Apoptosis* **2010**, *15*, 331–349. [CrossRef] [PubMed]
45. Santoriello, C.; Zon, L.I. Hooked! Modeling human disease in zebrafish. *J. Clin. Investig.* **2012**, *122*, 2337–2343. [CrossRef] [PubMed]
46. Langheinrich, U. Zebrafish: A new model on the pharmaceutical catwalk. *BioEssays* **2003**, *25*, 904–912. [CrossRef]
47. Letrado, P.; Miguel, I.D.; Lamberto1, I.; Díez-Martínez, R.; Oyarzabal, J. Zebrafish: Speeding Up the Cancer Drug Discovery Process. *Cancer Res.* **2018**, *78*, 6048–6058. [CrossRef]

48. Loibl, S.; Poortmans, P.; Morrow, M.; Denkert, C.; Curigliano, G. Breast cancer. *Lancet* **2021**, *397*, 1750–1769. [CrossRef]
49. Wang, S.; Li, X.M.; Teuscher, F.; Li, D.L.; Diesel, A.; Ebel, R.; Proksch, P.; Wang, B.G. Chaetopyranin, a benzaldehyde derivative, and other related metabolites from Chaetomium globosum, an endophytic fungus derived from the marine red alga Poly-siphonia urceolata. *J. Nat. Prod.* **2006**, *69*, 1622–1625. [CrossRef]

Disclaimer/Publisher's Note: The statements, opinions and data contained in all publications are solely those of the individual author(s) and contributor(s) and not of MDPI and/or the editor(s). MDPI and/or the editor(s) disclaim responsibility for any injury to people or property resulting from any ideas, methods, instructions or products referred to in the content.

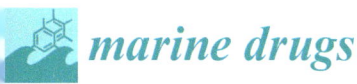

Article

Echinochrome Ameliorates Physiological, Immunological, and Histopathological Alterations Induced by Ovalbumin in Asthmatic Mice by Modulating the Keap1/Nrf2 Signaling Pathway

Islam Ahmed Abdelmawgood [1], Noha Ahmed Mahana [1], Abeer Mahmoud Badr [1], Ayman Saber Mohamed [1,*], Abdeljalil Mohamed Al Shawoush [2], Tarek Atia [3], Amir Elhadi Abdelrazak [4] and Hader I. Sakr [4,5]

1 Zoology Department, Faculty of Science, Cairo University, Giza 12613, Egypt
2 Zoology Department, Faculty of Science, Sirte University, Sirte 128123, Libya; sedra200713@yahoo.com
3 Department of Medical Laboratory Sciences, College of Applied Medical Sciences, Prince Sattam bin Abdulaziz University, Al-Kharj 11942, Saudi Arabia; t.mohamed@psau.edu.sa
4 Department of Medical Physiology, Medicine Program, Batterjee Medical College, Jeddah 21442, Saudi Arabia; physiology10.jed@bmc.edu.sa (A.E.A.); hadersakr@kasralainy.edu.eg (H.I.S.)
5 Department of Medical Physiology, Faculty of Medicine, Cairo University, Cairo 11562, Egypt
* Correspondence: ayman81125@cu.edu.eg

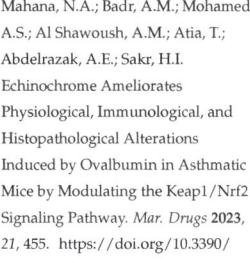

Citation: Abdelmawgood, I.A.; Mahana, N.A.; Badr, A.M.; Mohamed, A.S.; Al Shawoush, A.M.; Atia, T.; Abdelrazak, A.E.; Sakr, H.I. Echinochrome Ameliorates Physiological, Immunological, and Histopathological Alterations Induced by Ovalbumin in Asthmatic Mice by Modulating the Keap1/Nrf2 Signaling Pathway. *Mar. Drugs* 2023, 21, 455. https://doi.org/10.3390/md21080455

Academic Editor: Chang-Lun Shao

Received: 22 July 2023
Revised: 15 August 2023
Accepted: 16 August 2023
Published: 18 August 2023

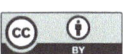

Copyright: © 2023 by the authors. Licensee MDPI, Basel, Switzerland. This article is an open access article distributed under the terms and conditions of the Creative Commons Attribution (CC BY) license (https:// creativecommons.org/licenses/by/ 4.0/).

Abstract: Asthma is a persistent inflammatory disease of the bronchi characterized by oxidative stress, airway remodeling, and inflammation. Echinochrome (Ech) is a dark-red pigment with antioxidant and anti-inflammatory activities. In this research, we aimed to investigate the effects of Ech against asthma-induced inflammation, oxidative stress, and histopathological alterations in the spleen, liver, and kidney in mice. Mice were divided into four groups (n = 8 for each): control, asthmatic, and asthmatic mice treated intraperitoneally with 0.1 and 1 mg/kg of Ech. In vitro, findings confirmed the antioxidant and anti-inflammatory activities of Ech. Ech showed antiasthmatic effects by lowering the serum levels of immunoglobulin E (IgE), interleukin 4 (IL-4), and interleukin 1β (IL-1β). It attenuated oxidative stress by lowering malondialdehyde (MDA) and nitric oxide (NO) contents and increasing reduced glutathione (GSH), superoxide dismutase (SOD), glutathione-s-transferase (GST), and catalase (CAT) in the liver, spleen, and kidney. Moreover, it protected asthma-induced kidney and liver functions by increasing total protein and albumin and decreasing aspartate aminotransferase (AST), alanine aminotransferase (ALT), creatinine, urea, and uric acid levels. Additionally, it ameliorated histopathological abnormalities in the lung, liver, spleen, and kidney. Additionally, molecular docking studies were used to examine the interactions between Ech and Kelch-like ECH-associated protein 1 (Keap1). PCR and Western blot analyses confirmed the association of Ech with Keap1 and, consequently, the regulatory role of Ech in the Keap1-(nuclear factor erythroid 2-related factor 2) Nrf2 signaling pathway in the liver, spleen, and kidney. According to our findings, Ech prevented asthma and its complications in the spleen, liver, and kidney. Inhibition of inflammation and oxidative stress are two of echinochrome's therapeutic actions in managing asthma by modulating the Keap1/Nrf2 signaling pathway.

Keywords: echinochrome; asthma; ovalbumin; oxidative stress; inflammation; Keap1; Nrf2

1. Introduction

Asthma is a common chronic lung condition characterized by bronchial hyperreactivity, inflammation, and structural and functional alterations of the airways. Asthma affects approximately 235 million individuals globally [1]. Asthma development has been reported to be significantly influenced by differences in Th1/Th2 responses. Increased production of Th2-type cytokines, such as interleukin (IL)-4, IL-5, and IL-13, has been associated with uncontrolled Th2 immune responses. These cytokines cause tissue structure and function changes, eosinophil infiltration, bronchial inflammation, mucus hyperproduction, and immunoglobulin E (IgE) synthesis [2,3]. IL-4 drives the polarization of T lymphocytes towards Th2 cells, which in turn triggers the generation of more IL-4, which stimulates the switch of B cells to IgE release and the infiltration of mast cells and eosinophils [4]. Combining these effects results in airway constriction and hyperresponsiveness. Therefore, reducing the levels of these cytokines may alleviate asthmatic symptoms.

Additionally, the pathogenesis of asthma is greatly affected by oxidative stress, and the asthmatic condition is frequently associated with oxidative stress [5]. Oxidative stress harms liver and kidney function [6,7]. Oxidative stress, an essential contributor to liver disorders, develops when there are elevated levels of reactive oxygen species (ROS), and this will finally result in the loss of homeostasis [8]. The pathophysiology of kidney diseases has been associated with excessive ROS production and depletion of antioxidant defense mechanisms, resulting in tissue injury through various processes, including the propagation of lipid peroxidation [9]. The spleen is an essential supporting organ for maintaining bodily homeostasis. The spleen, as an essential part of the body's immune system, is a barrier and blood filter [10]. Although it is the most fundamental organ to experience stress, there are no longer any statistics on it when oxidative stress is present. Therefore, it is critical to attenuate oxidative stress and its deleterious impact on the body's organs.

One of the most crucial defensive systems against oxidative stress intimately linked to inflammatory illnesses is the Kelch-like ECH-associated protein 1/nuclear factor erythroid 2-related factor 2 (Keap1/Nrf2) pathway [11]. By controlling Keap1, Nrf2 exerts potent anti-inflammatory effects. Since many diseases are characterized by oxidative stress and inflammation, pharmacological stimulation of Nrf2 is a potentially effective therapeutic method for treating and preventing many conditions [12]. Echinochrome (Ech)'s possible binding mechanism with Keap1 is to disrupt the Keap1/Nrf2 protein–protein interaction and activate Nrf2 signaling, which was investigated using molecular docking simulations.

To manage symptoms, enhance pulmonary function, and improve patient outcomes, inhaled corticosteroids (ICS) and bronchodilators are the recommended primary medications for respiratory problems. Nevertheless, prolonged ICS administration has been linked to evident harmful effects [13]. Surprisingly, most marine species have various pharmacological actions, including antibacterial, antiviral, antiparasitic, anti-inflammatory, and antidiabetic properties [14]. Ech, a naturally occurring pigment extracted from the shells and spines of sea urchins, has been shown to have antioxidant properties and to be helpful in various diseases [15]. A previous study showed that Ech possesses antifibrotic and anti-inflammatory properties by suppressing fibroblast stimulation and proinflammatory cytokine expression [16]. It has been reported that Ech treatment showed protective effects on the kidney and liver by eliminating the production of ROS in these tissues [17,18]. Therefore, the purpose of the current research was to determine the antiasthmatic mechanisms of Ech on the liver, kidney, and spleen of asthmatic mice.

2. Results

2.1. High-Performance Liquid Chromatography (HPLC)

As illustrated in Figure 1, the HPLC analyses of separated Ech showed a notable peak with a retention period of 7.11 min, which is the same as the standard Ech with a total concentration of 85.5%.

2.2. In Vitro Antioxidant and Anti-Inflammatory Activities

In vitro studies confirmed the antioxidant and anti-inflammatory properties of Ech. Ech's antioxidant properties were dose-dependent (Figure 2a). The anti-inflammatory activity of Ech was validated by its ability to protect the membrane of red blood cells from heat-induced hemolysis at a range of concentrations (Figure 2b).

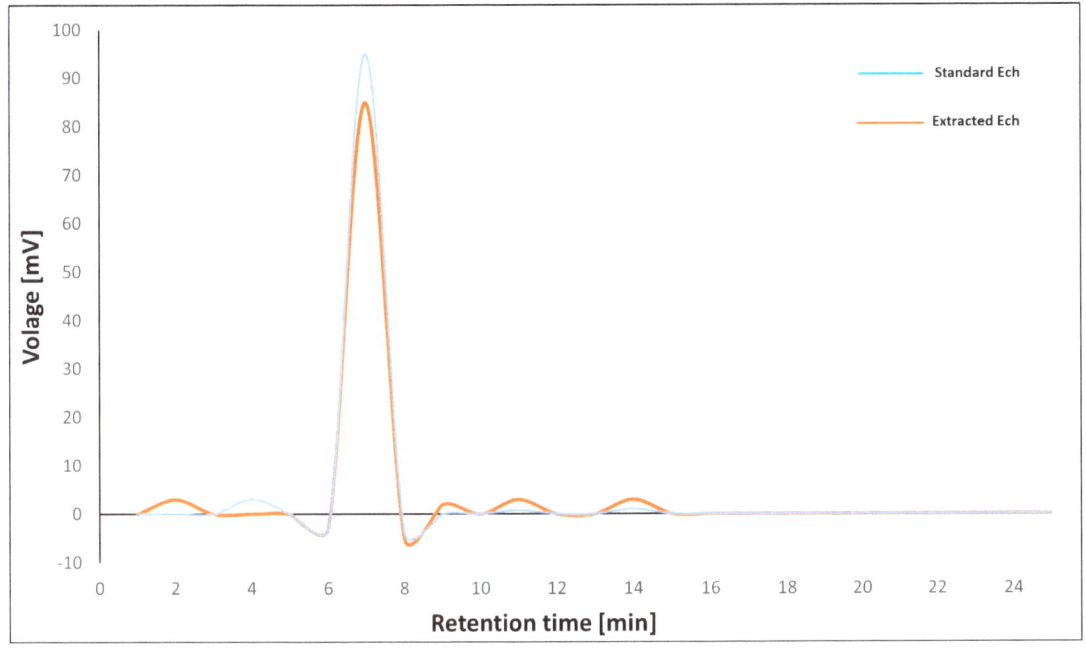

Figure 1. HPLC chromatograph of standard Ech and extracted Ech from sea urchin.

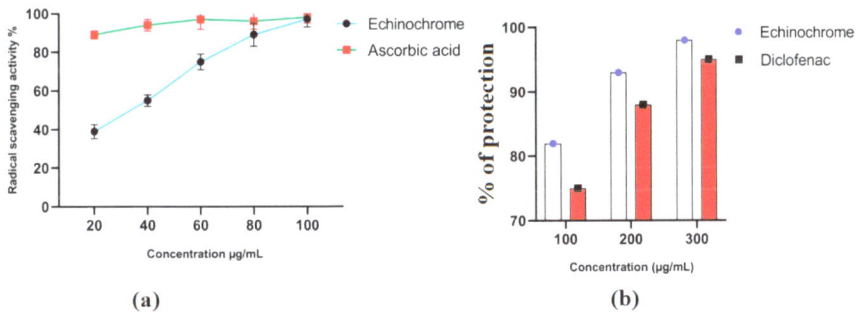

Figure 2. In vitro biological activities of Ech. (**a**) Antioxidant activity measured using 2,2-Diphenyl-1-picrylhydrazyl (DPPH) assay. (**b**) Anti-inflammatory activity using heat-induced hemolysis.

2.3. Molecular Docking Interaction between Ech and Keap1

Grid box dimensions in Table 1 were used in the docking of Ech to Keap1. The docking score of Ech binding with Keap1 was −7.9 kcal/mol. Ech three-dimensional visualization showcased several favorable interactions in the binding site of the target protein, including several hydrogen bonds, hydrophobic interactions, and π-stacking. Visualization of the protein–ligand complex revealed a total of six hydrogen bonds with target residues Y334, S363, N382, N387, N414, and S602; it exhibited strong hydrophobic interactions with Y334, Y572, and F577. Ech's aromatic ring forms π–π stacking with the aromatic ring of Y334 (Figure 3). Two-dimensional visualization of the protein–ligand complex confirmed the three-dimensional results (Figure 4). Ech formed two hydrogen bonds with residues S363 and S602 in addition to seven hydrophobic interactions with residues R380, N382, N387, N414, R415, A556, and G603. Pi-stacking was also present between the aromatic rings of Ech and Y334.

Table 1. The docking interaction data calculations of Ech and Keap1.

Protein–Ligand Interactions Profile					
Index	Residue	Amino Acid	Distance (Å)	Ligand Atom	Type of Interaction
1	334B	TYR	3.54 (3.08)	19 O [O3]	Hydrogen bond acceptor
2	363B	SER	2.95 (2.06)	16 H [O2]	Hydrogen bond acceptor
3	382B	ASN	3.88 (3.36)	21 O [O3]	Hydrogen bond acceptor
4	387A	ASN	3.08 (2.15)	19 O [O3]	Hydrogen bond donor
5	414B	ASN	4.04 (3.24)	16 H [O2]	Hydrogen bond donor
6	602B	SER	2.88 (2.35)	17 O [O3]	Hydrogen bond acceptor
7	334B	TYR	3.85	1 O	Hydrophobic interaction
8	572B	TYR	3.79	2 O	Hydrophobic interaction
9	577B	PHE	3.63	1 O	Hydrophobic interaction
10	334 B	TYR	3.88	5 C, 6 C, 7 C, 8 C, 9 C, 10 C	π-Stacking

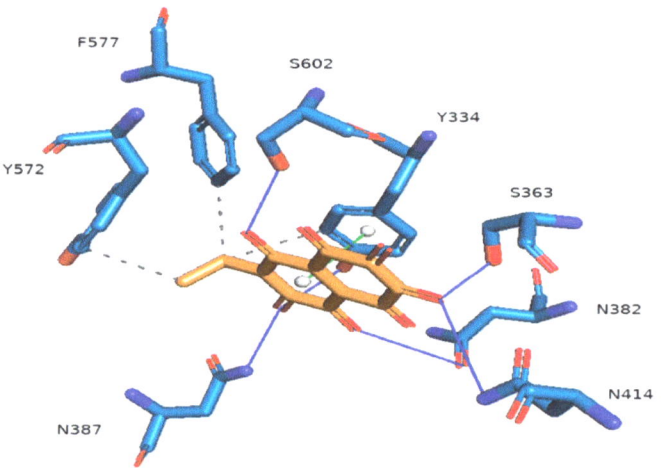

Figure 3. Three-dimensional visualization of Keap1–Ech binding complex showcasing favorable steric interactions, including a total of six hydrogen bonds with target residues Y334, S363, N382, N387, N414, and S602, strong hydrophobic interactions with Y334, Y572, and F577, and π–π stacking interaction with the aromatic ring of Y334.

2.4. Effect of Ech on Morphology, Body Weight, and Nasal Scratching

The lung, liver, spleen, and kidney weights in OVA-challenged animals increased significantly compared to control animals. Remarkably, treatment with Ech (1 mg/kg) significantly ($p > 0.05$) improved the weight of the organs (Figure 5). Moreover, the OVA group had a significantly ($p < 0.05$) higher nasal scratching score than the control groups. Compared to the OVA group, the nasal scratching score significantly decreased after treatment with the high dose of Ech. The overall organ morphologies are represented in Figure 6.

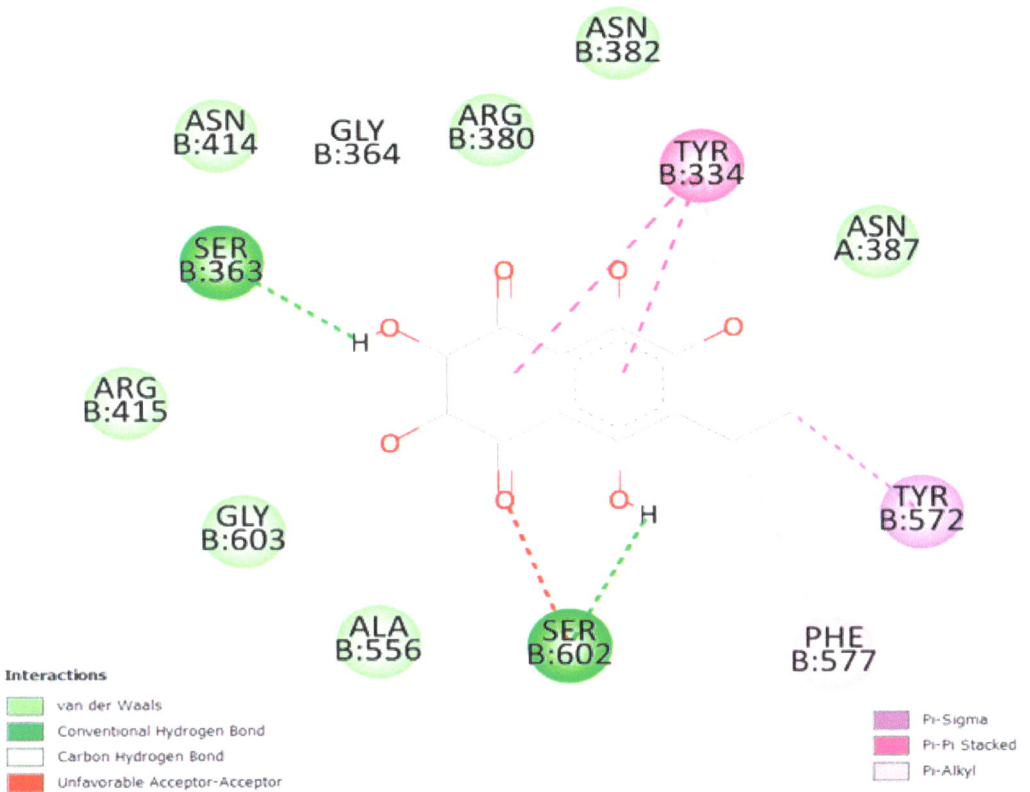

Figure 4. Two-dimensional visualization of the Keap1–Ech complex showcasing a total of two hydrogen bonds with binding site residues S363 and S602 as well as a total of seven hydrophobic interactions with residues N382, N387, N414, R415, A556, and G603, and pi-stacking with the aromatic ring of Y334.

2.5. Ech Reduced the Serum Levels of IgE, IL-4, and IL-1β

IgE, IL-4, and IL-1β levels increased significantly ($p < 0.05$) in OVA mice. However, Ech treatment dose-dependently reduced their concentrations, as shown in Figure 7.

2.6. Effect of Ech on Liver and Kidney Function

As shown in Figure 8, the OVA-challenged mice showed significantly higher levels of aspartate aminotransferase (AST), alanine aminotransferase (ALT), creatinine, uric acid, and urea compared to the control animals, with significantly lower levels of albumin and total protein. No noticeable difference was observed after treatment with 0.1 mg/kg Ech. In contrast to the OVA group, 1 mg/kg of Ech treatment significantly improved the liver and kidney function biomarkers ($p < 0.05$).

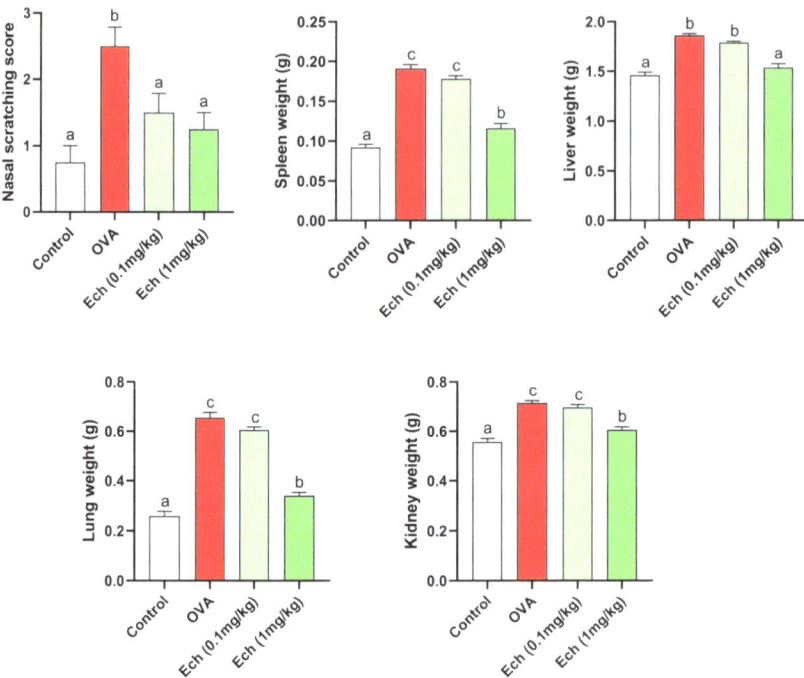

Figure 5. The effect of Ech on nasal scratching, lung, liver, kidney, and spleen weights. Values are given as means for 8 mice in each group ± standard error of the mean (SEM). The value that does not share a common letter superscript is significantly different ($p < 0.05$).

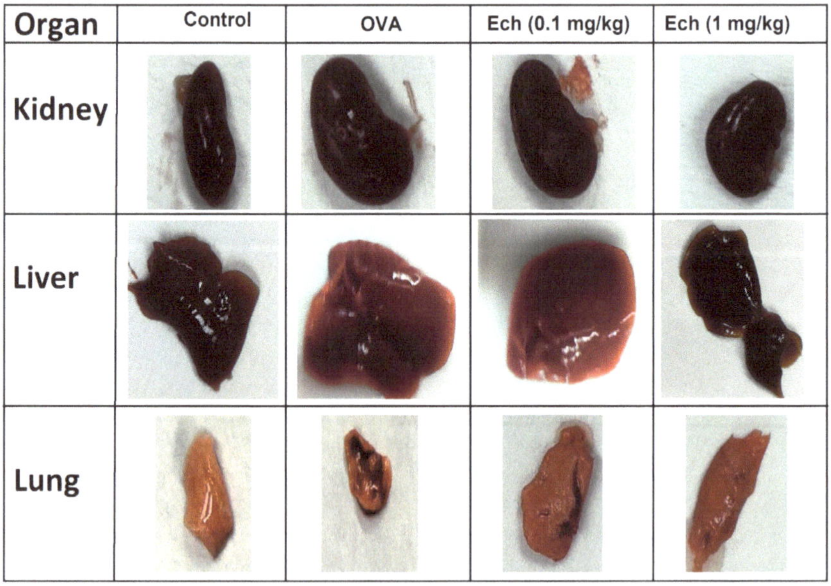

Figure 6. Organ morphology of the different groups.

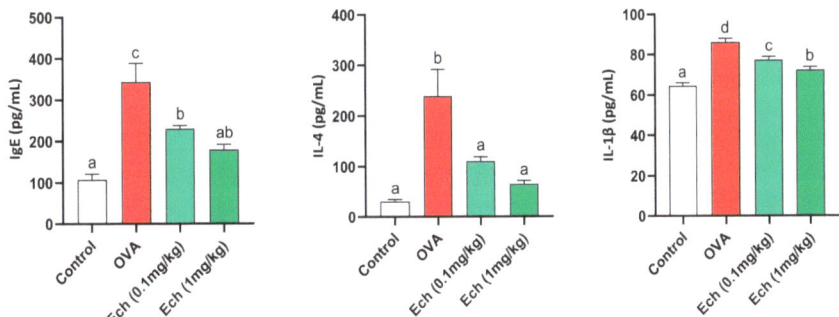

Figure 7. The effect of Ech on the serum levels of IgE, IL-4, and IL-1β. Values are given as means for 8 mice in each group ± standard error of the mean (SEM). The value that does not share a common letter superscript is significantly different ($p < 0.05$).

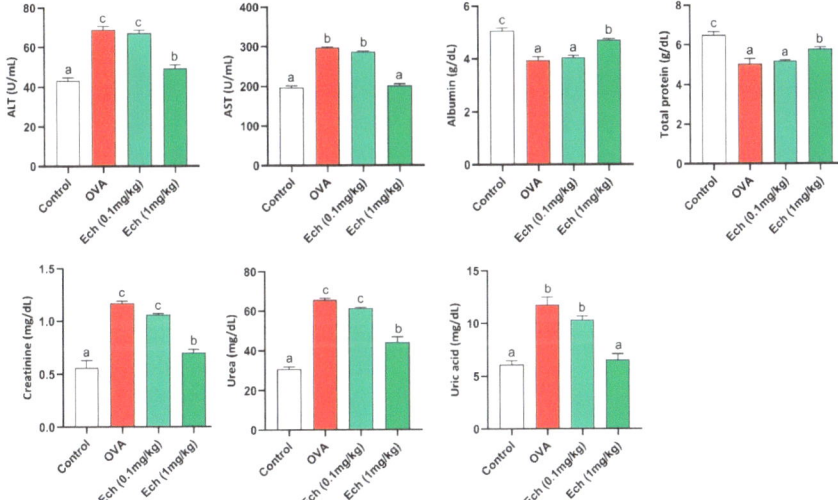

Figure 8. The effect of Ech on the liver functions parameters (AST, ALT, total protein, and albumin) and kidney function parameters (creatinine, urea, and uric acid). Values are given as means for 8 mice in each group ± standard error of the mean (SEM). The value that does not share a common letter superscript is significantly different ($p < 0.05$).

2.7. Effect of Ech on Keap1 and Nrf2 Protein Levels in the Liver, Kidney, and Spleen of Asthmatic Mice

To further evaluate the therapeutic effect of Ech, we measured the expression of Keap1 and Nrf2 in the liver, kidney, and spleen (Figure 9). In the OVA group, Keap1 expression was considerably upregulated ($p < 0.05$), but Nrf2 expression was significantly downregulated ($p < 0.05$). Keap1 protein levels were significantly decreased, and Nrf2 levels were significantly increased after administering Ech (high dose). These findings suggested that Ech could regulate the Keap1/Nrf2 signaling pathway with anti-inflammatory and antioxidant properties.

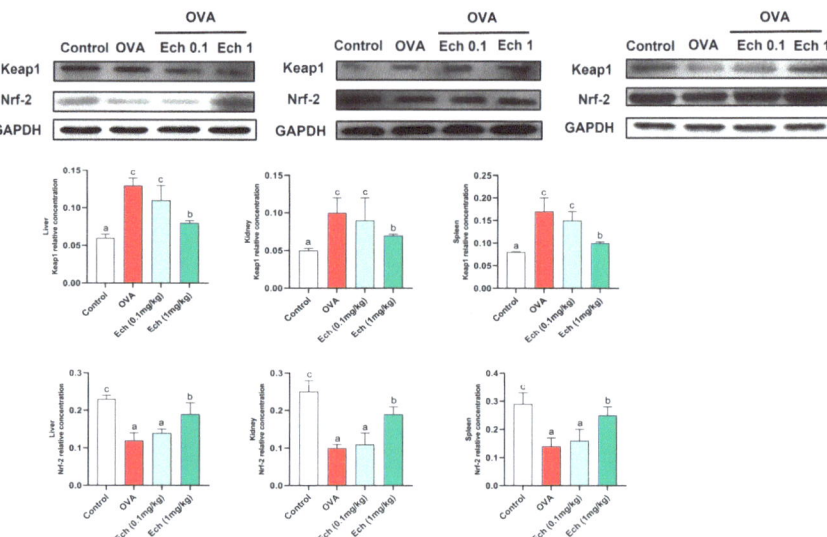

Figure 9. The effect of Ech on Keap1 and Nrf2 expression in the liver, kidney, and spleen of mice. The levels of Keap1 and Nrf2 proteins in the liver, kidney, and spleen were evaluated using Western blot with anti-GAPDH as a loading control. Values are given as means for 8 mice in each group ± standard error of the mean (SEM). The value that does not share a common letter superscript is significantly different ($p < 0.05$).

2.8. Effects of Ech on the Expression of Keap1 and Nrf2 Genes in the Liver, Kidney, and Spleen of Asthmatic Mice

According to real-time PCR results, the Nrf2 mRNA level in the OVA-challenged group was significantly ($p < 0.05$) lower than in the control group, whereas the Keap1 mRNA level was increased. Keap1 expression was suppressed, whereas Nrf2 expression was greatly boosted by the high dose of Ech (Figure 10).

2.9. Effect of Ech on Kidney Antioxidants and Oxidative Stress Markers

Data concerning kidney antioxidants and oxidative stress markers such as MDA, NO, GSH, GST, and CAT are illustrated in Figure 11. The amounts of MDA, GSH, and NO were elevated in the OVA group. Also, the activity levels of GST and CAT were reduced in the OVA mice. No significant change was observed after treatment with 0.1 mg/kg Ech compared to the asthmatic mice. However, 1 mg/kg Ech treatment significantly decreased their levels ($p < 0.05$) compared to the OVA group.

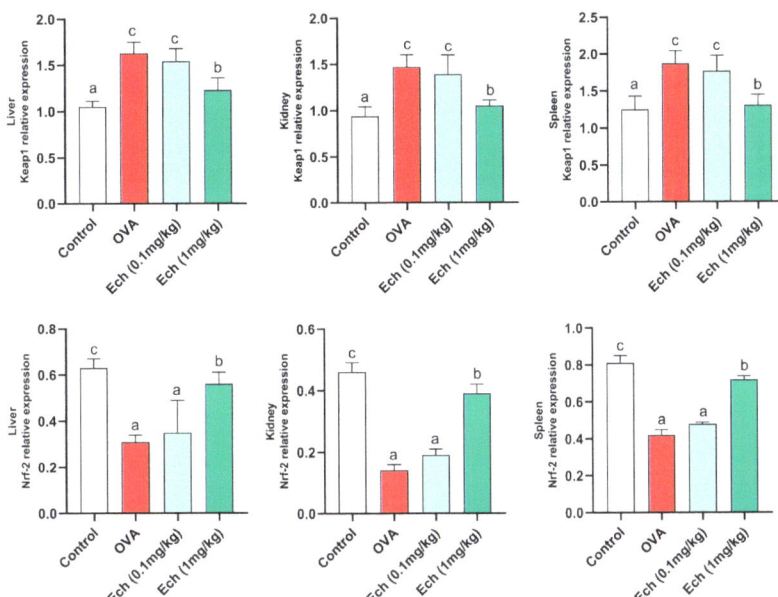

Figure 10. The effect of Ech on Keap1/Nrf2 pathway expression. The Keap1 and Nrf2 mRNA levels in the liver, kidney, and spleen were evaluated using RT-PCR with β-actin as an internal standard. Values are given as means for 8 mice in each group ± standard error of the mean (SEM). The value that does not share a common letter superscript is significantly different ($p < 0.05$).

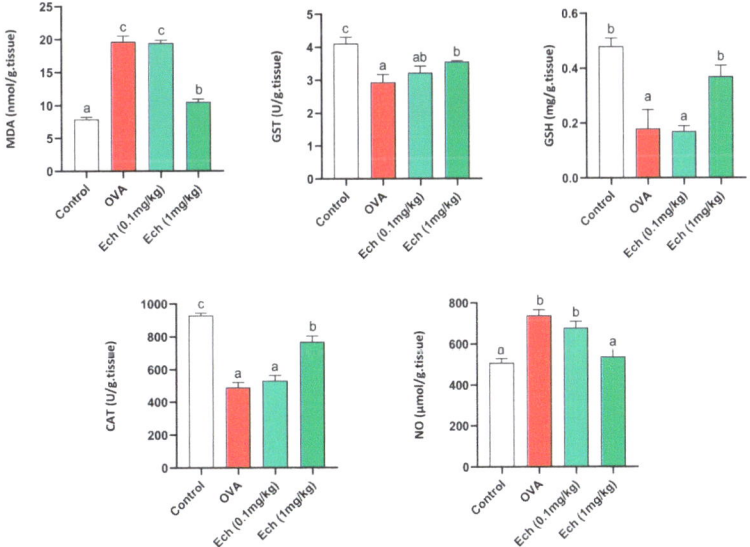

Figure 11. The effect of Ech on the kidney MDA, NO, and GSH levels and GST and CAT activity levels. Values are given as means for 8 mice in each group ± standard error of the mean (SEM). The value that does not share a common letter superscript is significantly different ($p < 0.05$).

2.10. Effect of Ech on Liver Antioxidants and Oxidative Stress Markers

Data concerning liver antioxidants and oxidative stress markers such as MDA, GSH, CAT, and SOD are shown in Figure 12. MDA and GSH were elevated in the OVA group compared to the control. Furthermore, the activity of CAT and SOD was reduced in the OVA group. Treatment with 0.1 mg/kg Ech showed no significant change in the OVA group. However, 1 mg/kg Ech treatment significantly decreased their concentrations compared to the OVA-challenged group ($p < 0.05$).

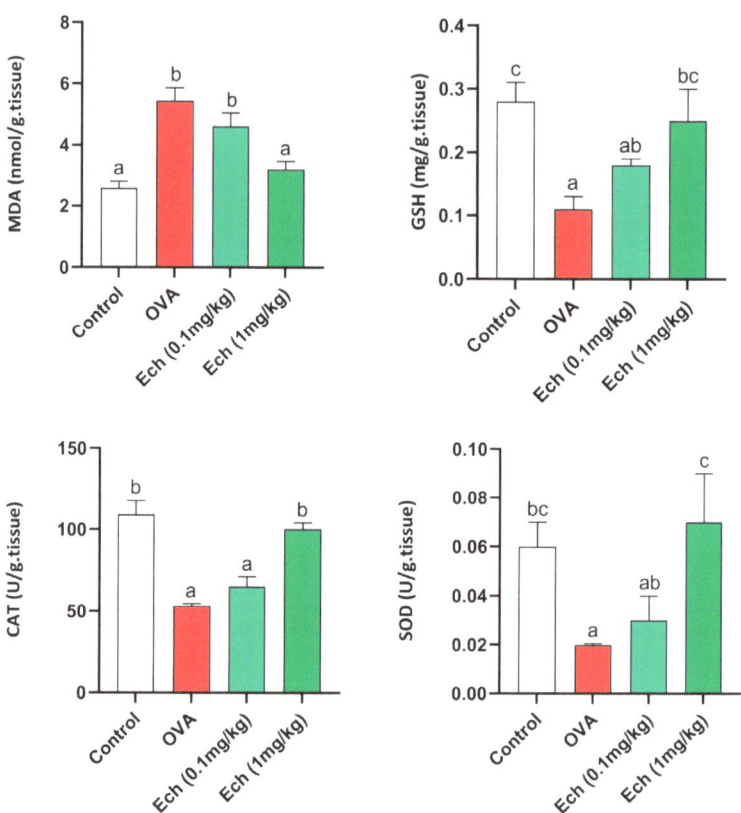

Figure 12. The effect of Ech on the liver's MDA and GSH levels and SOD and CAT activity levels. Values are given as means for 8 mice in each group ± standard error of the mean (SEM). The value that does not share a common letter superscript is significantly different ($p < 0.05$).

2.11. Effect of Ech on Spleen Antioxidants and Oxidative Stress Markers

Data concerning spleen antioxidants and oxidative stress markers (MDA, NO, GSH, GST, and CAT) are shown in Figure 13. The MDA, GSH, and NO levels were elevated in the OVA group. Moreover, the activity levels of GST and CAT were diminished in the OVA group. Intraperitoneal injection of 0.1 mg/kg Ech showed no significant change in the OVA-challenged group. However, 1 mg/kg Ech treatment notably diminished their levels ($p < 0.05$) compared to the OVA-challenged mice.

2.12. Effect of Ech on Lung Histopathology

The lung sections of control mice showed normal lung morphology. At the same time, the OVA challenge resulted in the marked recruitment of inflammatory cells, thickening of the bronchial epithelium, and smooth muscle thickening. Treatment with Ech in OVA-challenged mice ameliorated the lung morphology in a dose-dependent way, as seen in Figure 14.

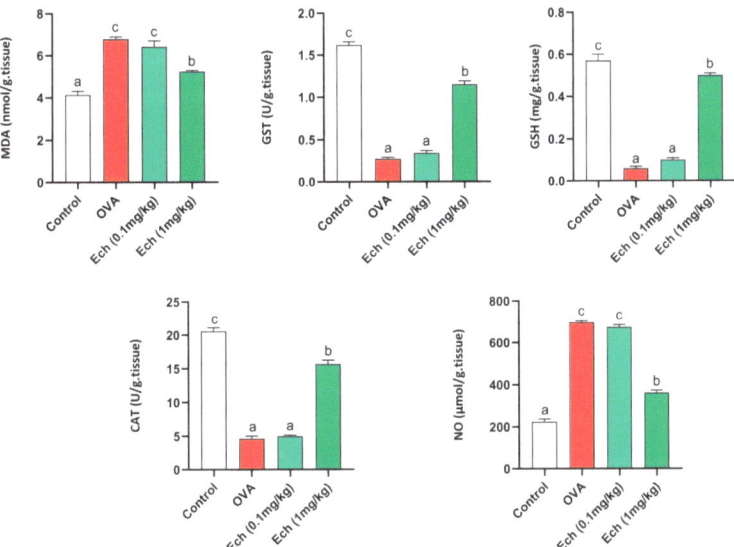

Figure 13. The effect of Ech on the spleen's MDA, NO, and GSH levels and GST and CAT activity levels. Values are given as means for 8 mice in each group ± standard error of the mean (SEM). The value that does not share a common letter superscript is significantly different ($p < 0.05$).

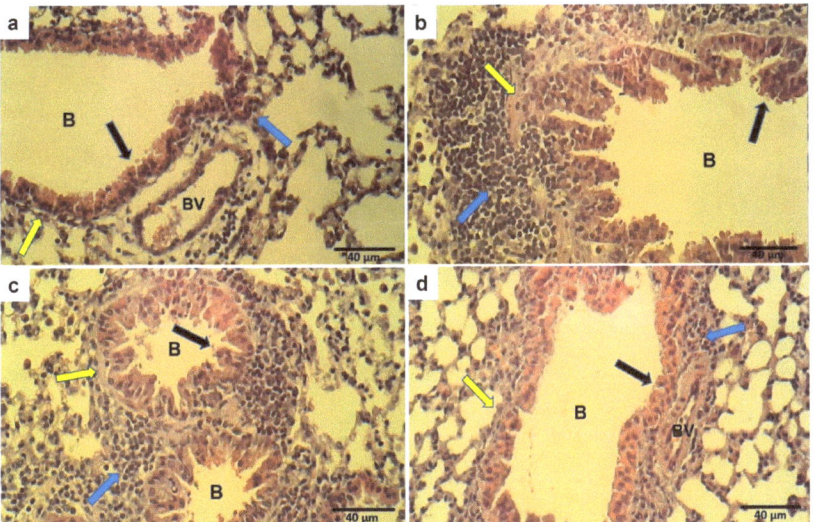

Figure 14. Lung sections of the control group (**a**) showed normal bronchi (B) with average epithelial lining (black arrow), average airway smooth muscles (yellow arrow), and minimal infiltrating immune cells (blue arrow). Sections from a mouse in the OVA group showed thickness in the bronchial epithelium (black arrow) and smooth muscle (yellow arrow) with marked infiltrating inflammatory cells (blue arrow) (**b**). Moderate cell infiltration, bronchial epithelium, and smooth muscle thickness were noticed in the 0.1 mg/kg Ech-treated group (**c**). Mild cell infiltration and average airway epithelium and smooth muscle were observed in the 1 mg/kg Ech-treated mice (**d**).

2.13. Effect of Ech on Liver Histopathology

The normal liver architecture of control mice was observed. In contrast, the OVA challenge resulted in marked cytoplasmic vacuolation with inflammatory cell infiltrations.

Treatment with Ech in OVA-challenged mice attenuated these changes in tissue morphology in a dose-dependent way, as demonstrated in Figure 15.

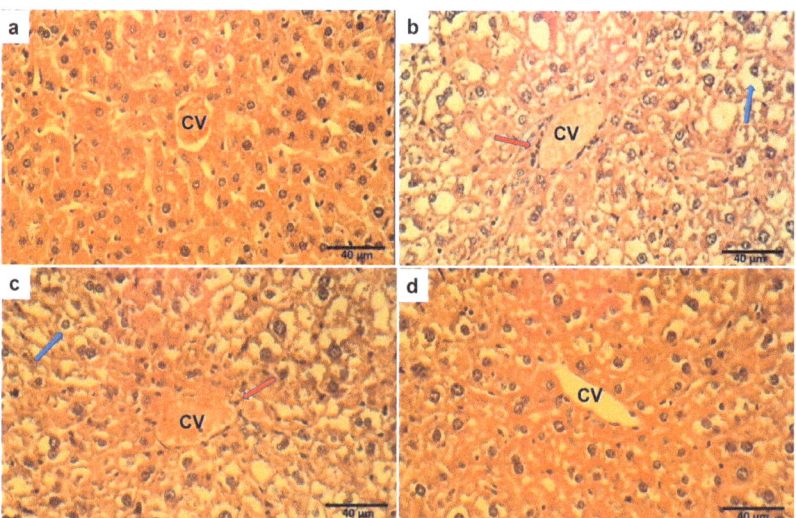

Figure 15. The control group (**a**) showed normal liver histology. Sections from a mouse in the OVA group (**b**) showed marked cytoplasmic vacuolation (blue arrow) with inflammatory cell infiltrations around the central vein (CV) (red arrow). Mild immune cell infiltration and vacuolation were noticed in the 0.1 mg/kg Ech-treated group (**c**). Normal liver tissue structure was observed in the 1 mg/kg Ech-treated mice (**d**).

2.14. Effect of Ech on Kidney Histopathology

The sections of control mice showed normal kidney structure. However, the OVA challenge resulted in structural abnormalities in the kidney tissue. Treatment with Ech (0.1 mg/kg) did not improve these alterations. However, treatment with 1 mg/kg Ech restored the normal kidney architecture, as shown in Figure 16.

2.15. Effect of Ech on Spleen Histopathology

The sections of control mice showed normal spleen structure. On the other hand, the OVA challenge resulted in structural changes in the spleen's morphology. Treatment with Ech in OVA-challenged mice reduced these changes in a dose-dependent way, as described in Figure 17.

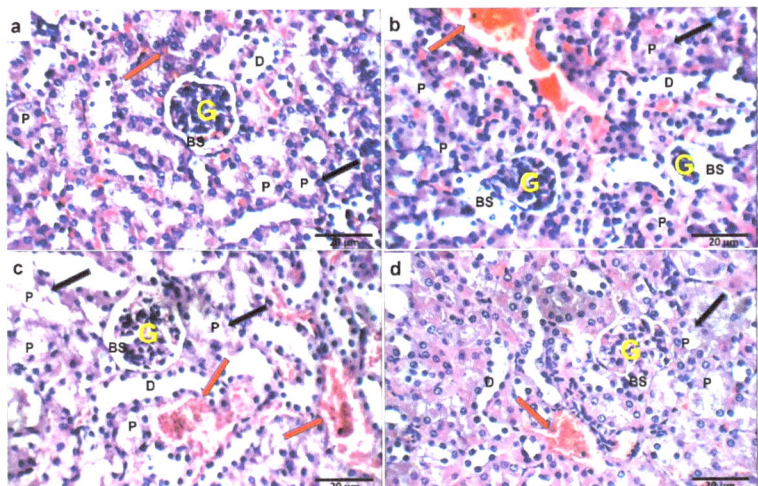

Figure 16. Kidneys from mice in the control group (**a**) showed normal-sized glomeruli (G) with average Bowman's spaces (BS), proximal tubules (P) with average epithelial lining and preserved brush borders (black arrow), average distal tubules (D), and average interstitial blood vessels (red arrow). Sections from a mouse in the OVA group showed small-sized glomeruli with widened Bowman's spaces, proximal tubules with scattered apoptotic epithelial lining and preserved brush borders, average distal tubules, and mildly congested interstitial blood vessels (**b**). No changes were observed after 0.1 mg/kg Ech treatment (**c**). Ameliorated kidney structure was observed in the 1 mg/kg Ech-treated mice (**d**).

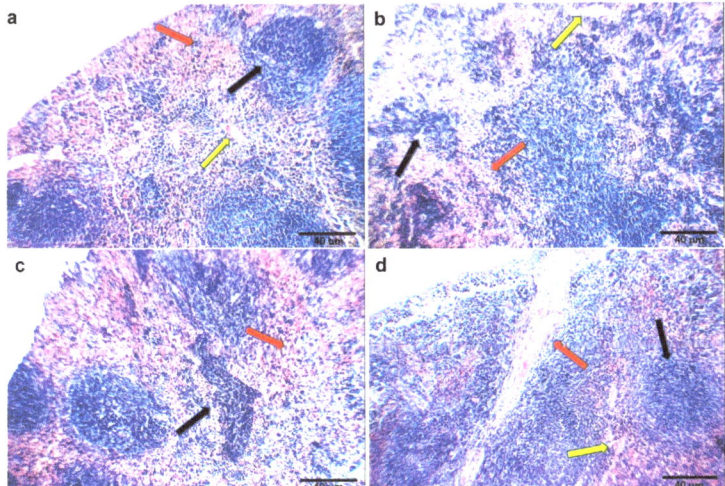

Figure 17. Sections of the spleens of mice in the control group (**a**) showed normal lymphoid follicles (white bulb) (black arrow), normal blood sinusoids (red bulb) (red arrow), and normal blood vessels (yellow arrow). Sections from a mouse in the OVA group showed small-sized lymphoid follicles (white bulb) (black arrow), expanded blood sinusoids (red bulb) (red arrow), and average blood vessels (yellow arrow). (**b**) Small-sized lymphoid follicles (black arrow) and markedly expanded congested blood sinusoids with many giant cells (red arrow) were observed after treatment with 0.1 mg/kg Ech. (**c**) Normal lymphoid follicles (white bulb) (black arrow), average blood sinusoids (red bulb) (red arrow), and mildly congested blood vessels (yellow arrow) were observed after treatment with 1 mg/kg Ech (**d**).

3. Discussion

Allergic asthma is a chronic respiratory condition that affects many people and is caused by exposure to allergens. Lung inflammation increases the level of immune cell infiltration, increases the production of inflammatory mediators, and causes structural and functional alterations in the airways [19]. Currently, corticosteroids are among the primary medications used to manage asthma. However, these drugs can have notable negative consequences upon prolonged consumption [20]. Therefore, discovering a reliable asthma treatment is essential. The in vitro DPPH assay results demonstrated that Ech has antioxidant activity linked to its radical scavenging action. The heat-induced hemolysis assays also supported the anti-inflammatory properties of Ech. The in vitro findings showed that Ech possesses both antioxidant and anti-inflammatory activities.

Multiple irregularities in biological processes contribute to lung weight gain during persistent airway irritation. Numerous investigations have demonstrated that lung expansion results from increased smooth muscle in the lung during airway remodeling [21]. The lung weight can be utilized as a sign of tissue edema brought on by asthmatic inflammation and overproduction of mucus [22]. This study demonstrated a significant increase in the weights of the kidney, liver, spleen, and lung of OVA animals, which may be related to these organs' oxidative stress and inflammation. On the other hand, administration of the Ech treatment restored the organs' weight.

Typical clinical signs of asthma include wheezing, sneezing, and shortness of breath. Although it might be challenging to spot these symptoms in rodents, they exhibit symptoms like nasal scratching and fast breathing. The present study found that the comprehensive score of nasal scratching significantly increased in the untreated asthmatic group. However, following Ech treatment (1 mg/kg), the nasal scratching scores significantly decreased, showing the ameliorative effect of Ech on asthma symptoms.

Keap1 inhibitors impair the covalent link between Keap1 and Nrf2 to release Nrf2 transcriptional machinery that regulates its cellular antioxidant, cytoprotective, and detoxifying functions, protecting cells from oxidative-stress-mediated diseases [23]. Thus, Nrf2 activation offers cytoprotection against various pathologies, such as chronic lung and liver illnesses, autoimmune, neurological, and metabolic disorders, and cancer [24]. According to the outcomes of our molecular docking, Ech could stabilize Keap1. Our findings imply that Ech's binding to Keap1 and disruption of the protein–protein interaction between Keap1 and Nrf2 may cause the nuclear translocation of Nrf2, which upregulates the expression of antioxidant molecules. Keap1 is an actin-binding protein with a molecular weight of 69.7 kD and 625 amino acid residues, 27 of which are cysteine residues [25]. Electrophilic drugs were initially developed to induce nuclear accumulation of Nrf2 by targeting its natural repressor protein Keap1 via covalent modifications on cysteine residues [26]. Quinones are a well-studied class of Nrf2 inducers [26]. Echinochrome A (7-ethyl-2,3,5,6,8-pentahydroxy-1,4-naphthoquinone) is a natural quinone that is oxidized to electrophilic quinones with a Michael acceptor group, permitting the thiol of Keap1 reactivity to bind to it [27,28]. Using RT-PCR and Western blot techniques, the gene and protein expressions of Keap1 and Nrf2 confirm molecular docking results.

The pathogenesis of asthma is mainly due to a disparity in the polarization of CD4+ Th cells. Increased Th2 cell activation is believed to play a pivotal role in asthmatic immunological responses, triggering and expanding inflammation through the secretion of a variety of Th2 mediators, including IL-4, IL-5, and IL-13 [29]. In our research, IgE, IL-4, and IL-1β serum levels increased significantly in the OVA-challenged mice. It has been reported that asthma is associated with a rise in IgE, IL-4, and IL-1β levels [30]. The increased level of these cytokines causes IgE synthesis and the infiltration of inflammatory immune cells, particularly eosinophils, that induce the release of ROS [31]. However, Ech's treatment notably reduced their levels in a dose-dependent way.

Although asthma is a well-known lung condition, it also has a negative impact on other organs. More recent research has revealed the epidemiological association between asthma and a metabolic disorder [32]. Serum transaminases are sensitive biomarkers of liver cell destruction [33]. According to the study's findings, the OVA group had significantly higher serum levels of AST and ALT and lower levels of total proteins and albumin than the control group. These results are consistent with previous investigations where OVA challenge led to higher AST and ALT levels and decreased levels of albumin and total proteins [34]. This rise in AST and ALT levels has been used as a sign of the severity of asthma, and it has been linked to the inadequate exchange of gases, which leads to hepatic oxygen deficiency and hepatocyte destruction [35]. Treatment with 1 mg/kg Ech has a significant protective effect against liver injury, as demonstrated by the lowering of serum AST and ALT levels and the elevation of albumin and total protein levels.

Asthma affects many chronic disorders, including chronic renal disease [36]. In the current study, kidney damage was shown by a significant rise in creatinine, urea, and uric acid in the mice that were given OVA compared to the control group. These findings align with previous research where the OVA challenge resulted in greater creatinine, uric acid, and urea concentrations [34]. It is possible to explain this increase in creatinine, urea, and uric acid due to the inflammatory response that can result in renal injury and dysfunction [37]. The current study further shows that treatment with 1 mg/kg Ech has a robust protective impact against kidney injury by decreasing the serum levels of creatinine, uric acid, and urea.

Oxidative stress plays a key role in the pathogenesis of multiple respiratory conditions, such as asthma [38,39]. It results from the disparity between the formation of free radicals and the antioxidant system. Elevated concentrations of free radicals in the lungs can cause functional and structural alterations and initiate biochemical cascades that are important in the pathogenesis of asthma [40]. Additionally, it promotes inflammation by increasing the secretion of proinflammatory cytokines and lowering antioxidant activity [41]. This study confirmed oxidative stress in different organs by increasing MDA and NO while GSH, SOD, GST, and CAT levels decreased. Collectively, it is possible to explain this increase in MDA and NO and the decline in GSH, SOD, GST, and CAT after OVA exposure as a result of disruption of the redox system and impaired antioxidant defenses, leading to the production of highly reactive free radicals, peroxidation of lipids, and cell destruction [42]. However, Ech treatment restored the balance between the oxidant and antioxidant defense mechanisms. Our study's findings agree with a previous study, where the treatment with Ech reduced the level of oxidative stress parameters (MDA and NO) while increasing the concentration of GSH and the activity of CAT, SOD, and GST [43]. Furthermore, a recent study revealed that Ech-A inhibits sulfide catabolism and H_2S/HS^- formation in hypoxic and inflammatory cells [44]. Thiyl radicals, disulfides, sulfenic acids, and disulfide oxides are reactive sulfur species that rapidly oxidize and inhibit thiolproteins and enzymes [45].

4. Materials and Methods

4.1. Reagents

Standard Echinochrome (Ech) (Vladivostok, Russia) and Dulbecco's phosphate buffer saline (PBS) 10× (SEROX GmbH®, Mannheim, Germany) were used. Ovalbumin (OVA), aluminum hydroxide, dimethyl sulfoxide (DMSO), tris ethylenediaminetetraacetic acid (EDTA), bovine serum albumin (BSA), hydrochloric acid (HCl), diethyl ether, and anhydrous sodium sulfate were obtained from Sigma-Aldrich (St. Louis, MO, USA). Biochemical kits were obtained from Bio-diagnostics Company (Giza, Egypt). Total IgE (Cat No. E-20550Mo) (Houston, TX, USA), IL-4 (Cat No. BMS613), and IL-1β (Cat No. BMS6002) (Invitrogen by Thermo Fisher Scientific, Waltham, MA, USA) were obtained. TaqMan probes and TaqMan Gene Expression Mastermix (Thermo Fisher Scientific) were obtained. Antibodies against Nrf2, Keap1, and HRP-conjugated goat anti-rabbit secondary antibody were obtained from (Abclonal Technology, Wuhan, China). Antibody against GAPDH was obtained from Cell Signaling Technology (Danvers, MA, USA).

4.2. Ech Extraction

Sea urchins (*Paracentrotus lividus*) were gathered from the Mediterranean shore of Alexandria (Egypt) and transferred to the lab on ice. The samples were properly cleaned with seawater to remove sand and overgrown organisms at the collection location and transferred to the lab. Taxonomic guides recognized the specimens [46]. The specimens were shade-dried immediately. Ech was extracted according to the method adopted by Amarowicz et al. [47] with modifications. Spines were removed, and then the shells were opened into 2 pieces using scissors to remove the animal's internal structures under constant tap water flow. The spines and shells were allowed to air-dry for three days in a cold, dark place. Dried samples were ground into powder. After this, the obtained powder was slowly added to a certain amount of 6 M HCl. Then, the obtained solution was filtrated before extracting the echinochrome pigment several times with diethyl ether. Then, a suitable amount of sodium sulfate (anhydrous) was added to remove the water before evaporating the ether using a rotatory evaporator. Ech was eventually obtained and kept at -20 °C. Detailed information about FTIR and mass spectroscopy, UV, ^{1}H NMR, and ^{13}C NMR spectra of Ech is described in the Supplementary File.

4.3. HPLC Analysis

A Shimadzu HPLC system (Kyoto, Japan) was used, which included two LC20AD pumps, a DGU-20 A3 degasser, and an SPD-M20 A diode-array detector. With a 1.0 mL/min flow rate, a Zorbax Eclipse Plus C18 column (250 mm 4.6 mm, 5 m) was employed for chromatographic separation with acetonitrile/methanol (5:9 v/v) and 0.1% formic acid as the binary mobile phase. An elution profile was as follows: formic acid containing 40–70% acetonitrile for 0–25 min (linear gradient). The volume of the injection was 20 µL. Between 200 and 800 nm, the detection was noted. The LC Solution (Shimadzu) was the data analysis system. DMSO was used to dissolve Ech at a of 5 mg/mL concentration.

4.4. In Vitro Biological Studies

4.4.1. Antioxidant Activity Using DPPH Radical Scavenging Protocol

Ech (20, 40, 60, and 100 µg/mL) in ethanol was combined with 1500 µL of 0.1 mM DPPH–ethanol solution. After 30 min of incubation at ambient temperature, the DPPH free radical was reduced by reading the absorbance at 517 nm [48,49]. Positive control included ascorbic acid. The following equation calculated the inhibition ratio (percent):

% RSA = (absorbance of control − absorbance of sample)/(absorbance of control) × 100.

4.4.2. Anti-Inflammatory Activity Using Heat-Induced Hemolysis Protocol

Venipuncture blood from healthy volunteers was centrifuged at 3000 rpm for 10 min at 4 °C in heparinized tubes. RBCs were washed three times in PBS after plasma removal. RBCs were resuspended in 10 mL PBS. The assay combination included 0.5 mL of RBC suspension and 0.5 mL of Ech (100, 200, 300, 50 µg). A UV–visible spectrophotometer at 560 nm evaluated supernatant hemoglobin [50]. Diclofenac was used as the control. This equation estimates hemolysis percentage:

Protection % = 100 − [(Optical density of sample)/(Optical density of control) × 100]

4.5. Molecular Docking Interaction between Ech and Keap1

The crystal structure of the Kelch-like ECH-associated protein 1 (Keap1) was obtained from the Protein Data Bank with PDB ID: 4L7B. Using the molecular visualization software, Pymol [51], solvent molecules, heteroatoms, and other experimental inhibitors were removed from the target macromolecule. Hydrogen bonds were added, and the file was extracted in PDB format. The grid box dimensions of the binding site were then determined with Keap1's cocrystallized ligand as its center [52]. The structures of the target protein file and the cocrystallized ligand were converted into the PDBQT format using Auto-Dock

(MGL Tools) [53]. Ech structure was downloaded in sdf format from PubChem and converted into the PDBQT using Open Babel software [54]. Virtual docking was performed using Auto-Dock Vina [55]. The results were exported as comma-separated files (CSV). The mean lowest binding energy was used to predict the binding affinity of echinochrome with Keap1. Pymol and the Protein–Ligand Interaction Profiler were used to visualize three-dimensional hydrophobic interactions [56]. Two-dimensional interactions were viewed with Discovery Studio (BIOVIA, San Diego, CA, USA).

4.6. Experimental Animals

The National Research Center (Giza, Egypt) provided 32 female BALB/c mice (Mus musculus) weighing (18–22 g). They were fed, kept in groups in sterile enclosures, and had free access to water *ad libitum*. The Institutional Animal Care and Use Committee (IACUC) at Cairo University in Egypt approved this research with the number CU/I/F/32/22. The instructions for the care and use of laboratory animals were used in all of the experiments in accordance with international guidelines.

4.7. Animal Grouping and Experiment Design

The experimental procedure used in this research to induce asthma was established according to Bai et al. [57], with some modifications. For sensitization, the mice were intraperitoneally injected with 20 µg of OVA mixed with 1 mg aluminum hydroxide gel in sterile PBS (pH 7.4) (200 µL final volume). For the challenge, the mice were exposed once daily to inhalations with 2.5% OVA on days 21, 22, and 23. After two weeks of acclimatization, mice were randomly assigned to 4 groups—a control group, an OVA group, a low-dose group of Ech (0.1 mg/kg) [58], and a high-dose group of Ech (1 mg/kg)—each of which contained 8 mice. One hour before the challenge, Ech (0.1 and 1 mg/kg) was intraperitoneally administered. Mice received the same volume of PBS as the control group. Mice were sacrificed after the last challenge.

4.8. Evaluation of Body Weight and Nasal Scratching

Body weight gain and the weight of the lung, spleen, kidney, and liver of all mice were recorded at the end of the experiment. Nasal scratching was assessed and scored for 10 min following the final challenge, with 2.5% OVA on the final day. The results were as follows: Mice who scratched their noses 0–2 times received a score of 0, 3–5 times received a score of 1, 6–8 times received a score of 2, and 9 or more times received a score of 3 [59] (an illustration video is attached as Supporting Material).

4.9. Sample Collection

Twenty-four hours after the last OVA challenge, mice were isoflurane-anesthetized and blood was taken from the retro-orbital plexus to assess the liver (ALT, AST, albumin, and total protein) and kidney (creatinine, urea, and uric acid) function biomarkers and measure the serum concentrations of IgE, IL-4, and IL-1β. The spleen, kidney, and liver were removed, weighed, and homogenized for evaluating Nrf2, Keap1, and oxidative stress biomarkers. At the same time, the lung, liver, kidney, and spleen were utilized for evaluating OVA-induced histopathological alterations using H&E.

4.10. Measurement of Serum Levels of IgE, IL-4, and IL-1β

IgE, IL-4, and interleukin 1β (IL-1β) were quantified according to the instructions of the kits and expressed as pg/mL using an ELISA plate reader (DAS Instruments, model A3, Rome, Italy).

4.11. Evaluation of Serum Biochemical Parameters

The serum levels of ALT, AST, total protein, albumin, creatinine, uric acid, and urea were evaluated according to the kit's instructions.

4.12. Western Blot Assays

The tissue homogenates were mixed with protein lysis buffer (50 mM Tris-HCl pH 7.5, 150 mM NaCl, 5 mM EDTA, 0.5% Triton X-100, and protease inhibitor). Samples were sonicated and centrifuged for ten minutes at a speed of 10,000 rpm at 4 °C. The samples were then subjected to 10% SDS-PAGE gel electrophoresis (50 µg of protein per lane), and the Bradford technique assay was used to determine the protein content. After transferring proteins to PVDF membranes, they were blocked for 1 h at room temperature with blocking buffer (TBST buffer with 5% skim milk powder), followed by the addition of the primary antibodies Keap1, Nrf-2 (1:1000), and GAPDH (1:2000), which were then incubated overnight at 4 °C. After washing with TBST, secondary antibodies (1:5000) were applied to the membranes. They were incubated for 1 h at room temperature. Enhanced chemiluminescence (ECL; Thermo Scientific; Shanghai, China) was used to observe the blots. All reactions were performed in triplicate and the blots were quantified and assessed using ImageJ (version 1.8.0, Bethesda, MD, USA).

4.13. Real-Time Reverse Transcriptase-Polymerase Chain Reaction (RT-PCR)

RT-PCR was used to analyze the amount of mRNA expression for both Nrf2 and Keap1. The liver, kidney, and spleen homogenates were treated with the triazole reagent and subjected to the standard protocol for isolating total RNA. A Sensi-Script Reverse Transcriptase Kit (Qiagen Hilden, Germany) was used to convert RNA to cDNA. With the use of TaqMan probes, we were able to conduct quantitative PCR. TaqMan Gene Expression Master Mix was used for qPCR using TaqMan primers for mouse Nrf2 and Keap1. The CFX384 Touch Real-Time PCR Detection System (BioRad, Mississauga, ON, Canada) was used for the quantitative RT-PCR. Using the delta–delta Ct technique, we calculated the abundance of each transcript. All reactions were performed in triplicate and the mean value was used to calculate expression levels after normalization against β-actin.

4.14. Determination of Liver, Kidney, and Spleen Oxidative Stress Biomarkers

The kidney, spleen, and liver tissues were homogenized in an ice-cold 0.1 M Tris HCl buffer, pH 7.4, and centrifuged for 15 min at 3000 rpm [60,61]. The supernatant was utilized for evaluating the concentration of GSH and the activities of CAT, SOD, and GST enzymes in the liver, kidney, and spleen tissues. Additionally, the MDA and NO were measured according to the instructions of commercial kits.

4.15. Histopathological Examination of Lung, Kidney, Liver, and Spleen

Mice were dissected, and the lung, kidney, spleen, and liver were removed entirely and fixed in 10% formalin for 24 h. Sample sections were cut, stained with hematoxylin and eosin (H&E), and examined under a light microscope [62].

4.16. Statistical Analysis

For the statistical analyses, IBM's Statistical Package for the Social Sciences (SPSS) was utilized. Mean and SEM were used to express values. A one-way analysis of variance (ANOVA) was used to determine group differences. The graphs were made utilizing the 8th version of GraphPad Prism. The group means were compared using Duncan's post hoc test, and $p < 0.05$ was regarded as statistically significant.

5. Conclusions

We found that Ech reduced the severity of asthma-induced immunological and physiological alterations in mice. Treatment with Ech also improves the histology of the spleen, lungs, kidneys, and liver of asthmatic mice. Inhibition of inflammation and oxidative stress are two of Ech's therapeutic actions in managing asthma by modulating the Keap1/Nrf2 signaling pathway.

Supplementary Materials: The following supporting information can be downloaded at: https://www.mdpi.com/article/10.3390/md21080455/s1, Video S1: Nasal Scratching.

Author Contributions: Conceptualization, A.S.M.; methodology, I.A.A.; software, T.A.; validation, H.I.S.; formal analysis, N.A.M.; investigations, A.M.A.S.; resources, A.E.A.; data curation, I.A.A.; writing—original draft preparation I.A.A.; writing—review and editing, A.S.M.; visualization, A.M.B.; supervision, H.I.S. All authors have read and agreed to the published version of the manuscript.

Funding: This research received no external funding.

Institutional Review Board Statement: The experimental techniques and practices of the study were approved by the Faculty of Science Institutional Animal Care and Use Committee (IACUC) at Cairo University, Egypt. All the experimental procedures followed the international guidelines for laboratory animal care and use (CU/I/F/32/22).

Data Availability Statement: Not applicable.

Conflicts of Interest: The authors declare no conflict of interest.

References

1. Zhu, Y.; Sun, D.; Liu, H.; Sun, L.; Jie, J.; Luo, J.; Peng, L.; Song, L. Bixin protects mice against bronchial asthma though modulating PI3K/Akt pathway. *Int. Immunopharmacol.* **2021**, *101*, 108266. [CrossRef]
2. Zheng, M.; Guo, X.; Pan, R.; Gao, J.; Zang, B.; Jin, M. Hydroxysafflor Yellow A Alleviates Ovalbumin-Induced Asthma in a Guinea Pig Model by Attenuateing the Expression of Inflammatory Cytokines and Signal Transduction. *Front. Pharmacol.* **2019**, *10*, 328. [CrossRef] [PubMed]
3. Zou, B.; Fu, Y.; Cao, C.; Pan, D.; Wang, W.; Kong, L. Gentiopicroside ameliorates ovalbumin-induced airway inflammation in a mouse model of allergic asthma via regulating SIRT1/NF-κB signaling pathway. *Pulm. Pharmacol. Ther.* **2021**, *68*, 102034. [CrossRef] [PubMed]
4. Liang, Z.; Luo, Z.; Chen, J.; Li, B.; Li, L.; Shen, C. Bavachin inhibits IL-4 expression by downregulating STAT6 phosphorylation and GATA-3 expression and ameliorates asthma inflammation in an animal model. *Immunobiology* **2022**, *227*, 152182. [CrossRef]
5. Zhu, Y.; Wang, C.; Luo, J.; Hua, S.; Li, D.; Peng, L.; Liu, H.; Song, L. The protective role of Zingerone in a murine asthma model via activation of the AMPK/Nrf2/HO-1 pathway. *Food Funct.* **2021**, *12*, 3120–3131. [CrossRef]
6. Daenen, K.; Andries, A.; Mekahli, D.; Van Schepdael, A.; Jouret, F.; Bammens, B. Oxidative stress in chronic kidney disease. *Pediatr. Nephrol.* **2019**, *34*, 975–991. [CrossRef]
7. Muriel, P.; Gordillo, K.R. Role of Oxidative Stress in Liver Health and Disease. *Oxidative Med. Cell. Longev.* **2016**, *2016*, 9037051. [CrossRef]
8. Li, A.-N.; Li, S.; Zhang, Y.-J.; Xu, X.-R.; Chen, Y.-M.; Li, H.-B. Resources and Biological Activities of Natural Polyphenols. *Nutrients* **2014**, *6*, 6020–6047. [CrossRef] [PubMed]
9. Ozbek, E. Induction of Oxidative Stress in Kidney. *Int. J. Nephrol.* **2012**, *2012*, 465897. [CrossRef]
10. Mebius, R.E.; Kraal, G. Structure and function of the spleen. *Nat. Rev. Immunol.* **2005**, *5*, 606–616. [CrossRef]
11. Lu, M.-C.; Ji, J.-A.; Jiang, Z.-Y.; You, Q.-D. The Keap1–Nrf2–ARE Pathway As a Potential Preventive and Therapeutic Target: An Update. *Med. Res. Rev.* **2016**, *36*, 924–963. [CrossRef] [PubMed]
12. Hassanein, E.H.M.; Sayed, A.M.; Hussein, O.E.; Mahmoud, A.M. Coumarins as Modulators of the Keap1/Nrf2/ARE Signaling Pathway. *Oxidative Med. Cell. Longev.* **2020**, *2020*, 1675957. [CrossRef] [PubMed]
13. Tang, W.; Dong, M.; Teng, F.; Cui, J.; Zhu, X.; Wang, W.; Wuniqiemu, T.; Qin, J.; Yi, L.; Wang, S.; et al. TMT-based quantitative proteomics reveals suppression of SLC3A2 and ATP1A3 expression contributes to the inhibitory role of acupuncture on airway inflammation in an OVA-induced mouse asthma model. *Biomed. Pharmacother.* **2021**, *134*, 111001. [CrossRef]
14. Mayer, A.M.S.; Guerrero, A.J.; Rodríguez, A.D.; Taglialatela-Scafati, O.; Nakamura, F.; Fusetani, N. Marine Pharmacology in 2016-2017: Marine Compounds with Antibacterial, Antidiabetic, Antifungal, Anti-Inflammatory, Antiprotozoal, Antituberculosis and Antiviral Activities; Affecting the Immune and Nervous Systems, and Other Miscellaneous Mechanisms of Action. *Mar. Drugs* **2021**, *19*, 49.
15. Anderson, H.A.; Mathieson, J.W.; Thomson, R.H. Distribution of spinochrome pigments in echinoids. *Comp. Biochem. Physiol.* **1969**, *28*, 333–345. [CrossRef]
16. Park, G.-T.; Yoon, J.-W.; Yoo, S.-B.; Song, Y.-C.; Song, P.; Kim, H.-K.; Han, J.; Bae, S.-J.; Ha, K.-T.; Mishchenko, N.P.; et al. Echinochrome A Treatment Alleviates Fibrosis and Inflammation in Bleomycin-Induced Scleroderma. *Mar. Drugs* **2021**, *19*, 237. [CrossRef]
17. Fedoreyev, S.A.; Krylova, N.V.; Mishchenko, N.P.; Vasileva, E.A.; Pislyagin, E.A.; Iunikhina, O.V.; Lavrov, V.F.; Svitich, O.A.; Ebralidze, L.K.; Leonova, G.N. Antiviral and Antioxidant Properties of Echinochrome A. *Mar. Drugs* **2018**, *16*, 509. [CrossRef] [PubMed]
18. Mohamed, A.S.; Sadek, S.A.; Hassanein, S.S.; Soliman, A.M. Hepatoprotective Effect of Echinochrome Pigment in Septic Rats. *J. Surg. Res.* **2019**, *234*, 317–324. [CrossRef]

19. Han, J.; Zhang, S.; Jiang, B.; Wang, J.; Ge, X.; Wu, B.; Zhang, S.; Wang, D. Sesquiterpene lactones from Xanthium sibiricum Patrin alleviate asthma by modulating the Th1/Th2 balance in a murine model. *Phytomedicine* 2022, *99*, 154032. [CrossRef]
20. Yang, Z.; Li, X.; Fu, R.; Hu, M.; Wei, Y.; Hu, X.; Tan, W.; Tong, X.; Huang, F. Therapeutic Effect of Renifolin F on Airway Allergy in an Ovalbumin-Induced Asthma Mouse Model In Vivo. *Molecules* 2022, *27*, 3789. [CrossRef]
21. Dai, R.; Niu, M.; Wang, N.; Wang, Y. Syringin alleviates ovalbumin-induced lung inflammation in BALB/c mice asthma model via NF-κB signaling pathway. *Environ. Toxicol.* 2021, *36*, 433–444. [CrossRef]
22. Zhang, Q.; Wang, L.; Chen, B.; Zhuo, Q.; Bao, C.; Lin, L. Propofol inhibits NF-κB activation to ameliorate airway inflammation in ovalbumin (OVA)-induced allergic asthma mice. *Int. Immunopharmacol.* 2017, *51*, 158–164. [CrossRef] [PubMed]
23. Adelusi, T.I.; Abdul-Hammed, M.; Idris, M.O.; Oyedele, Q.K.; Adedotun, I.O.J.H. Molecular dynamics, quantum mechanics and docking studies of some Keap1 inhibitors–An insight into the atomistic mechanisms of their antioxidant potential. *Heliyon* 2021, *7*, e07317. [CrossRef]
24. Cuadrado, A.; Rojo, A.I.; Wells, G.; Hayes, J.D.; Cousin, S.P.; Rumsey, W.L.; Attucks, O.C.; Franklin, S.; Levonen, A.-L.; Kensler, T.W.; et al. Therapeutic targeting of the NRF2 and KEAP1 partnership in chronic diseases. *Nat. Rev. Drug Discov.* 2019, *18*, 295–317. [CrossRef]
25. Crisman, E.; Duarte, P.; Dauden, E.; Cuadrado, A.; Rodríguez-Franco, M.I.; López, M.G.; León, R.J.M.R.R. KEAP1-NRF2 protein–protein interaction inhibitors: Design, pharmacological properties and therapeutic potential. *Med. Res. Rev.* 2023, *43*, 237–287. [CrossRef] [PubMed]
26. Magesh, S.; Chen, Y.; Hu, L.J.M. Small molecule modulators of Keap1-Nrf2-ARE pathway as potential preventive and therapeutic agents. *Med. Res. Rev.* 2012, *32*, 687–726. [CrossRef]
27. Lee, S.; Hu, L. Nrf2 activation through the inhibition of Keap1-Nrf2 protein-protein interaction. *Med. Chem. Res. Int. J. Rapid Commun. Des. Mech. Action Biol. Act. Agents* 2020, *29*, 846–867. [CrossRef]
28. Mishchenko, N.P.; Vasileva, E.A.; Gerasimenko, A.V.; Grigorchuk, V.P.; Dmitrenok, P.S.; Fedoreyev, S.A. Isolation and Structure Determination of Echinochrome A Oxidative Degradation Products. *Molecules* 2020, *25*, 4778. [CrossRef]
29. Cho, K.-S.; Park, M.-K.; Kang, S.-A.; Park, H.-Y.; Hong, S.-L.; Park, H.-K.; Yu, H.-S.; Roh, H.-J. Adipose-Derived Stem Cells Ameliorate Allergic Airway Inflammation by Inducing Regulatory T Cells in a Mouse Model of Asthma. *Mediat. Inflamm.* 2014, *2014*, 436476. [CrossRef] [PubMed]
30. Yan, G.H.; Choi, Y.H. Salidroside Attenuates Allergic Airway Inflammation Through Negative Regulation of Nuclear Factor-Kappa B and p38 Mitogen–Activated Protein Kinase. *J. Pharmacol. Sci.* 2014, *126*, 126–135. [CrossRef]
31. Lambrecht, B.N.; Hammad, H. The immunology of asthma. *Nat. Immunol.* 2015, *16*, 45–56. [CrossRef]
32. Roh, J.-H.; Lee, H.; Yun-Jeong, B.; Park, C.S.; Kim, H.-J.; Yoon, S.-Y. A nationwide survey of the association between nonalcoholic fatty liver disease and the incidence of asthma in Korean adults. *PLoS ONE* 2022, *17*, e0262715. [CrossRef] [PubMed]
33. Ozer, J.; Ratner, M.; Shaw, M.; Bailey, W.; Schomaker, S. The current state of serum biomarkers of hepatotoxicity. *Toxicology* 2008, *245*, 194–205. [CrossRef] [PubMed]
34. Khaldi, T.; Chekchaki, N.; Rouibah, Z.; Chouala, K.; Cheniti, H.; Boumendjel, M.; Taibi, F.; Messarah, M.; Boumendjel, A. Preventive effects of oral administration of Nigella sativa oil against smokeless tobacco induced toxicity and oxidative stress in the liver and kidney of allergic asthma induced rats. *Toxicol. Environ. Health Sci.* 2022, *14*, 291–300. [CrossRef]
35. Iribarren, C.; Sidney, S.; Lydick, E.; Sorel, M.E.; Eisner, M.D. The association between asthma, asthma therapeutic classes and hepatic enzyme elevation among adult HMO members. *Compr. Ther.* 2001, *27*, 133–139. [CrossRef]
36. Huang, H.-L.; Ho, S.-Y.; Li, C.-H.; Chu, F.-Y.; Ciou, L.-P.; Lee, H.-C.; Chen, W.-L.; Tzeng, N.-S. Bronchial asthma is associated with increased risk of chronic kidney disease. *BMC Pulm. Med.* 2014, *14*, 80. [CrossRef]
37. Small, I.; Moreira, A.; Couto, M. Practical approach to managing exercise-induced asthma in children and adults. *Prim. Care Respir. J.* 2013, *22*, 126–129. [CrossRef] [PubMed]
38. Assayag, M.; Goldstein, S.; Samuni, A.; Kaufman, A.; Berkman, N. The nitroxide/antioxidant 3-carbamoyl proxyl attenuates disease severity in murine models of severe asthma. *Free Radic. Biol. Med.* 2021, *177*, 181–188. [CrossRef]
39. Rawash, M.A.; Mohamed, A.S.; El-Zayat, E.M. The Concurrent Therapeutic Potential of Adipose-derived Mesenchymal Stem Cells on Gentamycin-induced Hepatorenal Toxicity in Rats. *Curr. Stem. Cell Res. Ther.* 2022, *17*, 808–814.
40. Ajayi, B.O.; Olajide, T.A.; Olayinka, E.T. 6-gingerol attenuates pulmonary inflammation and oxidative stress in mice model of house dust mite-induced asthma. *Adv. Redox Res.* 2022, *5*, 100036. [CrossRef]
41. Malaquias, M.A.S.; Oyama, L.A.; Jericó, P.C.; Costa, I.; Padilha, G.; Nagashima, S.; Lopes-Pacheco, M.; Rebelatto, C.L.K.; Michelotto, P.V.; Xisto, D.G.; et al. Effects of mesenchymal stromal cells play a role in the oxidant/antioxidant balance in a murine model of asthma. *Allergol. Immunopathol.* 2018, *46*, 136–143. [CrossRef]
42. Tiwari, M.; Dwivedi, U.N.; Kakkar, P. Tinospora cordifolia extract modulates COX-2, iNOS, ICAM-1, pro-inflammatory cytokines and redox status in murine model of asthma. *J. Ethnopharmacol.* 2014, *153*, 326–337. [CrossRef] [PubMed]
43. Sadek, S.A.; Hassanein, S.S.; Mohamed, A.S.; Soliman, A.M.; Fahmy, S.R. Echinochrome pigment extracted from sea urchin suppress the bacterial activity, inflammation, nociception, and oxidative stress resulted in the inhibition of renal injury in septic rats. *J. Food Biochem.* 2022, *46*, e13729. [CrossRef]
44. Tang, X.; Nishimura, A.; Ariyoshi, K.; Nishiyama, K.; Kato, Y.; Vasileva, E.A.; Mishchenko, N.P.; Fedoreyev, S.A.; Stonik, V.A.; Kim, H.K.; et al. Echinochrome Prevents Sulfide Catabolism-Associated Chronic Heart Failure after Myocardial Infarction in Mice. *Mar. Drugs* 2023, *21*, 52. [CrossRef]

45. Giles, G.I.; Jacob, C. Reactive sulfur species: An emerging concept in oxidative stress. *Biol. Chem.* **2002**, *383*, 375–388. [CrossRef]
46. Clark, A.H. Monograph of shallow-water Indo-West Pacific echinoderms. *Br. Mus. (Nat. Hist.) Publ.* **1971**, *690*, 234.
47. Amarowicz, R.; Synowiecki, J.; Shahidi, F. Sephadex LH-20 separation of pigments from shells of red sea urchin (*Strongylocentrotus franciscanus*). *Food Chem.* **1994**, *51*, 227–229. [CrossRef]
48. Tung, Y.-T.; Wu, J.-H.; Kuo, Y.-H.; Chang, S.-T. Antioxidant activities of natural phenolic compounds from Acacia confusa bark. *Bioresour. Technol.* **2007**, *98*, 1120–1123. [CrossRef]
49. Abdelfattah, M.A.; Mohamed, A.S.; Ibrahim, S.A.; Fahmy, S.R. Allolobophora caliginosa coelomic fluid and extract alleviate glucocorticoid-induced osteoporosis in mice by suppressing oxidative stress and regulating osteoblastic/osteoclastic-related markers. *Sci. Rep.* **2023**, *13*, 2090. [CrossRef] [PubMed]
50. Parameswari, P.; Devika, R.; Vijayaraghavan, P. In vitro anti-inflammatory and antimicrobial potential of leaf extract from Artemisia nilagirica (Clarke) Pamp. *Saudi J. Biol. Sci.* **2019**, *26*, 460–463. [CrossRef]
51. DeLano, W.L. Pymol: An open-source molecular graphics tool. *CCP4 Newsl. Protein Crystallogr.* **2002**, *40*, 82–92.
52. Jnoff, E.; Albrecht, C.; Barker, J.J.; Barker, O.; Beaumont, E.; Bromidge, S.; Brookfield, F.; Brooks, M.; Bubert, C.; Ceska, T.; et al. Binding Mode and Structure–Activity Relationships around Direct Inhibitors of the Nrf2–Keap1 Complex. *ChemMedChem* **2014**, *9*, 699–705. [CrossRef]
53. Morris, G.M.; Huey, R.; Lindstrom, W.; Sanner, M.F.; Belew, R.K.; Goodsell, D.S.; Olson, A.J. AutoDock4 and AutoDockTools4: Automated docking with selective receptor flexibility. *J. Comput. Chem.* **2009**, *30*, 2785–2791. [CrossRef] [PubMed]
54. O'Boyle, N.M.; Banck, M.; James, C.A.; Morley, C.; Vandermeersch, T.; Hutchison, G.R. Open Babel: An open chemical toolbox. *J. Cheminf.* **2011**, *3*, 33. [CrossRef] [PubMed]
55. Trott, O.; Olson, A.J. AutoDock Vina: Improving the speed and accuracy of docking with a new scoring function, efficient optimization, and multithreading. *J. Comput. Chem.* **2010**, *31*, 455–461. [CrossRef] [PubMed]
56. Adasme, M.F.; Linnemann, K.L.; Bolz, S.N.; Kaiser, F.; Salentin, S.; Haupt, V.J.; Schroeder, M. PLIP 2021: Expanding the scope of the protein–ligand interaction profiler to DNA and RNA. *Nucleic Acids Res.* **2021**, *49*, W530–W534. [CrossRef] [PubMed]
57. Bai, D.; Sun, T.; Lu, F.; Shen, Y.; Zhang, Y.; Zhang, B.; Yu, G.; Li, H.; Hao, J. Eupatilin Suppresses OVA-Induced Asthma by Inhibiting NF-κB and MAPK and Activating Nrf2 Signaling Pathways in Mice. *Int. J. Mol. Sci.* **2022**, *23*, 1582.
58. Yun, H.R.; Ahn, S.W.; Seol, B.; Vasileva, E.A.; Mishchenko, N.P.; Fedoreyev, S.A.; Stonik, V.A.; Han, J.; Ko, K.S.; Rhee, B.D. Echinochrome A treatment alleviates atopic dermatitis-like skin lesions in NC/Nga mice via IL-4 and IL-13 suppression. *Mar. Drugs* **2021**, *19*, 622. [CrossRef]
59. Liu, C.; You, J.; Lu, Y.; Sun, J.; Pan, J.; Li, Y.; Liu, T.; Li, Y.; Wang, A.; Zhang, X. Protective effects on ovalbumin-induced mouse asthma models and qualitative and quantitative analysis of multiple compounds in Gerberae Piloselloidis Herba. *J. Sep. Sci.* **2022**, *45*, 990–1005. [CrossRef]
60. Abdelaziz, M.H.; El-Dakdoky, M.H.; Ahmed, T.A.; Mohamed, A.S. Biological impacts of the green synthesized silver nanoparticles on the pregnant albino rats and their fetuses. *Birth Defects Res.* **2023**, *115*, 441–457. [CrossRef]
61. Abdelaziz, M.H.; Abdelfattah, M.A.; Bahaaeldine, M.A.; Rashed, A.R.; Mohamed, A.S.; Ali, M.F.; Elbatran, M.M.; Saad, D.Y. Earthworm Extract Enhanced Organ Functions in Diabetic Rats by Ameliorating Physiological and Structural Changes. *Biointerface Res. Appl. Chem.* **2022**, *13*, 445.
62. Koura, R.A.A.; Mohamed, H.R.H.; Baiomy, A.A.; Bahaaeldine, M.A.; Mohamed, A.S. The Therapeutic Role of Chitosan-Saponin-Bentonite Nanocomposite on Acute Kidney Injury Induced by Chromium in Male Wistar Rats. *Biointerface Res. Appl. Chem.* **2023**, *13*, 595.

Disclaimer/Publisher's Note: The statements, opinions and data contained in all publications are solely those of the individual author(s) and contributor(s) and not of MDPI and/or the editor(s). MDPI and/or the editor(s) disclaim responsibility for any injury to people or property resulting from any ideas, methods, instructions or products referred to in the content.

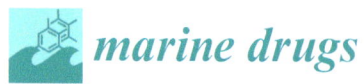
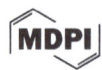

Article

Isaridin E Protects against Sepsis by Inhibiting Von Willebrand Factor-Induced Endothelial Hyperpermeability and Platelet–Endothelium Interaction

Yao-Sheng Liu [1,†], Wen-Liang Chen [2,†], Yu-Wei Zeng [1], Zhi-Hong Li [1], Hao-Lin Zheng [3], Ni Pan [4], Li-Yan Zhao [1], Shu Wang [1], Sen-Hua Chen [5,6], Ming-Hua Jiang [5,6], Chen-Chen Jin [1], Yu-Chen Mi [1], Zhao-Hui Cai [1], Xin-Zhe Fang [1], Yong-Jun Liu [7,8,*], Lan Liu [5,6,*] and Guan-Lei Wang [1,*]

[1] Department of Pharmacology, Zhongshan School of Medicine, Sun Yat-sen University, Guangzhou 510080, China; liuysh55@mail2.sysu.edu.cn (Y.-S.L.); zengyw25@mail2.sysu.edu.cn (Y.-W.Z.); l1352272780@163.com (Z.-H.L.); zhaoyan0809@hotmail.com (L.-Y.Z.); medpharm_ws@163.com (S.W.); 18826478932@163.com (C.-C.J.); miych@mail2.sysu.edu.cn (Y.-C.M.); caizhh28@mail2.sysu.edu.cn (Z.-H.C.); fangxzh3@mail.sysu.edu.cn (X.-Z.F.)

[2] Scientific Research Center, The Medical Interdisciplinary Science Research Center of Western Guangdong, College of Women and Children, The Second Affiliated Hospital of Guangdong Medical University, Zhanjiang 524023, China; febright@126.com

[3] Division of Biosciences, University College London, London WC1E 6BT, UK; leo.zheng.22@ucl.ac.uk

[4] Department of Pharmacy, The Second Clinical College, Guangzhou Medical University, Guangzhou 510261, China; pann@mail2.sysu.edu.cn

[5] School of Marine Sciences, Sun Yat-sen University, Guangzhou 510006, China; chensenh@mail.sysu.edu.cn (S.-H.C.); jiangmh23@mail2.sysu.edu.cn (M.-H.J.)

[6] Southern Marine Sciences and Engineering Guangdong Laboratory (Zhuhai), Zhuhai 519000, China

[7] Guangdong Provincial Clinical Research Center of Critical Care Medicine, Guangzhou 510080, China

[8] Department of Critical Care Medicine, The First Affiliated Hospital of Sun Yat-sen University, Guangzhou 510080, China

* Correspondence: liuyjun3@mail.sysu.edu.cn (Y.-J.L.); cesllan@mail.sysu.edu.cn (L.L.); wangglei@mail.sysu.edu.cn (G.-L.W.)

† These authors contributed equally to this work.

Citation: Liu, Y.-S.; Chen, W.-L.; Zeng, Y.-W.; Li, Z.-H.; Zheng, H.-L.; Pan, N.; Zhao, L.-Y.; Wang, S.; Chen, S.-H.; Jiang, M.-H.; et al. Isaridin E Protects against Sepsis by Inhibiting Von Willebrand Factor-Induced Endothelial Hyperpermeability and Platelet–Endothelium Interaction. *Mar. Drugs* **2024**, *22*, 283. https://doi.org/10.3390/md22060283

Academic Editor: Chang-Lun Shao

Received: 25 April 2024
Revised: 14 June 2024
Accepted: 14 June 2024
Published: 16 June 2024

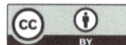

Copyright: © 2024 by the authors. Licensee MDPI, Basel, Switzerland. This article is an open access article distributed under the terms and conditions of the Creative Commons Attribution (CC BY) license (https:// creativecommons.org/licenses/by/ 4.0/).

Abstract: Endothelial hyperpermeability is pivotal in sepsis-associated multi-organ dysfunction. Increased von Willebrand factor (vWF) plasma levels, stemming from activated platelets and endothelium injury during sepsis, can bind to integrin αvβ3, exacerbating endothelial permeability. Hence, targeting this pathway presents a potential therapeutic avenue for sepsis. Recently, we identified isaridin E (ISE), a marine-derived fungal cyclohexadepsipeptide, as a promising antiplatelet and antithrombotic agent with a low bleeding risk. ISE's influence on septic mortality and sepsis-induced lung injury in a mouse model of sepsis, induced by caecal ligation and puncture, is investigated in this study. ISE dose-dependently improved survival rates, mitigating lung injury, thrombocytopenia, pulmonary endothelial permeability, and vascular inflammation in the mouse model. ISE markedly curtailed vWF release from activated platelets in septic mice by suppressing vesicle-associated membrane protein 8 and soluble N-ethylmaleide-sensitive factor attachment protein 23 overexpression. Moreover, ISE inhibited healthy human platelet adhesion to cultured lipopolysaccharide (LPS)-stimulated human umbilical vein endothelial cells (HUVECs), thereby significantly decreasing vWF secretion and endothelial hyperpermeability. Using cilengitide, a selective integrin αvβ3 inhibitor, it was found that ISE can improve endothelial hyperpermeability by inhibiting vWF binding to αvβ3. Activation of the integrin αvβ3-FAK/Src pathway likely underlies vWF-induced endothelial dysfunction in sepsis. In conclusion, ISE protects against sepsis by inhibiting endothelial hyperpermeability and platelet-endothelium interactions.

Keywords: sepsis; endothelial hyperpermeability; von Willebrand factor; isaridin E; acute lung injury

1. Introduction

Sepsis, a life-threatening disease caused by an excessive response to infection, manifests with multiple organ dysfunctions, notably acute lung injury [1]. Globally, there were approximately 48.9 million reported sepsis cases in 2017, contributing to 11.0 million deaths and constituting 19.7% of total deaths [2]. Despite its prevalence and high mortality, effective treatments remain elusive, underscoring the urgent need to develop intervention targets and therapeutic agents.

The progression of multiple organ failure is correlated with sepsis mortality. Endothelial hyperpermeability has emerged as a major cause of this phenomenon over the last two decades [3]. Early in septic infection, both exogenous pathogen-associated and endogenous damage-associated molecular patterns activate the vascular endothelium, leading to structural and/or functional damage to endothelial cells (ECs). This disruption causes decreased endothelial barrier integrity, interstitial oedema, and tissue hypoperfusion, which lead to sepsis-associated multi-organ failure. Several functional proteins, such as syndecan-1 and VE-cadherin, have been proposed as diagnostic and prognostic markers for sepsis due to their roles in regulating endothelial hyperpermeability. Strategies targeting endothelial hyperpermeability were able to attenuate sepsis in experimental models by limiting vascular leakage and inflammation and reversing maladaptive EC responses to infection during sepsis [3]. A deeper understanding of the molecular mechanisms regulating endothelial hyperpermeability will help to identify novel targets for sepsis treatment.

von Willebrand factor (vWF), crucial in hemostasis and thrombosis, bridges activated platelets and ECs and serves as a marker of endothelial damage and thrombotic risk in sepsis and other serious infectious diseases, particularly COVID-19 [4]. vWF is synthesized and stored exclusively in ECs and megakaryocytes in basal levels, and which is routinely used to stain or identify vascular ECs in tissue sections. The increased vWF is observed during endothelial damage [5]. Upon activation of platelets and/or injury of endothelium, there is a rapid, substantial local release of ultra-large vWF (ULvWF) at the site of injury. ADAMTS-13 (a disintegrin and metalloproteinase with a thrombospondin type 1 motif, member 13) is responsible for cleaving ULvWF into smaller pieces, thereby reducing its plasma levels and activity. Elevated vWF/ADAMTS-13 ratios have been observed in sepsis and COVID-19 and are positively correlated with high ICU mortality [6,7]. Recently, the vWF/ADAMTS-13 axis has emerged as a potential therapeutic target for both sepsis and COVID-19. The integrin $\alpha v \beta 3$ receptor in ECs facilitates the binding of acutely secreted vWF to ECs under fluid shear stress through the interaction between vWF and integrin $\alpha v \beta 3$ [8]. Additionally, integrin $\alpha v \beta 3$ has been implicated in sepsis-related endothelial injury in in vitro EC models of SARS-CoV-2 infection as well as infections with *Staphylococcus aureus* and *Escherichia coli* [9,10]. However, the pathological significance of vWF-integrin $\alpha v \beta 3$ interactions in sepsis-associated endothelial hyperpermeability and the underlying molecular mechanism remain unclear.

Platelet activation serving a catalytic spot for thrombin formation is associated with sepsis severity. Platelets that interplay with endothelium are essential for maintaining endothelium integrity in resting [11]. Platelet hyperactivity occurring during sepsis causes disruption or dysfunction of the endothelium, leading to intravascular coagulation, which is the critical stage of multiple organ failure [12]. Our previous investigation revealed that isaridin E (ISE), a cyclodepsipeptide derived from the marine fungus *Amphichorda felina* SYSU-MS7908 sourced from the South China Sea, displayed antiplatelet and antithrombotic effects in both in vitro and in vivo thrombosis formation models induced by adenosine diphosphate (ADP) and FeCl$_3$, respectively [13]. Notably, we observed that the bleeding risk of ISE in vivo was much lower compared to clopidogrel, and ISE did not exhibit cytotoxicity to mouse platelets at doses below 400 µM [13]. These findings motivated us to further explore its efficacy in a thrombotic disease animal model, specifically sepsis, wherein platelet hyperactivity is critical to its pathogenesis.

In this study, our objective was to investigate the therapeutic outcomes of ISE on sepsis and reveal the relevant underlying molecular mechanisms.

2. Results

2.1. ISE Increased the Survival Rate While Alleviating Acute Lung Injury and Systemic Inflammation in CLP-Induced Septic Mice

We examined the impact of ISE on sepsis-induced mortality. Mouse survival was monitored for 7 days post-CLP with or without ISE pretreatment (25, 50, and 100 mg/kg) (Figure 1B). Mice with CLP-induced sepsis had a 7-day survival rate of 20%, which increased to 30%, 50%, and 60% with pretreatment of 25, 50, and 100 mg/kg ISE, respectively (n = 10 per group, Figure 1C). Body weight is a crucial indicator of sepsis severity. Mice subjected to CLP-induced sepsis, with or without ISE pretreatment, experienced initial weight loss for the first three days, followed by weight recovery. Notably, 50 or 100 mg/kg ISE significantly alleviated sepsis-induced weight loss (Figure 1D).

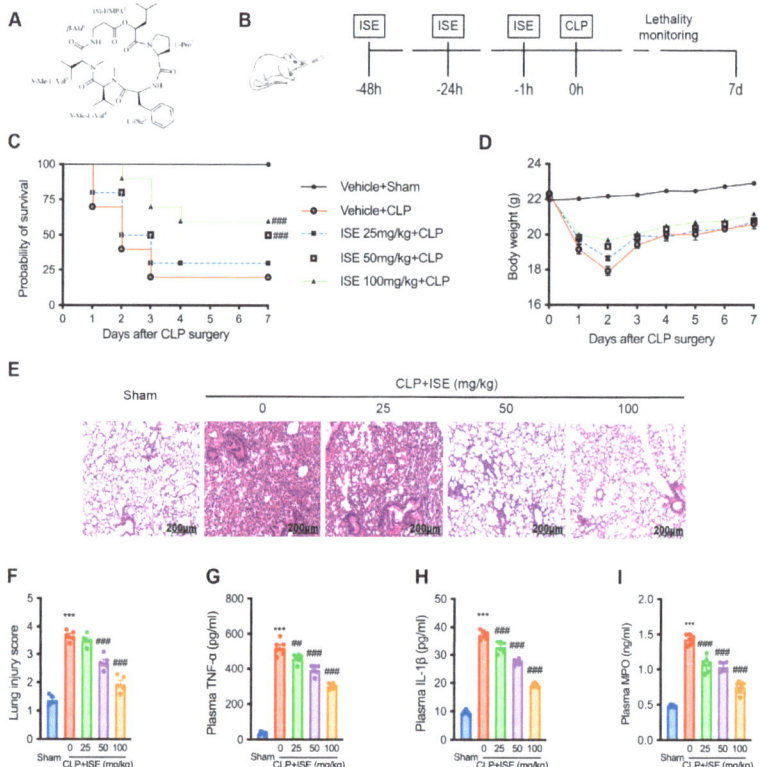

Figure 1. Effects of ISE on survival, lung injury, and systemic inflammation in septic mice. (**A**) Chemical structure of ISE. (**B**) Schematic overview of the experimental procedure. Mice were pretreated with multiple intragastric administrations of ISE (25, 50, or 100 mg/kg) or vehicle at 48 h, 24 h, and 1 h before the CLP operation. (**C**) Mice survival was monitored every 6 h for 7 consecutive days. Kaplan–Meier survival curves were used to analyze the data (n = 10 mice per group). The significance was evaluated by the log-rank (Mantel–Cox) test. (**D**) Body weights were measured and plotted every day for 7 days after the CLP surgery. (n = 2–10 mice per group). (**E**) Representative histological images of the lungs of control (vehicle-injected) and ISE-treated mice via H&E staining. Scale bar = 200 μm. (**F**) Lung tissue damage scores were evaluated in H&E-stained sections (five randomly chosen sections per mice, n = 5 mice per group). (**G–I**) Plasma inflammatory cytokine levels of TNF-α, IL-1β, and MPO after 12 h CLP surgery were determined using ELISA (n = 6 mice per group). *** $p < 0.001$ vs. the sham group; ## $p < 0.01$; ### $p < 0.001$ vs. the vehicle + CLP group.

We assessed the effects of ISE on lung injury in septic mice. Hematoxylin and eosin-stained sections of lung tissues revealed significant interalveolar septal thickening, interstitial hemorrhage, and microvascular thrombus formation in CLP-induced septic mice, indicative of CLP-induced acute lung injury (Figure 1E, F, *** $p < 0.001$). ISE pretreatment (50 and 100 mg/kg) significantly ameliorated sepsis-induced lung injury (Figure 1E) and reduced lung injury scores ($n = 5$ per group, ### $p < 0.001$; Figure 1F). Additionally, in CLP-induced septic mice, we observed a significant increase in the levels of TNF-α, IL-1β, and MPO in plasma, which were significantly reduced by ISE pretreatment. The levels of TNF-α, IL-1β, and MPO in CLP-induced septic mice were 520.3 ± 17.8 pg/mL, 37.3 ± 0.6 pg/mL, and 1.4 ± 0.03 ng/mL, respectively. ISE pretreatment at doses of 25, 50, and 100 mg/kg reduced the plasma levels of TNF-α by $10.9 \pm 4.1\%$, $23.6 \pm 3.5\%$, and $41.3 \pm 2.5\%$, IL-1β by $12.0 \pm 0.9\%$, $26.1 \pm 0.5\%$, and $48.0 \pm 1.6\%$, and MPO by $24.5 \pm 4.6\%$, $27.5 \pm 2.5\%$, and $47.3 \pm 2.7\%$, respectively. (## $p < 0.01$, ### $p < 0.001$ vs. the vehicle + CLP group, Figure 1G–I).

2.2. ISE Improved Pulmonary Vascular Permeability

Evans blue staining indicated significantly elevated pulmonary endothelial permeability in septic mice 12 h post-CLP ($n = 6$ per group, Figure 2A,B). As shown in Figure 2B, ISE at doses of 50 mg/kg and 100 mg/kg significantly decreased the CLP-induced maximum Evans blue penetration to $79.8 \pm 2.4\%$ and $66.7 \pm 4.3\%$ of the vehicle + CLP group. Moreover, CLP increased the levels of bronchoalveolar lavage fluid proteins and cells, which were reduced by ISE pretreatment ($n = 6$ per group, Figure 2C,D). These findings demonstrate that ISE may guard against sepsis-induced loss of endothelial barrier integrity.

CLP caused significant increases in plasma endoglin and syndecan-1 ($n = 6$ per group, Figure 2E,F) along with decreased tissue VE-cadherin and occludin levels ($n = 6$ per group, Figure 2G–I) in septic mice, which were ameliorated by ISE pretreatment. This suggests that ISE may have direct protective effects on lung vascular ECs, rendering the lungs less susceptible to sepsis-induced endothelial dysfunction. Furthermore, the effects of ISE on LPS-stimulated HUVECs were examined using an FITC-dextran assay. Incubation of HUVECs with 10 ng/mL LPS for 6 h substantially increased FITC-dextran permeability, while ISE significantly decreased this permeability with an IC_{50} of 21.5 μM ($n = 6$ per group, Figure 2J). Next, we chose the ISE concentration of 25 μM and 50 μM for the subsequent intervention experiments. Consistently, ISE pretreatment significantly reduced the LPS-induced increase in VE-cadherin and occludin protein expression in HUVECs ($n = 6$ per group, Figure 2K–M). Overall, these results suggest that ISE acts directly on vascular ECs, thereby mitigating increased pulmonary vascular permeability and lung injury induced by CLP sepsis.

2.3. ISE Suppressed Sepsis-Associated vWF Release

ISE significantly inhibited ATP release from activated platelets [8]. Activated platelets and injured endothelium are the primary sources of vWF, and vWF in injured endothelium plays an important role in the development of pulmonary embolism, platelet consumption, and multiple organ dysfunction during severe infectious diseases, such as sepsis and severe COVID-19 infection [14,15]. At doses of 25, 50, and 100 mg/kg, ISE reduced the plasma vWF level by $11.4 \pm 2.5\%$, $25.3 \pm 1.6\%$, and $39.4 \pm 2.4\%$, respectively, in comparison to the corresponding vehicle + CLP group ($n = 6$ per group, Figure 3A). Additionally, CLP-induced sepsis also decreased the platelet count from $(602.6 \pm 14.7) \times 10^9$/L to $(408.3 \pm 15.3) \times 10^9$/L, which was improved by ISE pretreatment ($n = 6$ per group, Figure 3B). Specifically, ISE (100 mg/kg) restored the decreased platelet count in CLP-septic mice to a level comparable to that in the sham group.

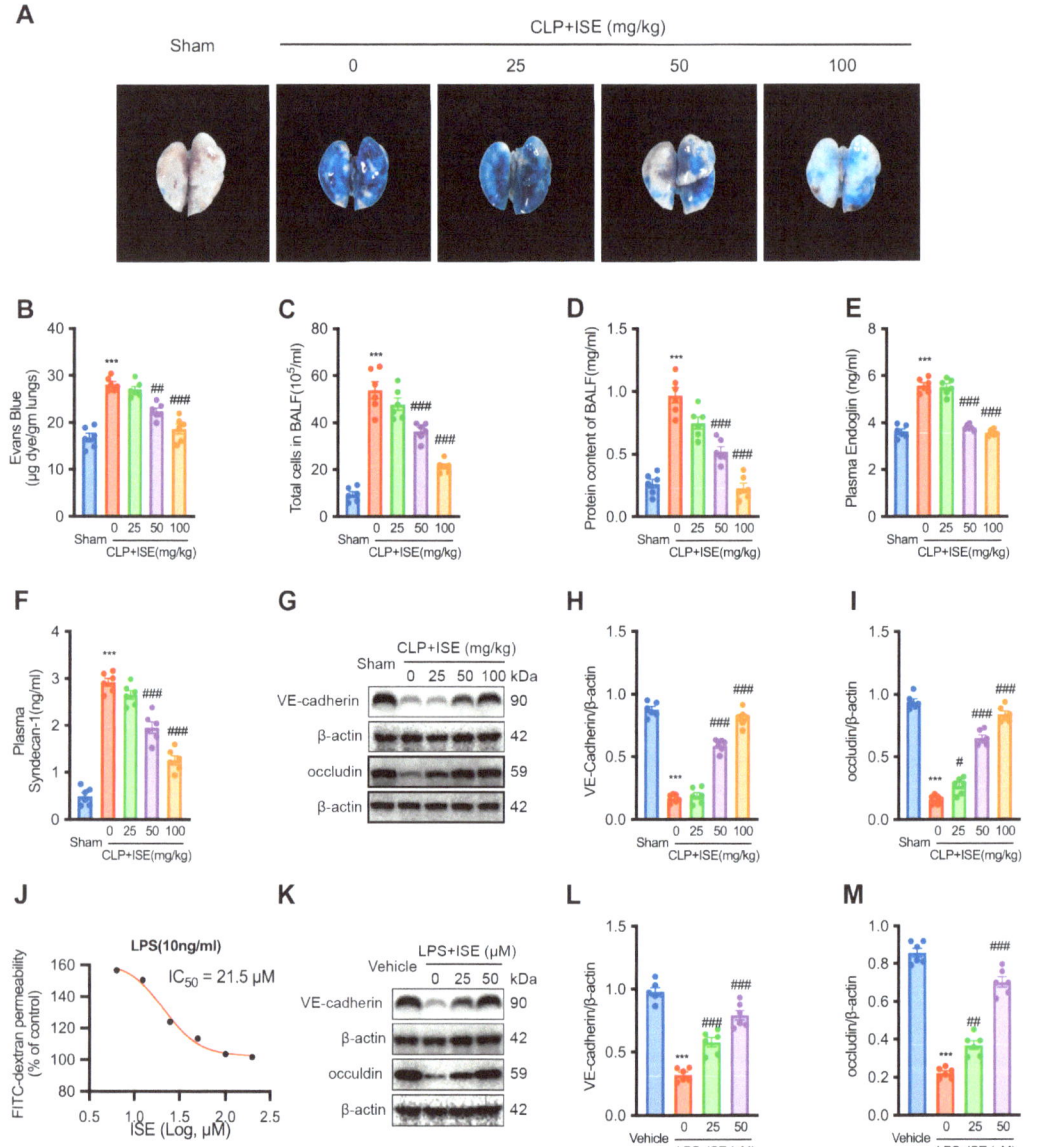

Figure 2. ISE significantly improved pulmonary endothelial permeability. (**A**) Representative images of lungs from mice treated via the tail vein with Evans blue staining. (**B**) Evans blue dye contents in the lungs. (**C,D**) The levels of cell count and protein content in bronchoalveolar lavage fluid. (**E,F**) The plasma levels of endoglin and syndecan-1 were determined by ELISA. (**G–I**) Western blot results of VE-cadherin and occludin expression in mouse lung tissue. (**J**) The IC$_{50}$ value of ISE for the increased endothelial permeability induced by 10 ng/mL LPS is 21.5 µM. (**K–M**) Western blot results of VE-cadherin and occludin expression in LPS-stimulated HUVECs. n = 6 independent experiments. *** $p < 0.001$ vs. the sham group (animal) or the control group (cell); # $p < 0.05$; ## $p < 0.01$, ### $p < 0.001$ vs. the vehicle + CLP group (animal) or LPS group (cell).

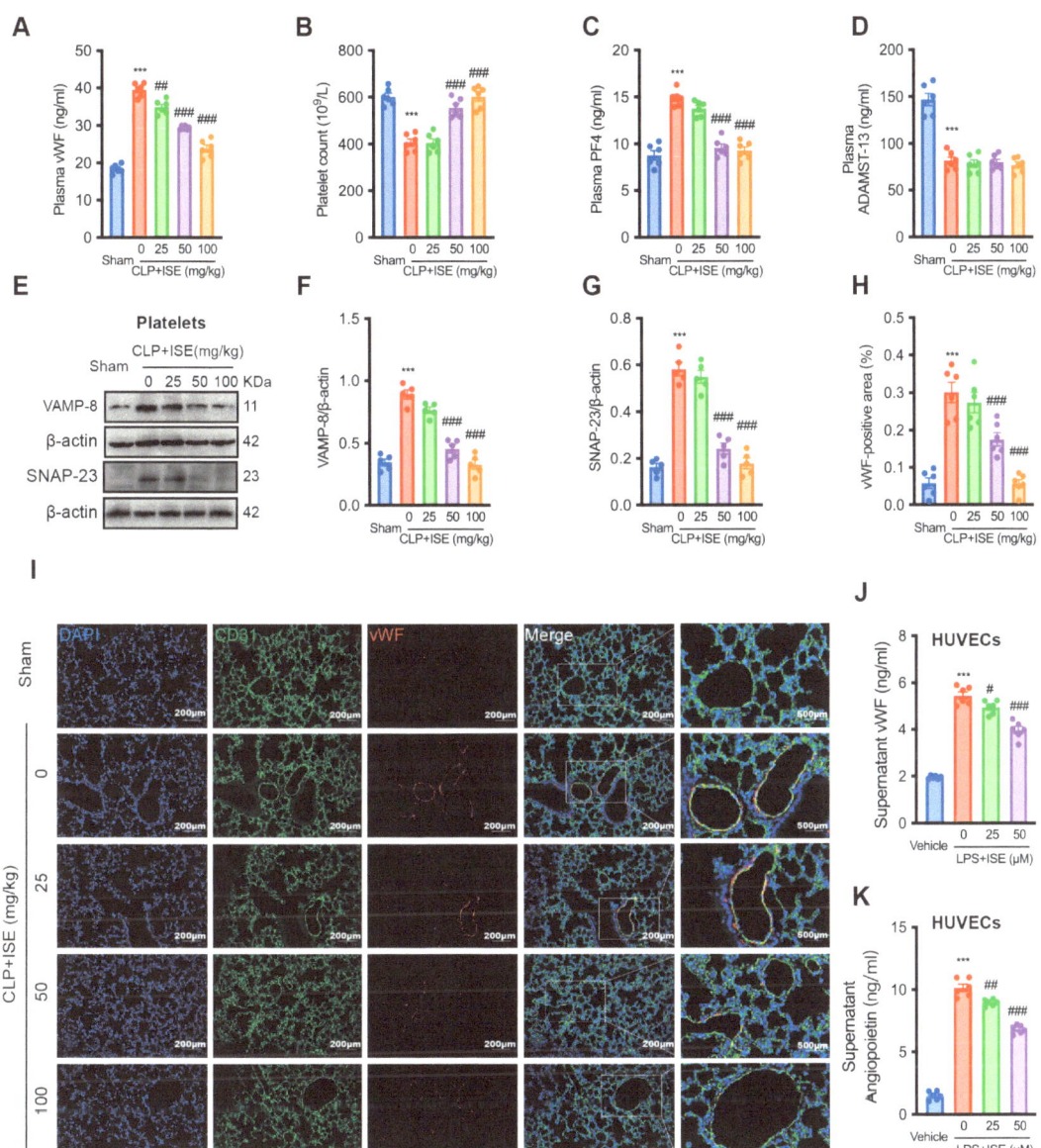

Figure 3. ISE inhibited vWF release under septic conditions. (**A**) The plasma levels of vWF were determined by ELISA. $n = 6$ mice per group. (**B**) Platelet count in mice. $n = 6$ mice per group. (**C,D**) The ELISA results of serum PF4 and ADAMST-13 in mice. $n = 6$ mice per group. (**E–G**) Western blot results of VAMP-8 and SNAP-23 expression in mouse platelets. $n = 5$ independent experiments. (**H,I**) Immunofluorescence staining results for vWF (red) expression in lung tissues and CD31 staining (green) were used as an endothelium marker. Scale bar = 200 μm and 500 μm, respectively. $n = 6$ mice per group. (**J,K**) VWF and angiopoietin 2 in the supernatant of HUVECs. $n = 6$ independent experiments. *** $p < 0.001$ vs. the sham group (animal) or the control group (cell); # $p < 0.05$; ## $p < 0.01$, ### $p < 0.001$ vs. the vehicle + CLP group (animal) or LPS group (cell).

Under diseased conditions, activated platelets and injured ECs are major sources of high levels of circulating vWF. We therefore examined whether ISE regulates the release of vWF from platelets and ECs during sepsis. ISE pretreatment significantly reduced elevated PF4 levels (n = 6 per group, Figure 3C), but did not affect the decreased ADAMST-13 levels in the plasma of CLP-septic mice (n = 6 per group, Figure 3D). Soluble N-ethylmaleide-sensitive factor attachment protein 23 (SNAP-23) and vesicle-associated membrane protein 8 (VAMP-8) are responsible for granule secretion during platelet activation. ISE pretreatment diminished enhanced SNAP-23 and VAMP-8 protein expression in the platelets of CLP-induced sepsis mice (n = 5 independent experiments, Figure 3E–G). Injured ECs are another important source of vWF in plasma. For a more intuitive observation, we used immunofluorescence to observe the effect of ISE on vWF derived from sepsis lung ECs. As shown in Figure 3H, I, pretreatment with 50 mg/kg and 100 mg/kg of ISE significantly reduced vWF expression in the pulmonary vascular endothelium of CLP-induced sepsis mice (vehicle + CLP group, 0.30 ± 0.03% vs. 50 mg/kg + ISE CLP, 0.18 ± 0.02%, ### $p < 0.001$; vs. 100 mg/kg ISE + CLP, 0.06 ± 0.01%, ### $p < 0.001$). The results in Figure 3H, I clearly show that ISE specifically reduced vWF synthesized in injured ECs under the CLP–sepsis condition. Moreover, preincubation with 25 μM and 50 μM ISE significantly suppressed LPS-induced vWF secretion in HUVECs to 91.9 ± 2.7% and 72.8 ± 2.0% of cells treated with vehicle + LPS. (n = 6 independent experiments, Figure 3J). Angiopoietin 2 serves as a marker of Weibel–Palade bodies during EC secretion, and its LPS-induced increase was inhibited by ISE pretreatment of HUVECs (n = 6 independent experiments, Figure 3K). Overall, these results suggest that ISE may reduce locally high accumulation of vWF by decreasing its secretion from activated platelets and injured ECs during sepsis.

2.4. ISE Inhibited LPS-Induced Platelet–EC Interaction

ISE pretreatment significantly decreased the increase in vWF caused by sepsis (Figure 3). Therefore, whether ISE affected vWF-mediated platelet–EC interactions was investigated. Fluorescence analysis showed that LPS stimulation of HUVECs increased the adhesion of platelets to HUVECs (n = 5 independent experiments, Figure 4A,B). This effect was inhibited by ISE in a concentration-dependent manner (LPS group, 1.3 ± 0.1% vs. LPS + 25 μM ISE group, 0.9 ± 0.1%, ### $p < 0.001$, LPS group 1.3 ± 0.1% vs. LPS + 50 μM ISE group 0.4 ± 0.1%, ### $p < 0.001$, Figure 4).

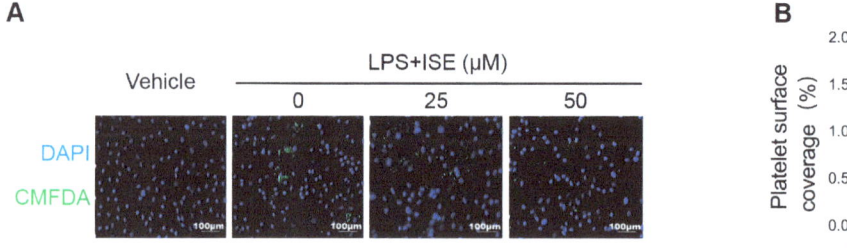

Figure 4. ISE inhibited LPS-induced platelet–EC interaction. (**A**) The representative fluorescent images of co-incubation experiments. Cultured HUVECs were pretreated with vehicle, LPS, or LPS + ISE, and the adhesion rate of isolated platelets (CellTracker™ Green CMFDA Dye, green) to HUVECs (DAPI, blue) was analyzed. Scale bar = 100 μm. (**B**) Quantitative analysis of platelet adhesion to HUVECs. n = 5 independent experiments. *** $p < 0.001$ vs. the control group; ### $p < 0.001$ vs. the LPS group.

2.5. Effects of ISE on the Integrin αvβ3-FAK/Src Signalling Pathway

Integrin αvβ3, an adhesion receptor for vWF, has emerged as a novel therapeutic target for treating sepsis and COVID-19 by lowering enhanced endothelial permeability [16]. Cilengitide, a selective αvβ3/αvβ5 integrin antagonist [17], was employed to assess αvβ3 protein expression in HUVECs upon LPS stimulation. ISE pretreatment inhibited αvβ3 protein expression in a concentration-dependent manner (n = 5 independent experiments, Figure 5A–C). Correspondingly, ISE pretreatment inhibited the LPS-induced increase in endothelial permeability (Figure 2J–M) and vWF release from ECs (n = 5 independent experiments, Figure 3J,K). These findings suggest that ISE may prevent LPS-induced endothelial dysfunction by inhibiting the vWF-αvβ3 interaction. Thereafter, vWF's concentration-dependent increase of endothelial permeability (n = 5 independent experiments, Figure 5D) and decrease of protein expression of VE-cadherin and occludin (n = 5 independent experiments, Figure 5E–G) were verified. The IC_{50} value of ISE protected against increased endothelial permeability induced by 100 ng/mL vWF was 37.5 μM (n = 5 independent experiments, Figure 5H). Endothelial permeability was significantly attenuated by pretreatment with 50 nM cilengitide or 50 μM ISE alone. However, the combination of 50 nM cilengitide and 50 μM ISE failed to enhance the inhibitory effect of ISE on endothelial injury compared to the 50 μM ISE pretreatment group (n = 5 independent experiments, Figure 5I–L).

Activation of the integrin αvβ3-FAK/Src signaling pathway is crucial for basic EC functions, such as cell adhesion and permeability [18]. VWF significantly increased both FAK (Y397) and Src (Try416) phosphorylation but not total protein expression levels. However, phosphorylated FAK and Src were concentration-dependently inhibited by ISE on vWF-induced HUVECs after 15 min of pretreatment (n = 5 independent experiments, Figure 5M–O). These results suggest that ISE can sustain the endothelial protective effects by blocking vWF-mediated integrin αVβ3-FAK/Src signaling pathways even after a 15 min pretreatment.

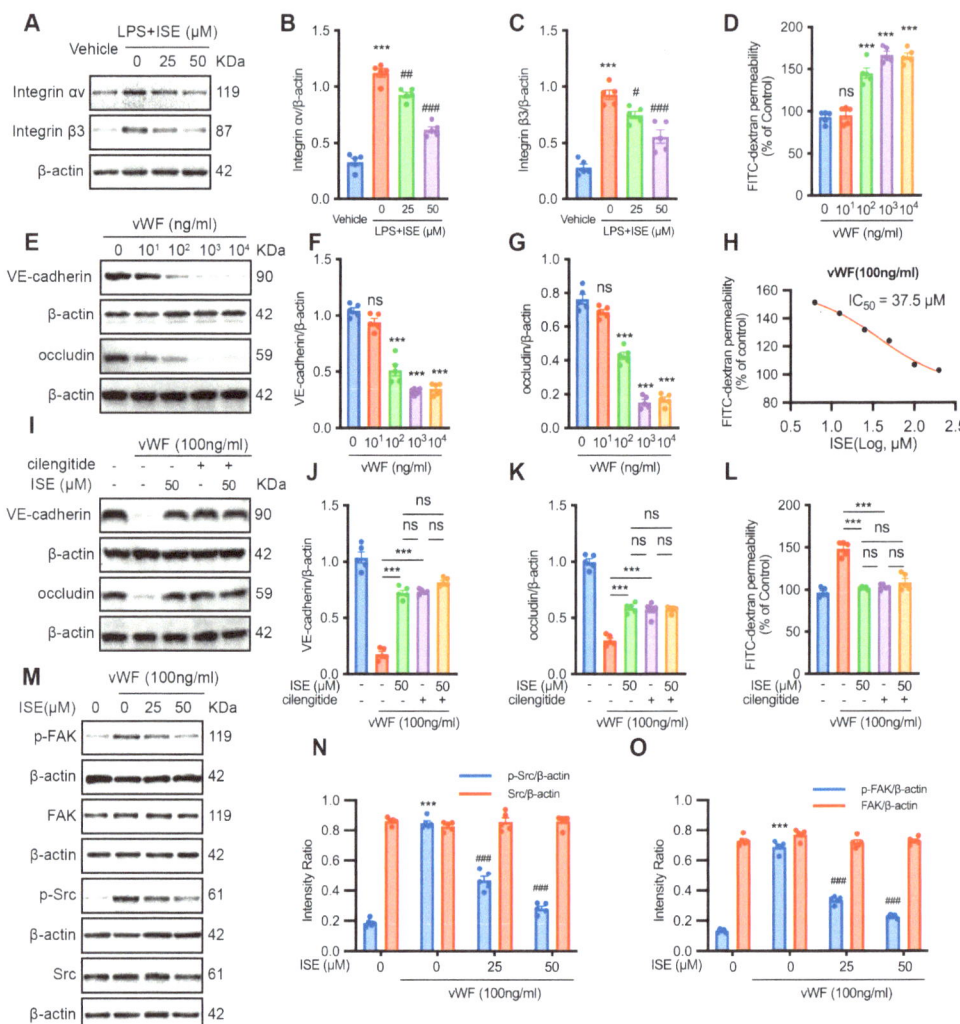

Figure 5. ISE inhibited the αVβ3-FAK/Src signaling pathway in vWF-stimulated HUVECs. (**A–C**) Western blotting analysis of integrin β3 and integrin αv expressions in HUVECs pretreated with LPS and different concentrations of ISE. $n = 5$ independent experiments. *** $p < 0.001$ vs. the vehicle group; # $p < 0.05$, ## $p < 0.01$, ### $p < 0.001$ vs. the LPS group. (**D**) Evaluation of endothelial permeability in vWF-stimulated HUVECs using the FITC-dextran assay. ns $p > 0.05$, *** $p < 0.001$ vs. the vehicle group. (**E–G**) Western blotting analysis of VE-cadherin and occludin expression in HUVECs pre-incubated with vehicle or different concentration of vWF. ns $p > 0.05$, *** $p < 0.001$ vs. the vehicle group. (**H**) The IC_{50} value of ISE for the increased endothelial permeability induced by 100 ng/mL vWF is 37.5 μM. (**I–K**) VE-cadherin and occludin expression in vWF-stimulated HUVECs following pretreatment with ISE or cilengitide alone or ISE + cilengitide. ns $p > 0.05$, *** $p < 0.001$. (**L**) Evaluation of endothelial permeability using the FITC-dextran assay. ns $p > 0.05$, *** $p < 0.001$. (**M–O**) Western blotting analysis of total and phosphorylated FAK (Y397) and Src (Try416) expressions in vWF-stimulated HUVECs pretreated with different concentrations of ISE. $n = 5$ independent experiments. *** $p < 0.001$ vs. the vehicle group; ### $p < 0.001$ vs. the vWF group.

3. Discussion

Endothelial hyperpermeability and subsequent vascular leakage are hallmarks of sepsis, contributing to microcirculatory blood flow damage, tissue hypoperfusion, and life-threatening multiple organ failure. Despite its significance, effectively targeting endothelial hyperpermeability remains a challenging aspect of sepsis treatment. This study provides compelling experimental evidence supporting the protective effects of ISE against sepsis through regulation of endothelial hyperpermeability and platelet–endothelial interactions. The findings indicate ISE has direct effects on activated ECs by inhibiting vWF secretion and the interaction between vWF-integrin $\alpha v \beta 3$ and downstream FAK/Src signaling. ISE also significantly reduced the increased release of vWF from activated platelets and platelet–EC interaction during sepsis.

According to the evidence, ISE, administered within a dose range between 25 mg/kg and 100 mg/kg, increases the survival rate and attenuates acute lung injury and systemic inflammation caused by CLP sepsis in a dose-dependent manner. Sepsis-induced platelet activation initiates microthrombus formation and rapid excessive platelet depletion, resulting in thrombocytopenia, a major cause of multiple organ failure [14,15]. Moreover, activated platelets secrete or generate agonists and cytokines, such as ADP, PF4, P-selectin, IL-1β, and vWF, which further amplify platelet activation and aggregation, fostering platelet–neutrophil interactions and NET formation, thereby fostering a proinflammatory and prothrombotic milieu during sepsis. Consequently, a reduced platelet count serves as a prognostic marker and predictor of poor outcomes in sepsis [16]. While antiplatelet and antithrombotic agents can improve survival and organ injury in animal models of sepsis, trials evaluating conventional antiplatelet drugs, such as $P2Y_{12}$ receptor antagonists, have yet to establish their efficacy in reducing sepsis mortality. Thus, there remains a critical need for novel antiplatelet agents with alternative mechanisms of action [15]. Although our previous investigation revealed the antiplatelet and antithrombotic effects of ISE in a mouse model of $FeCl_3$-induced carotid artery thrombosis [13], its effects in other thrombotic disease models remained unexplored. The present study found that ISE significantly attenuated CLP-induced sepsis by inhibiting pulmonary embolism and systemic inflammation and restoring depleted platelet counts, indicating its potential to protect against sepsis partly by mitigating platelet activation. The distinctive cyclodepsipeptides present in ISE may harbor novel antiplatelet molecular mechanisms and other undiscovered pharmacological effects against sepsis.

Notably, ISE pretreatment significantly ameliorated sepsis-induced pulmonary vascular permeability (Figure 2). During sepsis, enhanced pulmonary vascular permeability is mainly attributed to the disruption of endothelial barrier integrity. Syndecan-1 and endoglin are crucial components of the glycocalyx, the protective layer lining the luminal surface of ECs; their degradation contributes to microcirculatory dysfunction in sepsis [17]. VE-cadherin is expressed exclusively in ECs and maintains endothelial cell–cell junctions. Occludin is another critical transmembrane protein that is expressed at tight junctions in the endothelium. Both VE-cadherin and occludin expression are reduced in the lungs of CLP-induced septic mice [18]. Accumulating evidence shows that endothelial hyperpermeability is a key driver of sepsis pathology, and loss of endothelial barrier integrity contributes to vascular hyperpermeability development [3,19,20]. Experimental approaches targeting ECs specifically have yielded encouraging results. For instance, heparin (which protects against glycocalyx degradation), the Tie2 receptor agonist vasculotide (an angiopoietin-1 mimetic), and inhibitors of VE-cadherin internalization (via inhibition of the GTP-binding protein ARF6) are all promising therapies for reconstituting EC integrity during sepsis [3,21]. Moreover, ISE alleviated the disruption of pulmonary vascular permeability in septic mice, as evidenced by Evans blue dye extravasation assays and analysis of total protein and cells in bronchoalveolar lavage fluid. These findings support the hypothesis that ISE may prevent sepsis by acting directly on ECs. This was tested using LPS-stimulated ECs, which are a commonly used in vitro sepsis model. The results demonstrate the beneficial effects of ISE on LPS-induced disruption of endothelial permeability. This novel observation suggests that ISE acts directly on ECs, potentially contributing to its protective effects against sepsis-associated endothelial hyperpermeability.

vWF and vWF-mediated signaling pathways contribute to coagulation, platelet activation, adhesion, and endothelial activation, making them attractive therapeutic targets for various thrombotic and infectious diseases, including stroke, thrombotic thrombocytopenic purpura, sepsis, and COVID-19 [22–24]. Our previous research revealed that ISE specifically inhibits platelet activation and release with a relatively low IC_{50} value, suggesting that ISE affects vWF released from activated platelets during sepsis. Notably, the injured endothelium is another major source of elevated circulating vWF levels, especially under diseased conditions, such as vascular and infectious diseases [4,5,25–27]. For example, recent histological results in lung tissue from patients with COVID-19 have provided direct evidences showing clot formation with increased staining of EC-associated vWF [27]. Although a large amount of clinical evidence correlates the plasma levels of vWF with the severity and outcome of sepsis patients [28–30], there is no evidence of a correlation between local EC-vWF level with sepsis-induced lung injury. Here, we observed increased vWF in sepsis-induced lung sections, which was significantly reduced by ISE. Our results therefore supported the important role of EC-associated vWF in organ and tissue damage in many diseases. The significant inhibitory effect of ISE on EC-associated vWF levels may also provide an interesting direction for its application to other vascular and infectious diseases in the future.

High local concentrations of ULvWF strings can form net-like structures to capture platelets on injured ECs, resulting in increased platelet adhesion, aggregation, and initiation of the coagulation cascade. Given the high local concentration and unique network structure of vWF at vascular injury sites, drugs targeting vWF and vWF-mediated signaling pathways possess specific antithrombotic effects owing to their action at vascular injury sites, thereby reducing bleeding risk [31]. For instance, caplacizumab (ALX-0081), an anti-vWF A1 domain nanobody, is selectively used to treat acute thrombotic thrombocytopenic purpura by targeting the vWF-platelet glycoprotein 1bα interaction to inhibit microthrombosis formation [24]. In the present study, ISE reduced vWF release in LPS-stimulated HUVECs and inhibited platelet adhesion to LPS-stimulated HUVECs. Furthermore, the direct exposure of HUVECs caused impaired endothelial permeability, which was inhibited by ISE treatment. These findings suggest that the suppression of elevated vWF levels and increased platelet–EC interactions contribute to the protective effects of ISE against sepsis. Moreover, considering the emerging role of vWF as a selective antiplatelet target, the substantial inhibitory effect of ISE on elevated vWF levels resulting from activated platelets and injured endothelium might explain its significant antiplatelet effect and low bleeding risk.

Integrin $\alpha v \beta 3$, a heterodimeric transmembrane cell adhesion molecule composed of αv- and $\beta 3$-subunits, is prominently expressed on the surface of ECs [8]. It serves as a major vWF receptor on ECs [32] and is responsible for regulating endothelial permeability and angiogenesis [33,34]. Cilengitide, an integrin $\alpha v \beta 3$ inhibitor, has been shown to inhibit the disruption of endothelial permeability induced by bacterial attachment [35]. This study revealed that ISE inhibited integrin $\alpha v \beta 3$ expression in LPS-stimulated ECs. Notably, the combination of cilengitide and ISE produced comparable outcomes in mitigating vWF-mediated endothelial permeability disruption, underscoring the protective role of ISE against endothelial hyperpermeability during sepsis by suppressing the vWF–integrin $\alpha v \beta 3$ interaction. The FAK/Src signaling pathway serves as the downstream mediator of integrin $\alpha v \beta 3$ activation, regulating various biological processes, including angiogenesis [36,37]. Our findings demonstrate that vWF incubation significantly upregulated both phosphorylated FAK and Src protein expression, which was restored by ISE pretreatment without affecting their total protein expression. These results further reveal that ISE exerts its anti-sepsis effects by modulating the vWF/integrin $\alpha v \beta 3$/FAK/Src signaling pathway in ECs. As our focus was primarily on exploring the effects of ISE on endothelial hyperpermeability, further investigation of other functional phenotypes of ECs will provide valuable insights into the pharmacological effects of ISE on sepsis-induced endothelial responses.

NETs interact with platelets and the endothelium to activate matrix metalloproteinases, thereby impairing endothelial integrity. Therapeutic approaches that reduce NET formation, such as peptidylarginase deaminase 4 and TLR4 inhibitors, can improve lung injury and attenuate inflammation in sepsis [38]. In this study, ISE pretreatment significantly decreased MPO plasma levels, a marker of NET burden induced by CLP-induced sepsis. This suggests that ISE improves sepsis by inhibiting NET-associated mechanisms.

Endothelial hyperpermeability is the main driver of multiple organ failure and is associated with high morbidity and mortality rates in patients with sepsis. Thus, clinical drugs and novel compounds with beneficial effects on sepsis-associated endothelial hyperpermeability are promising avenues for sepsis therapy. In this study, we demonstrated that ISE pretreatment significantly increased the survival rate of mice with CLP-induced sepsis and attenuated sepsis-induced lung injury. Maintenance of EC integrity, improved thrombocytopenia, decreased vWF levels, and vWF-mediated platelet-EC interactions are responsible for these anti-sepsis effects. The regulation of vWF binding to integrin $\alpha v \beta 3$ and downstream FAK/Src signaling may explain the protective effects of ISE on endothelial hyperpermeability and warrant further investigation. The molecular mechanisms underlying the regulation of vWF release by ISE should also be investigated in future studies. Finally, given that ISE significantly improved sepsis-induced EC hyperpermeability and platelet activation with a low bleeding risk, it holds considerable potential for the development of new sepsis treatments.

4. Materials and Methods

4.1. Chemical Structure of Isaridin E

Isaridin E was obtained as a colorless crystal with a molecular formula of $C_{35}H_{54}O_7N_5$. The HR-ESIMS spectrum and NMR data of the molecule are described in our previous publication [13]. The chemical structure of ISE is depicted in Figure 1A. The HPLC data showed that the purity of ISE (Rt = 10.88 min) was >98.5% (Figure S1).

4.2. Preparations of ISE

For in vivo experiments, ISE was dissolved in a saline solution containing 10% Tween 80 and 15% propylene glycol (used as a vehicle control) at 2.5, 5, and 10 mg/mL [13]. For in vivo experiments, multiple intragastric administrations of ISE (25, 50, and 100 mg/kg/day) were applied at 48 h, 24 h, and 1 h before caecal ligation and puncture (CLP; Figure 1B). For in vitro experiments, ISE was dissolved in dimethyl sulfoxide (DMSO) and stored at 4 °C until use with a final concentration of DMSO < 0.1%.

4.3. Animals

The protocols for all experimental procedures were approved by the Sun Yat-sen University Animal Care and Use Committee (approval no. SYSU-IACUC-2020-B0112) and conducted in accordance with the "Guide for the Care and Use of Laboratory Animals" issued by the Ministry of Science and Technology of China.

Male C57BL/6 mice (6–8 weeks old, 21–23 g) were obtained from GemPharmatech, Nanjing, China, and housed under specific pathogen-free conditions. The CLP surgery was performed following established protocols [39]. Laparotomy was performed under anesthesia using 1.5% isoflurane (RWD, Shenzhen, China). Half the cecum was ligated and punctured twice with a 22-gauge needle, followed by resuscitation with an intraperitoneal injection of 1 mL of saline. Sham-operated mice underwent a similar laparotomy without ligation or double puncture. All mice were kept warm for 1 h post-surgery. Survival rates were monitored twice daily post-surgery, and mice were euthanized under anesthesia upon reaching the designed experimental endpoint. ISE pretreatment and CLP surgery were performed by different researchers to minimize the possible selection bias.

4.4. Hematoxylin and Eosin Staining

The lung samples were harvested and fixed in 4% paraformaldehyde (Sigma-Aldrich, St. Louis, MO, USA) for 48 h. Lung sections (5 µm) were stained with hematoxylin and eosin (H&E) following established procedures [40]. Pulmonary injury was evaluated using a lung injury grading system comprising four distinct categories: neutrophil infiltration, interstitial inflammation, oedema, and congestion. Five randomly selected tissue sections were used to calculate the average lung injury score, where scores assigned to four categories were averaged to acquire the overall lung injury score. The histological images were captured using Pannoramic MIDI (3DHISTECH, Budapest, Hungary).

4.5. Evans Blue Staining

Evans blue staining was employed to evaluate pulmonary vascular permeability [41]. Mice received an intravenous (*i.v.*) injection of 1% Evans blue dye (Sigma-Aldrich, St. Louis, MO, USA) diluted in normal saline. Lung tissues were harvested, and the dye was extracted by incubating the samples in 500 µL of formamide (Junsei, Tokyo, Japan) overnight at 60 °C. Subsequently, the samples were centrifuged at 14,000 rpm for 30 min, and Evans blue dye concentrations were determined by measuring absorbance at 630 nm.

4.6. Isolation and Culture of HUVECs

HUVECs were isolated and cultured following the protocol in our previous study [42]. The experimental protocol was approved by the Sun Yat-sen University Animal Care and Use Committee (No: SYSU-IACUC-2020-B0112). HUVECs were removed from human umbilical veins after collagenase type I digestion (Gibco, Grand Island, NY, USA) and cultured in 4 mL of ECM medium (Sciencell, Carlsbad, CA, USA) supplemented with 10% fetal bovine serum (Gibco, Grand Island, NY, USA) and 1% penicillin/streptomycin (Gibco, Grand Island, NY, USA) at 37 °C in 5% CO_2. Passage 3–6 HUVECs were utilized for experiments.

4.7. Platelet Preparation

Washed platelets followed previously established methods [43]. Whole blood was centrifuged at $300\times g$ for 10 min at room temperature to obtain platelet-rich plasma, which was then transferred to a fresh tube and centrifuged at $900\times g$ for 5 min. The platelet pellet was resuspended in Tyrode's buffer (134 mM NaCl, 12 mM $NaHCO_3$, 2.9 mM KCl, 0.34 mM Na_2HPO_4, 1 mM $MgCl_2$, 10 mM HEPES; pH 7.4) supplemented with 0.5 U/mL apyrase.

4.8. EC Permeability Assay

HUVECs were seeded at a density of 4×10^5 cells/well onto 12-well transwell semipermeable supports (0.4 µm pore size; Corning Incorporated, Corning, NY, USA) coated with 1% gelatin. Following treatment, FITC-dextran (30 mg/mL; Sigma–Aldrich, St. Louis, MO, USA) was added to the upper chamber, and the cells were incubated for an additional 30 min. Absorbance was measured at 492 nm (excitation) and 520 nm (emission) using the Victor Nivo 5S (PerkinElmer, Waltham, MA, USA).

4.9. Platelet Adhesion Experiment in HUVECs

HUVECs in 24-well plates were incubated with ISE for 1 h, followed by stimulation with 10 ng/mL LPS or PBS for 6 h. Freshly isolated platelets were labelled with 6 µM CellTracker™ Green CMFDA Dye (Invitrogen, Carlsbad, CA, USA) at 37 °C for 30 min. The dye-labelled platelets were added to stimulated HUVECs at a ratio of 100:1, and the cells were further incubated at 37 °C for 1 h. Images were acquired at 20-times and 40-times magnifications under a Leica DMI8 inverted fluorescence microscope (Leica, Wetzlar, Germany).

4.10. Measurement of Cytokine Levels

Elisa assays were performed following established protocols [44]. Briefly, ELISA kits for PF4, IL-1β, TNF-α, MPO (mibio, Shanghai, China), endoglin (MULTISCIENCES, Hangzhou, China), vWF, syndecan, and ADAMTS-13 (Cusabio, Wuhan, China) were used according to the manufacturer's protocol. Optical absorbance was measured at 450 nm using a Sunrise™ ELISA plate reader (Tecan, Zurich, Switzerland). Standard curves were generated by plotting the average optical density of the standard samples along the Y-axis against the corresponding concentration on the X-axis. Sample concentrations were performed with GraphPad Prism (Version 9.5.1, La Jolla, CA, USA).

4.11. Western Blot Analysis

For Western blot analysis, conventional or low-temperature SDS/PAGE were employed, as previously outlined [43]. Samples were separated on 8% SDS polyacrylamide gels and transferred onto nitrocellulose membranes. After incubation with primary antibodies, the membranes were kept at 4 °C overnight. Following this, nitrocellulose membranes were exposed to corresponding secondary antibodies conjugated with horseradish peroxidase (HRP) for 1.5 h at room temperature. Chemiluminescent signals emitted by protein bands were detected using an enhanced chemiluminescence (ECL) detection system (Millipore), and images were captured using an imaging system (Bio-Rad, Hercules, CA, USA). Optical densities were normalized to those of β-actin, and the fold difference for each target protein was calculated as the ratio of the target protein expression to β-actin expression using the ImageJ 2.1.0 software from the U.S. National Institutes of Health.

4.12. Statistical Analysis

The data are expressed as means ± SEM. All statistical analyses were performed using GraphPad Prism (Version 9.5.1, GraphPad Software, La Jolla, CA, USA). Student's t test was used to compare two groups. Three or more groups were compared using one-way analysis of variance, followed by Dunnett's multiple comparisons post-hoc test with a 95% confidence interval (CI). A p value of <0.05 was considered statistically significant.

Supplementary Materials: The following supporting information can be downloaded at: https://www.mdpi.com/article/10.3390/md22060283/s1, Figure S1: The HPLC diagram of sample of isaridin E. The analysis was performed on an Agilent ZORBAX Eclipse Plus C18 column (3.5 μm, 4.5 × 100 mm) using a linear gradient of MeCN and water (0–2 min: 30% MeCN, 2–15 min: 30% MeCN–100% MeCN, 15–25 min 100% MeCN, 25–26 min: 100% MeCN–30% MeCN, 26–30 min 30% MeCN, 0.8 mL/min; 210 nm; 30 °C; 10 μL).

Author Contributions: G.-L.W., Y.-S.L., W.-L.C. and L.L. designed the study. Y.-S.L., Y.-J.L., Y.-W.Z., Z.-H.L., S.-H.C. and M.-H.J. performed the experiments and analyzed the data. N.P., H.-L.Z., C.-C.J., S.W., L.-Y.Z., Y.-C.M., Z.-H.C. and X.-Z.F. assisted with the experiments. G.-L.W., Y.-S.L., W.-L.C., Y-J L. and H.-L.Z. wrote the manuscript. L.L. provided valuable suggestions. All authors have read and agreed to the published version of the manuscript.

Funding: This study was supported by the Key-Area Research and Development Program of Guangdong Province (No. 2023B1111050012; China); the National Natural Science Foundation of China (Nos. 82073848, 81773722, 82104160 and 81903687; China); the Natural Science Foundation of Guangdong Province (Nos. 2024A1515010479, 2021A1515012056); the Science and Technology Development Special Fund Competitive Allocation Project of Zhanjiang City (No: 2021A05086 to W.-L.C.).

Institutional Review Board Statement: The animal study protocol was approved by the Sun Yat-sen University Animal Care and Use Committee (approval no. SYSU-IACUC-2020-B0112, 3 April 2020).

Data Availability Statement: All data included in this study are available upon request by contact with the corresponding author.

Conflicts of Interest: The authors declare no conflicts of interest.

References

1. Cecconi, M.; Evans, L.; Levy, M.; Rhodes, A. Sepsis and Septic Shock. *Lancet* **2018**, *392*, 75–87. [CrossRef] [PubMed]
2. Rudd, K.E.; Johnson, S.C.; Agesa, K.M.; Shackelford, K.A.; Tsoi, D.; Kievlan, D.R.; Colombara, D.V.; Ikuta, K.S.; Kissoon, N.; Finfer, S.; et al. Global, Regional, and National Sepsis Incidence and Mortality, 1990-2017: Analysis for the Global Burden of Disease Study. *Lancet* **2020**, *395*, 200–211. [CrossRef] [PubMed]
3. Joffre, J.; Hellman, J.; Ince, C.; Ait-Oufella, H. Endothelial Responses in Sepsis. *Am. J. Respir. Crit. Care Med.* **2020**, *202*, 361–370. [CrossRef] [PubMed]
4. Birnhuber, A.; Fließer, E.; Gorkiewicz, G.; Zacharias, M.; Seeliger, B.; David, S.; Welte, T.; Schmidt, J.; Olschewski, H.; Wygrecka, M.; et al. Between Inflammation and Thrombosis: Endothelial Cells in COVID-19. *Eur. Respir. J.* **2021**, *58*, 2100377. [CrossRef]
5. Manz, X.D.; Bogaard, H.J.; Aman, J. Regulation of VWF (Von Willebrand Factor) in Inflammatory Thrombosis. *Arterioscler. Thromb. Vasc. Biol.* **2022**, *42*, 1307–1320. [CrossRef] [PubMed]
6. Levi, M.; Scully, M.; Singer, M. The Role of ADAMTS-13 in the Coagulopathy of Sepsis. *J. Thromb. Haemost. JTH* **2018**, *16*, 646–651. [CrossRef] [PubMed]
7. Madeeva, D.V.; Christian, J.; Goshua, G.; Chun, H.J.; Lee, A.I.; Pine, A.B. VWF/ADAMTS13 Ratios Are Potential Markers of Immunothrombotic Complications in Patients with COVID-19: A Cross-Sectional Study. *Blood* **2020**, *136*, 34–35. [CrossRef]
8. Huang, J.; Roth, R.; Heuser, J.E.; Sadler, J.E. Integrin Alpha(v)Beta(3) on Human Endothelial Cells Binds von Willebrand Factor Strings under Fluid Shear Stress. *Blood* **2009**, *113*, 1589–1597. [CrossRef] [PubMed]
9. Bugatti, A.; Filippini, F.; Bardelli, M.; Zani, A.; Chiodelli, P.; Messali, S.; Caruso, A.; Caccuri, F. SARS-CoV-2 Infects Human ACE2-Negative Endothelial Cells through an Avβ3 Integrin-Mediated Endocytosis Even in the Presence of Vaccine-Elicited Neutralizing Antibodies. *Viruses* **2022**, *14*, 705. [CrossRef]
10. McDonnell, C.J.; Garciarena, C.D.; Watkin, R.L.; McHale, T.M.; McLoughlin, A.; Claes, J.; Verhamme, P.; Cummins, P.M.; Kerrigan, S.W. Inhibition of Major Integrin αVβ3 Reduces Staphylococcus Aureus Attachment to Sheared Human Endothelial Cells. *J. Thromb. Haemost.* **2016**, *14*, 2536–2547. [CrossRef]
11. Ruggeri, Z.M. Von Willebrand Factor, Platelets and Endothelial Cell Interactions. *J. Thromb. Haemost. JTH* **2003**, *1*, 1335–1342. [CrossRef] [PubMed]
12. Dolmatova, E.V.; Wang, K.; Mandavilli, R.; Griendling, K.K. The Effects of Sepsis on Endothelium and Clinical Implications. *Cardiovasc. Res.* **2021**, *117*, 60–73. [CrossRef] [PubMed]
13. Pan, N.; Li, Z.-C.; Li, Z.-H.; Chen, S.-H.; Jiang, M.-H.; Yang, H.-Y.; Liu, Y.-S.; Hu, R.; Zeng, Y.-W.; Dai, L.-H.; et al. Antiplatelet and Antithrombotic Effects of Isaridin E Isolated from the Marine-Derived Fungus via Downregulating the PI3K/Akt Signaling Pathway. *Mar. Drugs* **2021**, *20*, 23. [CrossRef] [PubMed]
14. Wang, Y.; Ouyang, Y.; Liu, B.; Ma, X.; Ding, R. Platelet Activation and Antiplatelet Therapy in Sepsis: A Narrative Review. *Thromb. Res.* **2018**, *166*, 28–36. [CrossRef] [PubMed]
15. Giustozzi, M.; Ehrlinder, H.; Bongiovanni, D.; Borovac, J.A.; Guerreiro, R.A.; Gąsecka, A.; Papakonstantinou, P.E.; Parker, W.A.E. Coagulopathy and Sepsis: Pathophysiology, Clinical Manifestations and Treatment. *Blood Rev.* **2021**, *50*, 100864. [CrossRef] [PubMed]
16. Cheng, J.; Zeng, H.; Chen, H.; Fan, L.; Xu, C.; Huang, H.; Tang, T.; Li, M. Current Knowledge of Thrombocytopenia in Sepsis and COVID-19. *Front. Immunol.* **2023**, *14*, 1213510. [CrossRef] [PubMed]
17. Uchimido, R.; Schmidt, E.P.; Shapiro, N.I. The Glycocalyx: A Novel Diagnostic and Therapeutic Target in Sepsis. *Crit. Care Lond. Engl.* **2019**, *23*, 16. [CrossRef] [PubMed]
18. Yu, J.; Zhao, B.; Pi, Q.; Zhou, G.; Cheng, Z.; Qu, C.; Wang, X.; Kong, L.; Luo, S.; Du, D.; et al. Deficiency of S100A8/A9 Attenuates Pulmonary Microvascular Leakage in Septic Mice. *Respir. Res.* **2023**, *24*, 288. [CrossRef]
19. Bonaventura, A.; Vecchié, A.; Dagna, L.; Martinod, K.; Dixon, D.L.; Van Tassell, B.W.; Dentali, F.; Montecucco, F.; Massberg, S.; Levi, M.; et al. Endothelial Dysfunction and Immunothrombosis as Key Pathogenic Mechanisms in COVID-19. *Nat. Rev. Immunol.* **2021**, *21*, 319–329. [CrossRef]
20. Xu, S.-W.; Ilyas, I.; Weng, J.-P. Endothelial Dysfunction in COVID-19: An Overview of Evidence, Biomarkers, Mechanisms and Potential Therapies. *Acta Pharmacol. Sin.* **2023**, *44*, 695–709. [CrossRef]
21. Liu, Y.; Mu, S.; Li, X.; Liang, Y.; Wang, L.; Ma, X. Unfractionated Heparin Alleviates Sepsis-Induced Acute Lung Injury by Protecting Tight Junctions. *J. Surg. Res.* **2019**, *238*, 175–185. [CrossRef] [PubMed]
22. Chen, J.; Chung, D.W. Inflammation, von Willebrand Factor, and ADAMTS13. *Blood* **2018**, *132*, 141–147. [CrossRef] [PubMed]
23. Rostami, M.; Mansouritorghabeh, H.; Parsa-Kondelaji, M. High Levels of Von Willebrand Factor Markers in COVID-19: A Systematic Review and Meta-Analysis. *Clin. Exp. Med.* **2022**, *22*, 347–357. [CrossRef] [PubMed]
24. Joly, B.S.; Coppo, P.; Veyradier, A. An Update on Pathogenesis and Diagnosis of Thrombotic Thrombocytopenic Purpura. *Expert Rev. Hematol.* **2019**, *12*, 383–395. [CrossRef] [PubMed]
25. Hokama, L.T.; Veiga, A.D.M.; Menezes, M.C.S.; Sardinha Pinto, A.A.; de Lima, T.M.; Ariga, S.K.K.; Barbeiro, H.V.; Barbeiro, D.F.; de Lucena Moreira, C.; Stanzani, G.; et al. Endothelial Injury in COVID-19 and Septic Patients. *Microvasc. Res.* **2022**, *140*, 104303. [CrossRef] [PubMed]
26. Zhang, J.; Tecson, K.M.; McCullough, P.A. Endothelial Dysfunction Contributes to COVID-19-Associated Vascular Inflammation and Coagulopathy. *Rev. Cardiovasc. Med.* **2020**, *21*, 315–319. [CrossRef] [PubMed]

27. D'Agnillo, F.; Walters, K.-A.; Xiao, Y.; Sheng, Z.-M.; Scherler, K.; Park, J.; Gygli, S.; Rosas, L.A.; Sadtler, K.; Kalish, H.; et al. Lung Epithelial and Endothelial Damage, Loss of Tissue Repair, Inhibition of Fibrinolysis, and Cellular Senescence in Fatal COVID-19. *Sci. Transl. Med.* **2021**, *13*, eabj7790. [CrossRef] [PubMed]
28. Ware, L.B.; Eisner, M.D.; Thompson, B.T.; Parsons, P.E.; Matthay, M.A. Significance of von Willebrand Factor in Septic and Nonseptic Patients with Acute Lung Injury. *Am. J. Respir. Crit. Care Med.* **2004**, *170*, 766–772. [CrossRef] [PubMed]
29. Rubin, D.B.; Wiener-Kronish, J.P.; Murray, J.F.; Green, D.R.; Turner, J.; Luce, J.M.; Montgomery, A.B.; Marks, J.D.; Matthay, M.A. Elevated von Willebrand Factor Antigen Is an Early Plasma Predictor of Acute Lung Injury in Nonpulmonary Sepsis Syndrome. *J. Clin. Investig.* **1990**, *86*, 474–480. [CrossRef]
30. Hou, P.C.; Filbin, M.R.; Wang, H.; Ngo, L.; Huang, D.T.; Aird, W.C.; Yealy, D.M.; Angus, D.C.; Kellum, J.A.; Shapiro, N.I.; et al. Endothelial Permeability and Hemostasis in Septic Shock: Results From the ProCESS Trial. *Chest* **2017**, *152*, 22–31. [CrossRef]
31. Kim, D.; Bresette, C.; Liu, Z.; Ku, D.N. Occlusive Thrombosis in Arteries. *APL Bioeng.* **2019**, *3*, 041502. [CrossRef] [PubMed]
32. Hendrickson, C.M.; Matthay, M.A. Endothelial Biomarkers in Human Sepsis: Pathogenesis and Prognosis for ARDS. *Pulm. Circ.* **2018**, *8*, 2045894018769876. [CrossRef] [PubMed]
33. Ward, S.E.; Fogarty, H.; Karampini, E.; Lavin, M.; Schneppenheim, S.; Dittmer, R.; Morrin, H.; Glavey, S.; Ni Cheallaigh, C.; Bergin, C.; et al. ADAMTS13 Regulation of VWF Multimer Distribution in Severe COVID-19. *J. Thromb. Haemost. JTH* **2021**, *19*, 1914–1921. [CrossRef] [PubMed]
34. Claus, R.A.; Bockmeyer, C.L.; Budde, U.; Kentouche, K.; Sossdorf, M.; Hilberg, T.; Schneppenheim, R.; Reinhart, K.; Bauer, M.; Brunkhorst, F.M.; et al. Variations in the Ratio between von Willebrand Factor and Its Cleaving Protease during Systemic Inflammation and Association with Severity and Prognosis of Organ Failure. *Thromb. Haemost.* **2009**, *101*, 239–247. [PubMed]
35. McHale, T.M.; Garciarena, C.D.; Fagan, R.P.; Smith, S.G.J.; Martin-Loches, I.; Curley, G.F.; Fitzpatrick, F.; Kerrigan, S.W. Inhibition of Vascular Endothelial Cell Leak Following Escherichia Coli Attachment in an Experimental Model of Sepsis. *Crit. Care Med.* **2018**, *46*, e805–e810. [CrossRef] [PubMed]
36. Zhang, W.; Xu, Q.; Wu, J.; Zhou, X.; Weng, J.; Xu, J.; Wang, W.; Huang, Q.; Guo, X. Role of Src in Vascular Hyperpermeability Induced by Advanced Glycation End Products. *Sci. Rep.* **2015**, *5*, 14090. [CrossRef] [PubMed]
37. Cai, W.-J.; Li, M.B.; Wu, X.; Wu, S.; Zhu, W.; Chen, D.; Luo, M.; Eitenmüller, I.; Kampmann, A.; Schaper, J.; et al. Activation of the Integrins A5β1 and Avβ3 and Focal Adhesion Kinase (FAK) during Arteriogenesis. *Mol. Cell. Biochem.* **2009**, *322*, 161–169. [CrossRef] [PubMed]
38. Zou, S.; Jie, H.; Han, X.; Wang, J. The Role of Neutrophil Extracellular Traps in Sepsis and Sepsis-Related Acute Lung Injury. *Int. Immunopharmacol.* **2023**, *124*, 110436. [CrossRef] [PubMed]
39. Rittirsch, D.; Huber-Lang, M.S.; Flierl, M.A.; Ward, P.A. Immunodesign of Experimental Sepsis by Cecal Ligation and Puncture. *Nat. Protoc.* **2009**, *4*, 31–36. [CrossRef]
40. Matute-Bello, G.; Downey, G.; Moore, B.B.; Groshong, S.D.; Matthay, M.A.; Slutsky, A.S.; Kuebler, W.M. Acute Lung Injury in Animals Study Group An Official American Thoracic Society Workshop Report: Features and Measurements of Experimental Acute Lung Injury in Animals. *Am. J. Respir. Cell Mol. Biol.* **2011**, *44*, 725–738. [CrossRef]
41. Smith, P.; Jeffers, L.A.; Koval, M. Measurement of Lung Vessel and Epithelial Permeability In Vivo with Evans Blue. *Methods Mol. Biol. Clifton NJ* **2021**, *2367*, 137–148. [CrossRef] [PubMed]
42. Chen, W.-L.; Qian, Y.; Meng, W.-F.; Pang, J.-Y.; Lin, Y.-C.; Guan, Y.-Y.; Chen, S.-P.; Liu, J.; Pei, Z.; Wang, G.-L. A Novel Marine Compound Xyloketal B Protects against Oxidized LDL-Induced Cell Injury in Vitro. *Biochem. Pharmacol.* **2009**, *78*, 941–950. [CrossRef] [PubMed]
43. Yang, H.-Y.; Zhang, C.; Hu, L.; Liu, C.; Pan, N.; Li, M.; Han, H.; Zhou, Y.; Li, J.; Zhao, L.-Y.; et al. Platelet CFTR Inhibition Enhances Arterial Thrombosis via Increasing Intracellular Cl- Concentration and Activation of SGK1 Signaling Pathway. *Acta Pharmacol. Sin.* **2022**, *43*, 2596–2608. [CrossRef] [PubMed]
44. Han, H.; Liu, C.; Li, M.; Wang, J.; Liu, Y. S.; Zhou, Y.; Li, Z.-C.; Hu, R.; Li, Z.-H.; Wang, R.-M.; et al. Increased Intracellular Cl- Concentration Mediates Neutrophil Extracellular Traps Formation in Atherosclerotic Cardiovascular Diseases. *Acta Pharmacol. Sin.* **2022**, *43*, 2848–2861. [CrossRef] [PubMed]

Disclaimer/Publisher's Note: The statements, opinions and data contained in all publications are solely those of the individual author(s) and contributor(s) and not of MDPI and/or the editor(s). MDPI and/or the editor(s) disclaim responsibility for any injury to people or property resulting from any ideas, methods, instructions or products referred to in the content.

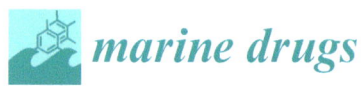 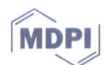

Article

A SIRT6 Inhibitor, Marine-Derived Pyrrole-Pyridinimidazole Derivative 8a, Suppresses Angiogenesis

Nannan Song [1], Yanfei Tang [1], Yangui Wang [1], Xian Guan [1], Wengong Yu [1,2], Tao Jiang [1,2], Ling Lu [1,2,*] and Yuchao Gu [2,3,*]

1. Key Laboratory of Marine Drugs, Ministry of Education, School of Medicine and Pharmacy, Ocean University of China, Qingdao 266003, China
2. Laboratory for Marine Drugs and Bioproducts of Laoshan Laboratory, Qingdao 266237, China
3. College of Marine Science and Biological Engineering, Qingdao University of Science and Technology, Qingdao 266042, China
* Correspondence: linglu@ouc.edu.cn (L.L.); guych@ouc.edu.cn (Y.G.); Tel.: +86-532-82032957 (L.L.); +86-0532-84022668 (Y.G.)

Abstract: Angiogenesis refers to the process of growing new blood vessels from pre-existing capillaries or post-capillary veins. This process plays a critical role in promoting tumorigenesis and metastasis. As a result, developing antiangiogenic agents has become an attractive strategy for tumor treatment. Sirtuin6 (SIRT6), a member of nicotinamide adenine (NAD^+)-dependent histone deacetylases, regulates various biological processes, including metabolism, oxidative stress, angiogenesis, and DNA damage and repair. Some SIRT6 inhibitors have been identified, but the effects of SIRT6 inhibitors on anti-angiogenesis have not been reported. We have identified a pyrrole-pyridinimidazole derivative **8a** as a highly effective inhibitor of SIRT6 and clarified its anti-pancreatic-cancer roles. This study investigated the antiangiogenic roles of **8a**. We found that **8a** was able to inhibit the migration and tube formation of HUVECs and downregulate the expression of angiogenesis-related proteins, including VEGF, HIF-1α, p-VEGFR2, and N-cadherin, and suppress the activation of AKT and ERK pathways. Additionally, **8a** significantly blocked angiogenesis in intersegmental vessels in zebrafish embryos. Notably, in a pancreatic cancer xenograft mouse model, **8a** down-regulated the expression of CD31, a marker protein of angiogenesis. These findings suggest that **8a** could be a promising antiangiogenic and cancer therapeutic agent.

Keywords: SIRT6 inhibitor; anti-angiogenesis; tube formation; anticancer

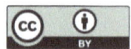

1. Introduction

Angiogenesis, which refers to the development of new blood vessels from existing capillaries or post-capillary veins, plays a critical role in tumor growth and metastasis [1,2]. As tumors grow, they consume nutrition and oxygen in the microenvironment, prompting the rapid development of new blood vessel networks to supply more nutrients and oxygen to the tumor, thereby promoting tumor growth and metastasis [3,4]. Therefore, the development of antiangiogenic inhibitors is of great value for the treatment of tumors, and antiangiogenic therapy has received widespread attention in the treatment strategy of solid tumors over the past few decades.

Sirtuin6 (SIRT6) is a member of the sirtuin family of nicotinamide adenine (NAD^+)-dependent histone deacetylases. SIRT6 has been proven to be involved in regulating diverse biological processes, including metabolism, oxidative stress, DNA damage, and repair, and plays a significant role in aging, cancer, inflammation, diabetes, and other diseases [5–8]. Several studies have reported that SIRT6 is involved in the regulation of angiogenesis. For instance, SIRT6 promotes angiogenesis by inhibiting the ubiquitination degradation of HIF-1α and promoting its expression in carotid artery plaque [9]. SIRT6 overexpression promotes angiogenesis and reduces cerebral ischemia and reperfusion (I/R)-induced injury through transcriptional inhibition of TXNIP [10]. In addition, recent reports have found that MDL-800, a highly efficient SIRT6 activator, can inhibit the NF-κB signaling pathway by activating SIRT6, promoting angiogenesis, and wound healing [11]. More importantly, in pancreatic cancer, SIRT6 could promote the expression of inflammatory factor IL-8, which could promote local inflammation and further promote angiogenesis, playing a key role in the occurrence and metastasis of pancreatic cancer [12–14]. These studies suggest that SIRT6 is a new anti-angiogenesis target, and inhibitors of SIRT6 may have a highly effective antiangiogenic effect.

Marine environments offer unique ecological conditions, making marine natural products a rich source of new bioactive agents [15–18]. Ageladine A (Figure 1A), a fluorescent pyrrol-2-aminoimidazole alkaloid extracted from the marine sponge *Agelas nakamurai* by Fusetani et al. has demonstrated significant activity as an inhibitor of matrix metalloproteinases (MMPs) such as MMP-1, 2, 8, 9, 12, and 13 at micromolar levels. These MMPs play crucial roles in apoptosis, metastasis, and angiogenesis of tumor cells [19,20]. In a prior study, we observed that the derivative of Ageladine A, **8a** (as shown in Figure 1B), displayed inhibitory effects on SIRT6 both in vivo and in vitro, while not affecting MMPs. Additionally, the derivative showed potential as an anti-pancreatic-cancer agent [21].

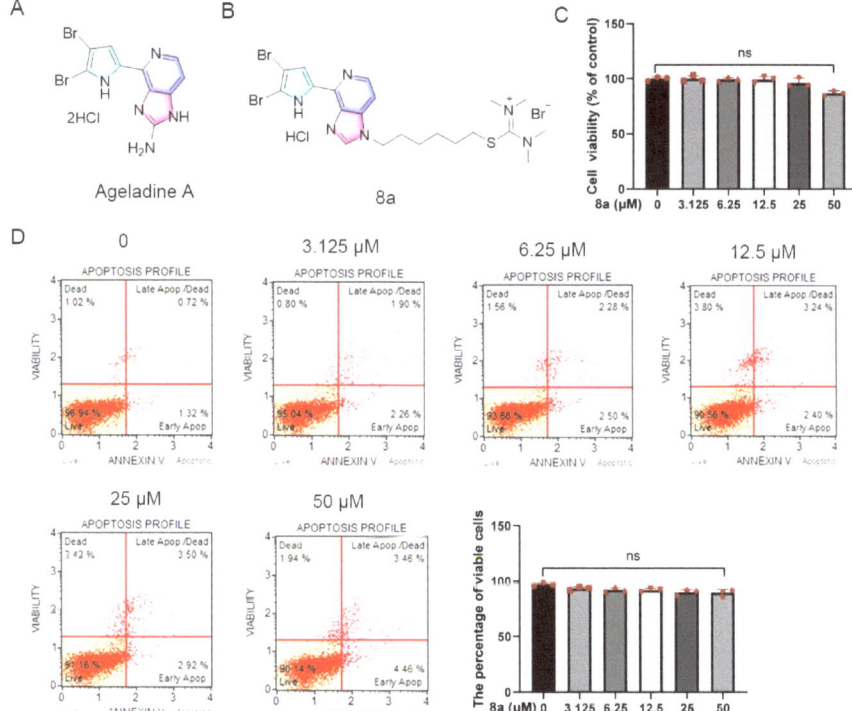

Figure 1. Compound **8a** did not induce toxicity in HUVECs. (**A**) Chemical structure of Ageladine A. (**B**) Chemical structure of **8a**. (**C**) HUVEC cells were treated with **8a** of 0, 3.125, 6.25, 12.5, 25, and 50 μM for 24 h; cell viability was determined by CCK8 assay. (**D**) The effect of **8a** on apoptosis was detected by flow cytometry. Data were presented as mean ± SD of three independent experiments.

The objective of this study was to investigate the antiangiogenic roles of SIRT6 inhibitor **8a** both in vivo and in vitro. Our findings demonstrated that **8a** suppressed the migration and angiogenesis of HUVECs without inducing apoptosis in these cells. The observed effects were linked to the downregulation of key angiogenic molecules, such as N-cadherin, VEGF, and HIF-1α. Moreover, we determined that **8a** inhibited intersegmental vessel formation in a zebrafish model. Most notably, our study revealed that **8a** significantly inhibited the expression of the angiogenic marker protein CD31 and suppressed angiogenesis in a pancreatic cancer xenograft model. Our results strongly suggest that SIRT6 inhibitors possess great potential as novel antiangiogenic agents.

2. Results

2.1. Compound **8a** Has No Obvious Toxicity in HUVECs

Initially, we assessed the potential impact of **8a** on HUVEC cell viability through the CCK8 assay (Figure 1C). HUVEC cells were treated with varying concentrations of **8a** (0, 3.125, 6.25, 12.5, 25, and 50 µM) for 24 h, and we observed that compound **8a** did not significantly affect the viability of HUVEC cells. Only at a concentration of 50 µM did we observe a slight reduction in HUVEC cell viability. Additionally, we evaluated the effect of compound **8a** on apoptosis via flow cytometry (Figure 1D). After HUVEC cells were treated with varying concentrations of **8a** (0, 3.125, 6.25, 12.5, 25, and 50 µM) for 24 h and stained with Annexin V and PI, we observed over 90% of viable cells in all samples, with no significant differences between **8a**-treated and untreated cells. Our findings suggested that **8a** did not exhibit any toxic effects on HUVEC cells at the selected concentration. As a result, the concentration of **8a** we used in subsequent experiments was below 25 µM and excluded any potential cytotoxicity of the compound.

2.2. Compound **8a** Inhibits Migration of HUVECs

Since vascular endothelial cell migration is a crucial step in angiogenesis, we evaluated the effect of **8a** on HUVEC cell migration using the scratch-wound assay. The results (Figure 2A) demonstrated that the migration of HUVECs was significantly reduced after 24 h treatment with 0, 3.125, 6.25, and 12.5 µM **8a**, with a wound healing percentage of 65.8, 51.6, and 43.2%. To further confirm the effect of **8a** on HUVEC cell migration, we conducted the transwell assay. The results (Figure 2B) showed that the number of migrated cells was significantly reduced after treatment with **8a**, providing further evidence that **8a** could inhibit the migration of HUVEC cells.

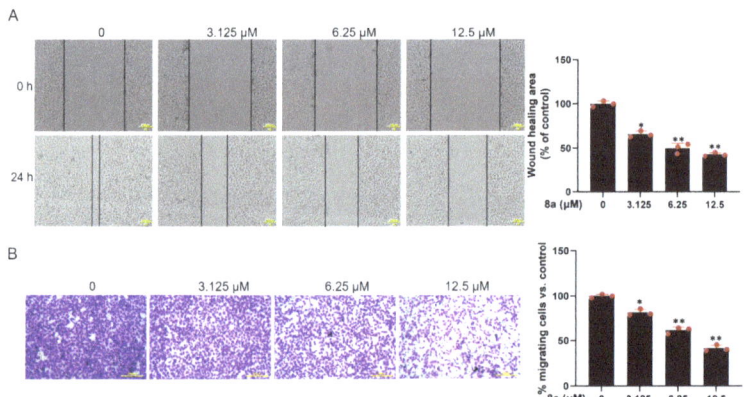

Figure 2. Compound **8a** inhibits the migration ability of HUVECs. (**A**) Representative images of wound healing assay of HUVECs at 0 and 24 h post-treatment with compound **8a** (magnification: ×200). The wound-healing area was determined using Image J software v1.53. Scale bar = 200 µm. (**B**) Transwell assay to detect the migration of HUVECs. Representative images of HUVECS traveling through membrane after treatment with different concentrations of **8a** were taken by a microscope. Scale bar = 200 µm. Data are presented as mean ± SD of three independent experiments. * $p < 0.05$, ** $p < 0.01$ versus control.

2.3. Compound 8a Inhibits Tube Formation Abilities of HUVECs

The ability of HUVEC cells to form capillary-like structures within 6 h on a Matrigel-coated culture plate makes them a suitable model for studying angiogenesis in vitro [22]. Therefore, we used HUVEC cells to investigate the antiangiogenic effects of **8a** in vitro. As illustrated in Figure 3, our findings revealed that **8a** significantly reduced both the number and length of tubes formed by HUVECs, indicating that it could significantly inhibit angiogenesis.

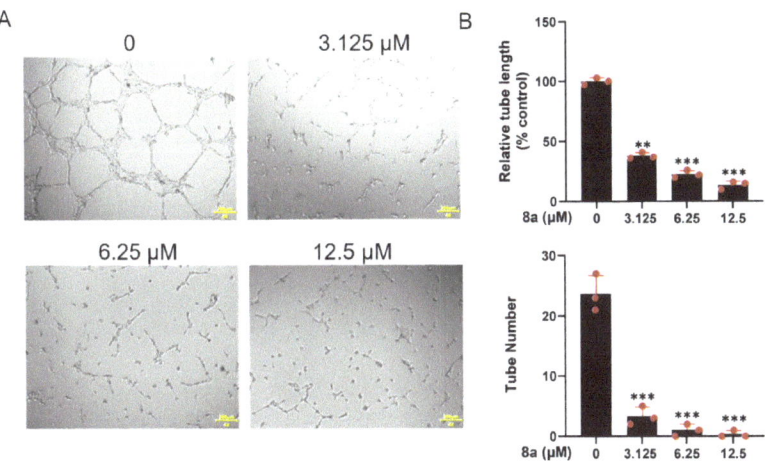

Figure 3. Compound **8a** inhibits the tube formation ability of HUVECs. (**A**) Tube formation ability of HUVECs treated with different concentrations of compound **8a** (0, 3.125, 6.25, and 12.5 µM) for 6 h. Scale bar = 200 µm. (**B**) Quantification of tube length and number. Data are presented as mean ± SD of three independent experiments. ** $p < 0.01$, *** $p < 0.001$ versus control.

2.4. Compound 8a Decreases the Expression of VEGF, p-VEGFR2, N-Cadherin, HIF-1α, p-AKT, and p-ERK in HUVECs

To further explore the effect of **8a** on the molecular mechanism related to angiogenesis, we detected the expression of angiogenesis-related proteins by Western blot. As shown in Figure 4A, we found that **8a** treatment of HUVEC cells significantly upregulated the acetylation level of SIRT6 downstream target protein H3, indicating that **8a** could inhibit the activity of SIRT6 in HUVEC cells. Vascular endothelial growth factor (VEGF) plays an important role in angiogenesis, causing the proliferation and migration of vascular endothelial cells and increasing vascular permeability by phosphorylating VEGF receptor-2 (VEGFR 2) [23–26]. We found that **8a** could significantly downregulate the expression of VEGF and p-VEGFR2 in a concentration-dependent manner. N-cadherin is a transmembrane glycoprotein that mediates vascular formation and structural integrity and is involved in the regulation of cell invasion and metastasis [27–30]. We examined the effect of **8a** on the expression level of N-cadherin by Western blot assay and found that **8a** could significantly inhibit the expression of N-cadherin in a concentration-dependent manner.

HIF-1α is an important transcription factor that can be involved in promoting angiogenesis by regulating VEGF [31]. SIRT6 promotes angiogenesis by inhibiting the ubiquitination degradation of HIF-1α and promoting its expression [9]. Therefore, we evaluated the effect of **8a** on HIF-1α and found that **8a** significantly inhibited the expression of HIF 1α (Figure 4B). Activation of pathways can also contribute to promoted angiogenesis by regulating the expression of factors such as VEGF [32,33]. Therefore, we also examined the effect of **8a** on the phosphorylation of AKT and ERK by Western blot, and we found that **8a** could downregulate the levels of p-AKT and p-ERK (Figure 4B). These results suggest that compound **8a** inhibits angiogenesis in HUVEC cells by suppressing the activation of AKT and ERK pathways and the expression of VEGF, N-cadherin, and HIF-1α.

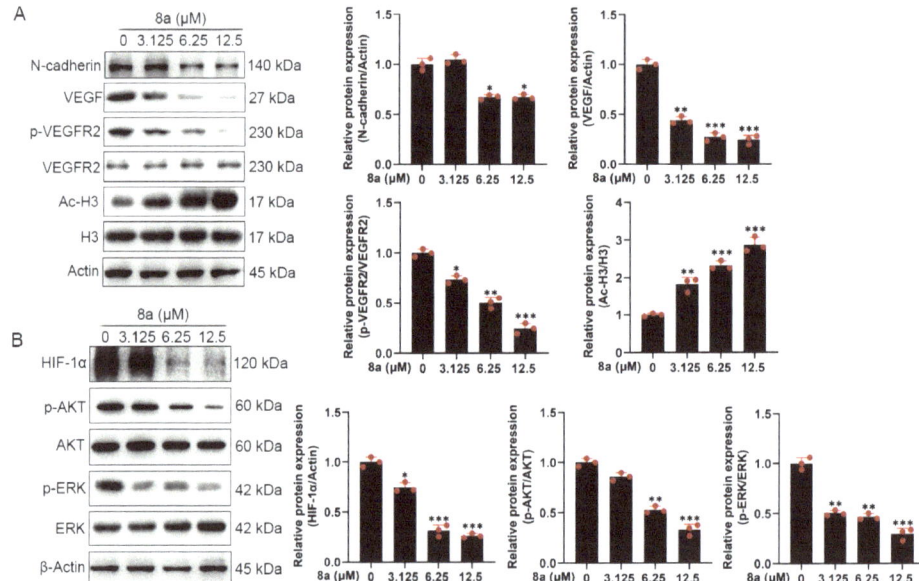

Figure 4. Compound **8a** decreases the expression of VEGF, p-VEGFR2, HIF-1α, and N-cadherin and the activation of AKT and ERK pathways which were associated with angiogenesis in HUVECs. (**A**) Western blot assay was used to detect the expression of VEGF, p-VEGFR2, VEGFR2, N-cadherin, H3, and Ac-H3 proteins after **8a** treatment for 24 h. (**B**) Western blot assay was used to detect the expression of HIF-1α, p-AKT, AKT, p-ERK, and ERK proteins after **8a** treatment for 24 h. Data are presented as mean ± SD of three independent experiments. * $p < 0.05$, ** $p < 0.01$, *** $p < 0.001$ versus control.

2.5. *Compound 8a Inhibits Intersegmental Vessel Formation in Zebrafish Model*

Zebrafish is an effective model organism for studying vascular development, owing to its highly characteristic vascular pattern and rapid vascular development [34,35]. Compared to other animal models, zebrafish offers several advantages [36,37]. The zebrafish genome has more than 95% similarity to human genes in function, particularly those related to angiogenesis. Angiogenesis in zebrafish starts at 12 hours post fertilization (hpf) and, by 20 hpf, its dorsal aorta (DA) and cardinal vein (CV) are already formed, with new vessels gradually extending towards the trunk and tail and intersegmental vessels (ISVs) sprouting from the aorta. By 48 hpf, the ISVs of the trunk and tail are largely formed and blood circulation is established [38–40]. Furthermore, various artificially mutated strains of zebrafish, such as the *Tg (flk1: EGFP)* zebrafish, allow for direct observation of vascular development dynamics via fluorescence microscopy [41–43]. Given the multiple advantages of zebrafish, this model organism has been successfully used to evaluate or screen different tissues for antiangiogenic agents on the vasculature [44,45]. Therefore, we employed *Tg (flk1: EGFP)* zebrafish to evaluate the effect of compound **8a** on angiogenesis in vivo. We treated *Tg (flk1: EGFP)* zebrafish with different concentrations of **8a** for 28 h and examined the formation of ISVs in zebrafish embryos. Our results (Figure 5) showed that **8a** inhibited ISV formation in zebrafish embryos by 34.57% and 59.87% at 100 and 150 μM, respectively. This illustrates that compound **8a** can inhibit angiogenesis in zebrafish and has no significant effect on mature vessels formed before drug treatment.

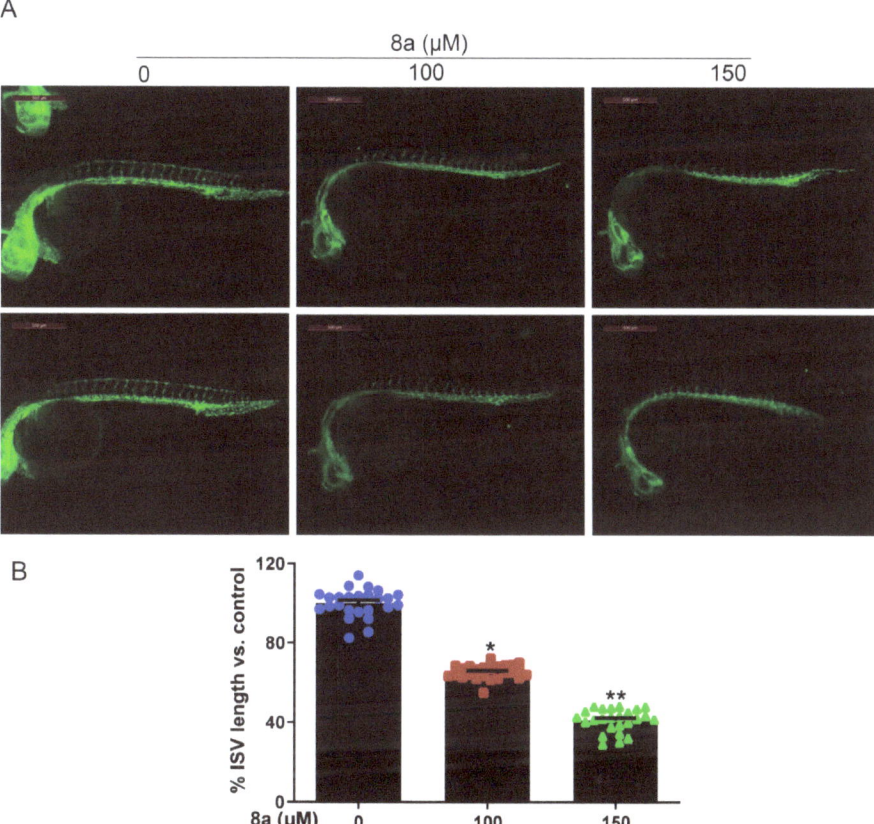

Figure 5. Compound **8a** blocks angiogenesis of intersegmental vessels in zebrafish embryos (N = 25, each group). (**A**) Representative vessel images of *Tg (flk1: EGFP)* zebrafish embryos treated with different concentrations of **8a**. Scale bar = 500 μm. (**B**) Quantitative analysis of intersegmental vessel formation induced by compound **8a**. Data are presented as mean ± SD of three independent experiments. * $p < 0.05$, ** $p < 0.01$ versus control.

2.6. Compound 8a Suppresses Tumor Angiogenesis in Pancreatic Cancer Xenograft Model

We conducted additional experiments to assess the impact of compound **8a** on angiogenesis in pancreatic cancer. CD31 is a marker protein that is commonly used to detect neovascularization and is localized at the border between vascular endothelial cells and newly formed blood vessels and lymphatic vessels [46,47]. HIF-1α can be involved in promoting angiogenesis by regulating VEGF [31]. In our previous research, we found that **8a** inhibited the growth of pancreatic tumors in the pancreatic cancer xenograft model and, on this basis, we evaluated the angiogenesis of pancreatic cancer by detecting the expression level of CD31 and HIF-1α using immunohistochemical staining. Our results (Figure 6) showed a reduction in the level of CD31 and HIF-1α protein expression after treatment with **8a**, indicating that compound **8a** inhibited angiogenesis in pancreatic cancer.

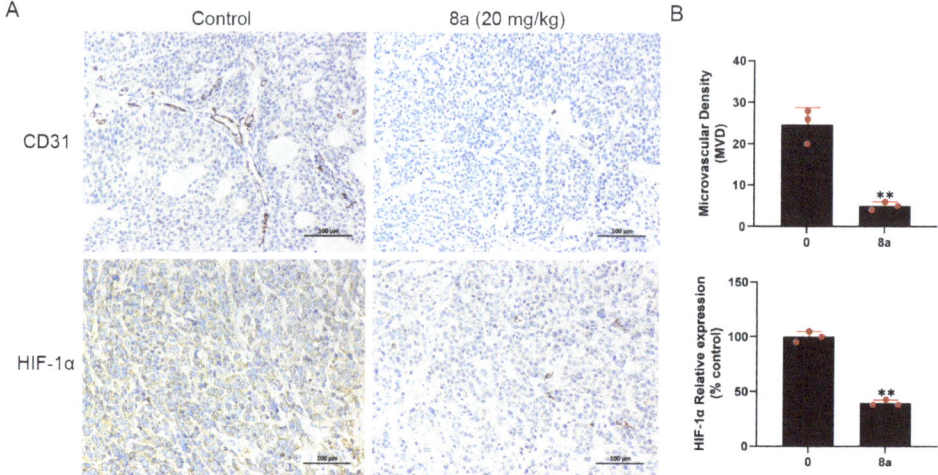

Figure 6. Compound **8a** suppressed tumor angiogenesis in pancreatic cancer xenograft model (N = 6, each group). (**A**) Representative tumor tissue sections from BXPC-3 xenograft tumors with CD31 and HIF-1α staining after treatment with compound **8a**. Scale bar = 100 μm. (**B**) Quantification analysis of newly formed vessels corresponding to immunohistochemical staining of CD31 and HIF-1α. Data are presented as mean ± SD. ** $p < 0.01$ versus control.

3. Discussion

Numerous studies have shown that the rapid growth and metastasis of tumors require blood vessels to provide oxygen and nutrients, without which they can only remain dormant [1,48,49]. Angiogenesis plays an important role in promoting tumorigenesis and metastasis; therefore, the development of antiangiogenic agents is an attractive strategy for tumor treatment. Previous research has demonstrated that SIRT6 promotes angiogenesis, suggesting that SIRT6 is an antiangiogenic target. We previously found that Ageladine A derivative **8a**, a novel and highly effective inhibitor of SIRT6, can inhibit the activity of SIRT6 and has anti-pancreatic-cancer activity in vivo and in vitro. However, its anti-angiogenesis activity has not been explored. In this study, we demonstrated for the first time that **8a**, a novel inhibitor of SIRT6, could inhibit angiogenesis both in vitro and in vivo. Molecular studies demonstrated that **8a** could downregulate the expression of angiogenesis-related proteins in HUVEC cells. Moreover, in pancreatic cancer, **8a** was able to downregulate the expression of CD31, a marker protein of angiogenesis, and inhibit angiogenesis. Therefore, **8a** could be used as a potential antiangiogenic and cancer therapeutic agent.

In the present study, compound **8a** showed significant inhibition of several angiogenic processes in HUVEC cells, including tube formation and migration, consistent with the clinical use of several antiangiogenic drugs such as monoclonal antibodies (bevacizumab and ramucirumab) [50,51]. Interestingly, **8a** induced almost no apoptosis in HUVEC cells in a short period at high doses (50 μM), indicating that **8a** has low cytotoxicity towards HUVEC cells and, therefore, the antiangiogenic effect of **8a** is not due to its cytotoxicity towards HUVEC cells.

We further investigated that **8a** could upregulate the acetylation level of histone H3, a downstream target protein of SIRT6, indicating that **8a** could inhibit the deacetylase activity of SIRT6 at the HUVEC cell level. VEGF is a key proangiogenic factor that plays an important role in angiogenesis and tumor metastasis [49,52]. It has been reported that SIRT6 promotes HUVEC cell migration, invasion, and angiogenesis under normoxic or hypoxic conditions by regulating HIF-1α and thereby promoting the expression of several angiogenic factors, including Ang1, Ang2, PDGF-BB, VEGF, and ET-1 [9]. Our results found that inhibitor **8a** of SIRT6 inhibits VEGF, p-VEGFR2, and HIF-1α expression and suppresses angiogenesis, consistent with the knockdown of SIRT6 in BMVEC and HUVEC cells [9,10]. N-cadherin is present in the adhesion complex between endothelial and pericytes, stabilizes cell–cell junctions, promotes cell migration, and is also involved in tumor progression and metastasis and is closely associated with the formation of blood vessels and the maintenance of vascular integrity [28,29,53]. We found that **8a** could inhibit the expression of N-cadherin. AKT and ERK pathways play an important role in the formation of blood vessels [32,33]. We also demonstrated that **8a** could inhibit the activation of AKT and ERK pathways. Thus, **8a** could exert an antiangiogenic effect by regulating AKT and ERK pathways and the expression of VEGF, N-cadherin, and HIF-1α. However, the explicit mechanism by which **8a** exerts its effect remains to be further explored.

Zebrafish embryos have become a very attractive model for studying vascular development due to their high genetic similarity to humans, external fertilization, rapid embryonic development, and high embryonic transparency [54–56]. Zebrafish embryos first develop to form the dorsal aorta and posterior main veins. Secondary vessels are then formed through sprouting angiogenesis, such as the intersegmental vessels [57]. We selected a transgenic zebrafish model *(Tg (flk1:EGFP))* to study the effect of **8a** on angiogenesis in vivo. We found that **8a** significantly inhibited the angiogenesis of intersegmental vessels in zebrafish, with no significant effect on mature vessels formed before **8a** treatment. This also suggests to us that **8a** may have a relatively small and safer effect on the blood vessels of normal organisms.

Pancreatic cancer is a highly aggressive malignancy with poor late-stage survival rates. The 5-year survival rate for patients with pancreatic cancer is the lowest, no more than 5%, and the median survival is only 6 months [58]. Angiogenesis is a key step in the growth and spread of malignant diseases, including pancreatic cancer [59]. These studies illustrate that targeting angiogenesis is an important strategy for tumor treatment. Previous reports have demonstrated that SIRT6 could promote the expression of inflammatory factor IL-8, which could promote local inflammation and further promote angiogenesis, playing a key role in the occurrence and metastasis of pancreatic cancer [12–14]. Thus, **8a**, an inhibitor of SIRT6, may inhibit angiogenesis in pancreatic cancer. In our study, we investigated the effect of **8a** on the angiogenesis of pancreatic cancer and found that **8a** could inhibit the expression of CD31 and HIF-1α, indicating that **8a** also has an inhibitory effect on angiogenesis in pancreatic cancer. Our previous study also demonstrated that **8a** inhibits the proliferation of pancreatic cancer and promotes the sensitivity of pancreatic cancer to gemcitabine in vivo and in vitro [21]. These results also suggest that the combination of **8a** with other drugs may be a promising antitumor strategy. For instance, the enzyme nicotinamide N-methyltransferase (NNMT) is overexpressed in pancreatic cancer, contributing to aggressiveness [60,61]. By methylating nicotinamide, NNMT can regulate the NAD levels reducing the amount of free nicotinamide, which could be converted into NAD through the NAD-salvage pathway, thus reducing the substrate for sirtuins activity [62]. In the light of these observations, coupling the antiangiogenic activity of **8a** with NNMT inhibitors [63–65] may be a promising strategy to improve the outcome of patients with pancreatic cancer, a malignancy that displays little therapeutic options. Taken together, these data suggest that **8a** has an antiangiogenic effect and is a potentially effective agent for cancer treatment.

4. Materials and Methods

4.1. Drugs and Reagents

Compound **8a** (purity > 95%) was synthesized as previously reported [21]. Compound **8a** was dissolved in double steaming water.

4.2. Cell Lines and Cell Culture

Human umbilical vein endothelial cells (HUVECs) were purchased from the Cell Resource Center of the Shanghai Institute for Biological Sciences, Chinese Academy of Sciences. HUVECs in passages 3 to 6 were used for experiments. HUVECs were cultured in Dulbecco's modified Eagle's medium (DMEM, GIBCO, Grand Island, NY, USA) supplemented with 10% (v/v) fetal bovine serum (FBS) (PAN-Biotech GmbH, Lot Number # ST200707), penicillin (50 units/mL), and streptomycin (50 µg/mL). Cells were cultured in a constant temperature incubator at 37 °C and 5% CO_2 concentration.

4.3. CCK8 Assay

The effect of compound **8a** on the viability of HUVEC cells was determined by the Cell Counting Kit-8 (CCK8, Beyotime, Shanghai, China). HUVEC cells were seeded in 96-well plates (Corning, New York, NY, USA) at a density of 1×10^4 cells/well. After incubation overnight, the HUVEC cells were incubated with different concentrations of **8a** (0, 3.125, 6.25, 12.5, 25, and 50 µM) for 24 h. The CCK8 solution was added to the well plates and incubated for 2–4 h in a 37 °C incubator. The absorbance was detected at 450 nm using a multifunctional enzyme marker (Bio-Tek, Winooski, VT, USA), and the cell viability (%) was calculated by the absorbance.

4.4. Cell Apoptosis Analysis

HUVEC cells were seeded in six-well culture plates at a density of 2×10^5 cells/well. After incubation overnight, HUVEC cells were added to fresh DMEM medium with different concentrations of **8a** (0, 3.125, 6.25, and 12.5 µM) for 24 h. After the treatment, cells were harvested into centrifuge tubes and washed three times using precooled PBS buffer. Apoptotic cells were stained with Muse™ Annexin V &Dead Cell assay kit (Muse TM Cell Analyzer, Millipore (catalog no. MCH100105)) according to the manufacturer's instruction. The cell samples were then analyzed by flow cytometry (Muse TM Cell Analyzer, Millipore, Bedford, MA, USA).

4.5. Scratch Wound-Healing Assay

A scratch wound-healing assay was used to detect cell migration. HUVEC cells were seeded in six-well culture plates at a density of 2×10^5 cells/well. When the HUVEC cell confluence reached 80%, scratch wounds were made by a 100 µL pipette tip in a sterile environment. After washing three times with PBS buffer, HUVEC cells were added to a fresh DMEM medium containing 1% FBS with different concentrations of **8a** (0, 3.125, 6.25, and 12.5 µM) for 24 h. Images were recorded at 0 and 24 h by microscope (NIB-100, Novel Optics, Ningbo, China) after the cells were scratched. Each wound area was measured by using Image J software version 1.53 (Medical Cybernetics, New York, NY, USA), and the cell migration rate was assessed as follows: wound healing area (%) = $(A_{0h}/A_{nh})/A_{0h} \times 100$, where A_0 represents the original wound area (t = 0 h) and A_n represents the area of the wound at the time of detection (t = n h).

4.6. Transwell Migration Assay

HUVEC migration assays were evaluated in transwell plates (8 µm pore size, Corning) as previously described [66]. Briefly, HUVEC cells were trypsinized and then counted with a Muse cell analyzer (Millipore, USA). Cells were diluted by DMEM medium supplemented with 1% bovine serum albumin (BSA) and different concentrations of **8a** (0, 3.125, 6.25, and 12.5 µM) and seeded into the upper chamber at a density of 2×10^4 cells/well. Then, the bottom chamber was added to DMEM medium containing 10% FBS as an attractant factor and different concentrations of **8a** (0, 3.125, 6.25, and 12.5 µM). After 24 h of incubation at 37 °C, the upper chambers were fixed with paraformaldehyde (4%) for 15 min, then washed three times with precooled PBS buffer and stained with crystal violet (0.1%) at room temperature for 15 min, the floating color washed off with PBS, and then the upper surface of the membrane cells was carefully removed by a cotton swab. Randomly selected fields of view were photographed using a microscope (NIB-100, CHN, original magnification). Then, the crystalline violet in the chambers was dissolved using acetic acid at a concentration of 33%, and the solution from each group was then added to a 96-well plate. The absorbance was detected at 570 nm using a multifunctional enzyme marker (Bio-Tek, USA).

4.7. In Vitro Tube Formation Assay

The tube formation assay on Matrigel (Corning (BD Biocoat), CA, USA) in vitro was used to assess the effect of compound **8a** on HUVEC tube formation capacity. In brief, the Matrigel was thawed overnight at 4 °C and added to 96-well plates with 60 µL per well. The plates were placed in a 37 °C incubator to solidify for 1 h. HUVEC cells were diluted by DMEM medium supplemented with 10% FBS and different concentrations of **8a** (0, 3.125, 6.25, and 12.5 µM), seeded into Matrigel at a density of 1×10^4 cells/well, and incubated at 37 °C in an incubator for 6 h. Moreover, the tube formation was recorded by a light microscope (NIB-100, CHN, original magnification). The total length of the tubes was quantitatively evaluated by Image J software v1.53.

4.8. Zebrafish Embryo Assay

Angiogenesis experiments in vivo were performed using the Tg(flk1:EGFP) transgenic zebrafish line that can be directed to express an enhanced green fluorescent protein (EGFP) via endothelial-specific flk1 promoter, which, in turn, labels vascular endothelial cells [67,68]. Adult zebrafish were kept in an environment with a water temperature of about 28.5 °C, pH in the range of 6.8–7.2, 14 h:10 h of light: dark cycle, and fed with the appropriate amount of food on time. Before fertilization, male and female zebrafish were placed on both sides of the tank in a ratio of 1:2. When they finished free mating, their fertilized embryos were collected and washed with embryo culture water (5.4 mol/L KCl, 0.137 mol/L NaCl, 0.44 mol/L K_2HPO_4, 0.25 mol/L Na_2HPO_4, 1.0 mol/L $MgSO_4$, 1.3 mol/L $CaCl_2$, and 4.2 mol/L $NaHCO_3$) and incubated in a constant temperature incubator at 28.5 °C. At about 20 hpf, the dorsal aorta (DA) and cardinal vein (CV) of zebrafish embryos were developed and new vessels started to extend towards their trunk and tail, and the intersegmental vessels were developed and blood circulation started to appear at about 48 hpf. To test the effect of compound **8a** on zebrafish angiogenesis, zebrafish embryos at 20 hpf were placed in 12-well plates with 25 embryos per well. The number of intersegmental vessels (ISVs) was counted after 48 h of administration of different concentrations of **8a** in the zebrafish culture medium. The ISVs formation was recorded by an inverted fluorescence microscope (DM6000, Leica, Wetzlar, Germany). The total length of ISVs was quantitatively evaluated by Image J software v1.53.

4.9. Western Blot Analysis

HUVEC cells were seeded in six-well culture plates at a density of 2×10^5 cells/well. After incubation overnight, HUVEC cells were added to fresh DMEM medium with different concentrations of **8a** (0, 3.125, 6.25, and 12.5 µM) for 24 h. Cells were harvested, then washed twice with PBS buffer and lysed in a lysis solution (solarbio, R0010) containing protease inhibitor (TargetMol, Boston, MA, USA) and 1 mM PMSF. Total protein concentrations were assessed with BCA Protein Assay Kit (NCM Biotech, Suzhou, China). Then, protein samples were boiled in loading buffer for 10 min and stored at 20 °C. Equal amounts of protein samples (30 µg) were separated in SDS-PAGE at a separation gel concentration of 12.5%, and then the proteins were transferred to 0.45 µm PVDF membranes (Merck Millipore, Bedford, MA, USA). The PVDF membranes were blocked by 5% BSA in TBST buffer (10 mM Tris–HCl, 100 mM NaCl, 0.1% Tween-20, pH 7.5) at room temperature for 1 h. The blocked PVDF membranes were incubated with primary antibodies: β-Actin (1:2000, Cell Signaling Technology, Danvers, MA, USA, Cat#4970S), Acetyl-Histone H3 (Lys9) (1:2000, Cell Signaling Technology, Cat#9649), VEGF (1:1000, ZEN-BIOSCIENCE, R26073), N-Cadherin (1:1000, Cell Signaling Technology, Cat#13116), VEGFR2 (1:1000, Cell Signaling Technology, Cat#9698), p-VEGFR2 (1:1000, Cell Signaling Technology, Cat#3770), Histone H3 (1:2000, Cell Signaling Technology, Cat#9715S), AKT (1:1000, Cell Signaling Technology, Cat#9272S), Phospho-AKT (Ser473) (D9E) (1:1000, Cell Signaling Technology, Cat#4060S), ERK1/2 (1:1000, Cell Signaling Technology, Cat#4695), Phospho-p44/42 MAPK (ERK1/2) (Thr202/Tyr204) (1:1000, Cell Signaling Technology, Cat#4370S), and HIF-1α (1:1000, Cell Signaling Technology, Cat#36169) at 4 °C overnight. The PVDF membranes were washed three times by TBST for 10 min each time. Subsequently, the PVDF membranes were incubated with the respective horseradish peroxidase-conjugated secondary antibodies at room temperature for 1–2 h. The PVDF membranes were washed three times again by TBST for 10 min each time. Finally, the bands were detected by an electrochemiluminescence detection system (Tanon, Beijing, China) and were quantified using Image J software v1.53.

4.10. Immunohistochemical Staining

Female BALB/c nude mice (5 weeks old) were obtained from Beijing Vital River Laboratories (Beijing, China). All procedures were performed in adherence with international ethical guidelines and approved by the Animal Ethics Committee of the Ocean University of China. All mice were placed under standard conditions with free access to food and water. BXPC-3 cells (2×10^6) were injected into the flank region of nude mouse. After the tumors' volume had grown to 100 mm^3, the mice were treated with **8a** (20 mg/kg) or vehicle every 2 days. Mice tumor tissues were removed. The tissue sections were dewaxed using xylene for 30 min and then rehydrated. The tissue sections were incubated with primary antibody of anti-CD31 (Cell Signaling Technology, Cat#77699) at 1:100 dilution at 4 °C overnight. Subsequently, the tissue sections were incubated with a universal secondary antibody (Maixin Biotechnology, Fuzhou, China, KIT-9707). The color development reaction was then performed using DAB solution and then counterstained with hematoxylin. Images were captured with inverted fluorescence microscope (DM6000, Leica, Wetzlar, Germany).

4.11. Statistical Analysis

All data are presented as the mean ± s.d. of at least three independent biological experiments (shown as error bars). Statistical differences were evaluated using one-way analysis of variance (ANOVA) or two-tailed Student's t-tests. All statistical analyses were conducted using GraphPad Prism 8 software. p values less than 0.05 were considered statistically significant (*, $p < 0.05$; **, $p < 0.01$; ***, $p < 0.001$).

5. Conclusions

In this study, we demonstrated for the first time that **8a**, a novel inhibitor of SIRT6, could inhibit HUVEC cell migration and tube formation. Molecular studies demonstrated that **8a** could inhibit angiogenesis by suppressing the activation of AKT and ERK pathways and the expression of VEGF, N-cadherin, p-VEGFR2, and HIF-1α in HUVEC cells. Moreover, **8a** significantly inhibited the angiogenesis of intersegmental vessels in zebrafish embryos. Importantly, in the pancreatic cancer xenograft mouse model, **8a** was able to downregulate the expression of CD31, a marker protein of angiogenesis, and inhibit angiogenesis. Therefore, these findings suggest that **8a** could be used as a potential antiangiogenic and cancer therapeutic agent.

Author Contributions: Y.G. and L.L. designed this study. N.S. conducted the main experiments and manuscript writing with the assistance of Y.G. and W.Y.; Y.T. and L.L. contributed to zebrafish embryo experiments. Y.W. conducted the IHC experiments. X.G. and T.J. synthesized compounds **8a**. N.S., L.L. and Y.G. were responsible for the accuracy of the study and the review of the article. All authors have read and agreed to the published version of the manuscript.

Funding: This work was supported by the Program of the National Natural Science Foundation of China (No. 82273846), the Qingdao Marine Science and Technology Centre (No. 2022QNLM030003-4, No. 8-01), the Fundamental Research Funds for the Central Universities (No. 202042011), and the Taishan Scholars Program (No. tsqn202211058).

Institutional Review Board Statement: All aspects of this study were approved by the Institutional Research Ethics Committee of Ocean University of China (Ethical Approval Numbers OUC-AE-2021-076).

Data Availability Statement: The data are contained within the article.

Conflicts of Interest: The authors declare no conflict of interest.

References

1. Folkman, J. Tumor angiogenesis: Therapeutic implications. *N. Engl. J. Med.* **1971**, *285*, 1182–1186. [CrossRef] [PubMed]
2. Bhat, T.A.; Singh, R.P. Tumor angiogenesis—A potential target in cancer chemoprevention. *Food Chem. Toxicol. Int. J. Publ. Br. Ind. Biol. Res. Assoc.* **2008**, *46*, 1334–1345. [CrossRef] [PubMed]
3. Carmeliet, P.; Jain, R.K. Principles and mechanisms of vessel normalization for cancer and other angiogenic diseases. *Nat. Rev. Drug Discov.* **2011**, *10*, 417–427. [CrossRef] [PubMed]
4. Viallard, C.; Larrivée, B. Tumor angiogenesis and vascular normalization: Alternative therapeutic targets. *Angiogenesis* **2017**, *20*, 409–426. [CrossRef] [PubMed]
5. Mostoslavsky, R.; Chua, K.F.; Lombard, D.B.; Pang, W.W.; Fischer, M.R.; Gellon, L.; Liu, P.; Mostoslavsky, G.; Franco, S.; Murphy, M.M.; et al. Genomic instability and aging-like phenotype in the absence of mammalian SIRT6. *Cell* **2006**, *124*, 315–329. [CrossRef] [PubMed]
6. Michishita, E.; McCord, R.A.; Berber, E.; Kioi, M.; Padilla-Nash, H.; Damian, M.; Cheung, P.; Kusumoto, R.; Kawahara, T.L.; Barrett, J.C.; et al. SIRT6 is a histone H3 lysine 9 deacetylase that modulates telomeric chromatin. *Nature* **2008**, *452*, 492–496. [CrossRef] [PubMed]
7. Li, Y.; Jin, J.; Wang, Y. SIRT6 Widely Regulates Aging, Immunity, and Cancer. *Front. Oncol.* **2022**, *12*, 861334. [CrossRef]
8. Liu, G.; Chen, H.; Liu, H.; Zhang, W.; Zhou, J. Emerging roles of SIRT6 in human diseases and its modulators. *Med. Res. Rev.* **2021**, *41*, 1089–1137. [CrossRef]
9. Yang, Z.; Huang, Y.; Zhu, L.; Yang, K.; Liang, K.; Tan, J.; Yu, B. SIRT6 promotes angiogenesis and hemorrhage of carotid plaque via regulating HIF-1α and reactive oxygen species. *Cell Death Dis.* **2021**, *12*, 77. [CrossRef]
10. Song, M.Y.; Yi, F.; Xiao, H.; Yin, J.; Huang, Q.; Xia, J.; Yin, X.M.; Wen, Y.B.; Zhang, L.; Liu, Y.H.; et al. Energy restriction induced SIRT6 inhibits microglia activation and promotes angiogenesis in cerebral ischemia via transcriptional inhibition of TXNIP. *Cell Death Dis.* **2022**, *13*, 449. [CrossRef]
11. Jiang, X.; Yao, Z.; Wang, K.; Lou, L.; Xue, K.; Chen, J.; Zhang, G.; Zhang, Y.; Du, J.; Lin, C.; et al. MDL-800, the SIRT6 Activator, Suppresses Inflammation via the NF-κB Pathway and Promotes Angiogenesis to Accelerate Cutaneous Wound Healing in Mice. *Oxidative Med. Cell. Longev.* **2022**, *2022*, 1619651. [CrossRef] [PubMed]
12. Bauer, I.; Grozio, A.; Lasiglè, D.; Basile, G.; Sturla, L.; Magnone, M.; Sociali, G.; Soncini, D.; Caffa, I.; Poggi, A.; et al. The NAD+-dependent histone deacetylase SIRT6 promotes cytokine production and migration in pancreatic cancer cells by regulating Ca^{2+} responses. *J. Biol. Chem.* **2012**, *287*, 40924–40937. [CrossRef] [PubMed]
13. Ebrahimi, B.; Tucker, S.L.; Li, D.; Abbruzzese, J.L.; Kurzrock, R. Cytokines in pancreatic carcinoma: Correlation with phenotypic characteristics and prognosis. *Cancer* **2004**, *101*, 2727–2736. [CrossRef] [PubMed]
14. Matsuo, Y.; Ochi, N.; Sawai, H.; Yasuda, A.; Takahashi, H.; Funahashi, H.; Takeyama, H.; Tong, Z.; Guha, S. CXCL8/IL-8 and CXCL12/SDF-1alpha co-operatively promote invasiveness and angiogenesis in pancreatic cancer. *Int. J. Cancer* **2009**, *124*, 853–861. [CrossRef] [PubMed]
15. Blunt, J.W.; Copp, B.R.; Keyzers, R.A.; Munro, M.H.; Prinsep, M.R. Marine natural products. *Nat. Prod. Rep.* **2013**, *30*, 237–323. [CrossRef] [PubMed]
16. Mayer, A.M.; Rodríguez, A.D.; Taglialatela-Scafati, O.; Fusetani, N. Marine pharmacology in 2009–2011: Marine compounds with antibacterial, antidiabetic, antifungal, anti-inflammatory, antiprotozoal, antituberculosis, and antiviral activities; affecting the immune and nervous systems, and other miscellaneous mechanisms of action. *Mar. Drugs* **2013**, *11*, 2510–2573. [CrossRef]
17. Hai, Y.; Wei, M.-Y.; Wang, C.-Y.; Gu, Y.-C.; Shao, C.-L. The intriguing chemistry and biology of sulfur-containing natural products from marine microorganisms (1987–2020). *Mar. Life Sci. Technol.* **2021**, *3*, 488–518. [CrossRef]
18. Xu, W.-F.; Wu, N.-N.; Wu, Y.-W.; Qi, Y.-X.; Wei, M.-Y.; Pineda, L.M.; Ng, M.G.; Spadafora, C.; Zheng, J.-Y.; Lu, L.; et al. Structure modification, antialgal, antiplasmodial, and toxic evaluations of a series of new marine-derived 14-membered resorcylic acid lactone derivatives. *Mar. Life Sci. Technol.* **2022**, *4*, 88–97. [CrossRef]
19. Fujita, M.; Nakao, Y.; Matsunaga, S.; Seiki, M.; Itoh, Y.; Yamashita, J.; Van Soest, R.W.; Fusetani, N. Ageladine A: An antiangiogenic matrixmetalloproteinase inhibitor from the marine sponge Agelas nakamurai. *J. Am. Chem. Soc.* **2003**, *125*, 15700–15701. [CrossRef]
20. Ando, N.; Terashima, S. Synthesis and matrix metalloproteinase-12 inhibitory activity of ageladine A analogs. *Chem. Pharm. Bull.* **2011**, *59*, 579–596. [CrossRef]
21. Song, N.; Guan, X.; Zhang, S.; Wang, Y.; Wang, X.; Lu, Z.; Chong, D.; Wang, J.Y.; Yu, R.; Yu, W.; et al. Discovery of a pyrrole-pyridinimidazole derivative as novel SIRT6 inhibitor for sensitizing pancreatic cancer to gemcitabine. *Cell Death Dis.* **2023**, *14*, 499. [CrossRef] [PubMed]
22. Grant, D.S.; Tashiro, K.; Segui-Real, B.; Yamada, Y.; Martin, G.R.; Kleinman, H.K. Two different laminin domains mediate the differentiation of human endothelial cells into capillary-like structures in vitro. *Cell* **1989**, *58*, 933–943. [CrossRef] [PubMed]
23. Melincovici, C.S.; Boşca, A.B.; Şuşman, S.; Mărginean, M.; Mihu, C.; Istrate, M.; Moldovan, I.M.; Roman, A.L.; Mihu, C.M. Vascular endothelial growth factor (VEGF)—Key factor in normal and pathological angiogenesis. *Rom. J. Morphol. Embryol. Rev. Roum. Morphol. Embryol.* **2018**, *59*, 455–467.
24. Ferrara, N. Vascular endothelial growth factor: Basic science and clinical progress. *Endocr. Rev.* **2004**, *25*, 581–611. [CrossRef] [PubMed]

25. Hicklin, D.J.; Ellis, L.M. Role of the vascular endothelial growth factor pathway in tumor growth and angiogenesis. *J. Clin. Oncol. Off. J. Am. Soc. Clin. Oncol.* **2005**, *23*, 1011–1027. [CrossRef]
26. Chen, T.T.; Luque, A.; Lee, S.; Anderson, S.M.; Segura, T.; Iruela-Arispe, M.L. Anchorage of VEGF to the extracellular matrix conveys differential signaling responses to endothelial cells. *J. Cell Biol.* **2010**, *188*, 595–609. [CrossRef]
27. Blaschuk, O.W. N-cadherin antagonists as oncology therapeutics. *Philos. Trans. R. Soc. London Ser. B Biol. Sci.* **2015**, *370*, 20140039. [CrossRef] [PubMed]
28. Blaschuk, O.W.; Devemy, E. Cadherins as novel targets for anti-cancer therapy. *Eur. J. Pharmacol.* **2009**, *625*, 195–198. [CrossRef]
29. Gerhardt, H.; Wolburg, H.; Redies, C. N-cadherin mediates pericytic-endothelial interaction during brain angiogenesis in the chicken. *Dev. Dyn. Off. Publ. Am. Assoc. Anat.* **2000**, *218*, 472–479. [CrossRef]
30. Gaengel, K.; Genové, G.; Armulik, A.; Betsholtz, C. Endothelial-mural cell signaling in vascular development and angiogenesis. *Arterioscler. Thromb. Vasc. Biol.* **2009**, *29*, 630–638. [CrossRef]
31. Bai, X.; Zhi, X.; Zhang, Q.; Liang, F.; Chen, W.; Liang, C.; Hu, Q.; Sun, X.; Zhuang, Z.; Liang, T. Inhibition of protein phosphatase 2A sensitizes pancreatic cancer to chemotherapy by increasing drug perfusion via HIF-1α-VEGF mediated angiogenesis. *Cancer Lett.* **2014**, *355*, 281–287. [CrossRef] [PubMed]
32. Karar, J.; Maity, A. PI3K/AKT/mTOR Pathway in Angiogenesis. *Front. Mol. Neurosci.* **2011**, *4*, 51. [CrossRef] [PubMed]
33. Srinivasan, R.; Zabuawala, T.; Huang, H.; Zhang, J.; Gulati, P.; Fernandez, S.; Karlo, J.C.; Landreth, G.E.; Leone, G.; Ostrowski, M.C. Erk1 and Erk2 regulate endothelial cell proliferation and migration during mouse embryonic angiogenesis. *PLoS ONE* **2009**, *4*, e8283. [CrossRef] [PubMed]
34. Childs, S.; Chen, J.N.; Garrity, D.M.; Fishman, M.C. Patterning of angiogenesis in the zebrafish embryo. *Development* **2002**, *129*, 973–982. [CrossRef] [PubMed]
35. Gore, A.V.; Monzo, K.; Cha, Y.R.; Pan, W.; Weinstein, B.M. Vascular development in the zebrafish. *Cold Spring Harb. Perspect. Med.* **2012**, *2*, a006684. [CrossRef] [PubMed]
36. McKinney, M.C.; Weinstein, B.M. Chapter 4. Using the zebrafish to study vessel formation. *Methods Enzymol.* **2008**, *444*, 65–97. [CrossRef] [PubMed]
37. Isogai, S.; Hitomi, J.; Yaniv, K.; Weinstein, B.M. Zebrafish as a new animal model to study lymphangiogenesis. *Anat. Sci. Int.* **2009**, *84*, 102–111. [CrossRef] [PubMed]
38. Schuermann, A.; Helker, C.S.; Herzog, W. Angiogenesis in zebrafish. *Semin. Cell Dev. Biol.* **2014**, *31*, 106–114. [CrossRef]
39. Serbedzija, G.N.; Flynn, E.; Willett, C.E. Zebrafish angiogenesis: A new model for drug screening. *Angiogenesis* **1999**, *3*, 353–359. [CrossRef]
40. Ma, C.; Wu, Z.; Wang, X.; Huang, M.; Wei, X.; Wang, W.; Qu, H.; Qiaolongbatu, X.; Lou, Y.; Jing, L.; et al. A systematic comparison of anti-angiogenesis efficacy and cardiotoxicity of receptor tyrosine kinase inhibitors in zebrafish model. *Toxicol. Appl. Pharmacol.* **2022**, *450*, 116162. [CrossRef]
41. Isogai, S.; Horiguchi, M.; Weinstein, B.M. The vascular anatomy of the developing zebrafish: An atlas of embryonic and early larval development. *Dev. Biol.* **2001**, *230*, 278–301. [CrossRef] [PubMed]
42. Lawson, N.D.; Weinstein, B.M. In vivo imaging of embryonic vascular development using transgenic zebrafish. *Dev. Biol.* **2002**, *248*, 307–318. [CrossRef] [PubMed]
43. Kamei, M.; Isogai, S.; Weinstein, B.M. Imaging blood vessels in the zebrafish. *Methods Cell Biol.* **2004**, *76*, 51–74. [CrossRef] [PubMed]
44. Kitambi, S.S.; McCulloch, K.J.; Peterson, R.T.; Malicki, J.J. Small molecule screen for compounds that affect vascular development in the zebrafish retina. *Mech. Dev.* **2009**, *126*, 464–477. [CrossRef]
45. Rezzola, S.; Paganini, G.; Semeraro, F.; Presta, M.; Tobia, C. Zebrafish (*Danio rerio*) embryo as a platform for the identification of novel angiogenesis inhibitors of retinal vascular diseases. *Biochim. Biophys. Acta* **2016**, *1862*, 1291–1296. [CrossRef] [PubMed]
46. Kim, M.; Park, H.J.; Seol, J.W.; Jang, J.Y.; Cho, Y.S.; Kim, K.R.; Choi, Y.; Lydon, J.P.; Demayo, F.J.; Shibuya, M.; et al. VEGF-A regulated by progesterone governs uterine angiogenesis and vascular remodelling during pregnancy. *EMBO Mol. Med.* **2013**, *5*, 1415–1430. [CrossRef] [PubMed]
47. Figueiredo, C.C.; Pereira, N.B.; Pereira, L.X.; Oliveira, L.A.M.; Campos, P.P.; Andrade, S.P.; Moro, L. Double immunofluorescence labeling for CD31 and CD105 as a marker for polyether polyurethane-induced angiogenesis in mice. *Histol. Histopathol.* **2019**, *34*, 257–264. [CrossRef]
48. Liotta, L.A.; Steeg, P.S.; Stetler-Stevenson, W.G. Cancer metastasis and angiogenesis: An imbalance of positive and negative regulation. *Cell* **1991**, *64*, 327–336. [CrossRef]
49. Folkman, J. Role of angiogenesis in tumor growth and metastasis. *Semin. Oncol.* **2002**, *29*, 15–18. [CrossRef]
50. Ferrara, N.; Hillan, K.J.; Gerber, H.P.; Novotny, W. Discovery and development of bevacizumab, an anti-VEGF antibody for treating cancer. *Nat. Rev. Drug Discov.* **2004**, *3*, 391–400. [CrossRef]
51. Poole, R.M.; Vaidya, A. Ramucirumab: First global approval. *Drugs* **2014**, *74*, 1047–1058. [CrossRef] [PubMed]
52. Ferrara, N. The role of VEGF in the regulation of physiological and pathological angiogenesis. *Mech. Angiogenesis* **2005**, *94*, 209–231. [CrossRef]
53. Paik, J.H.; Skoura, A.; Chae, S.S.; Cowan, A.E.; Han, D.K.; Proia, R.L.; Hla, T. Sphingosine 1-phosphate receptor regulation of N-cadherin mediates vascular stabilization. *Genes Dev.* **2004**, *18*, 2392–2403. [CrossRef] [PubMed]

54. Howe, K.; Clark, M.D.; Torroja, C.F.; Torrance, J.; Berthelot, C.; Muffato, M.; Collins, J.E.; Humphray, S.; McLaren, K.; Matthews, L.; et al. The zebrafish reference genome sequence and its relationship to the human genome. *Nature* **2013**, *496*, 498–503. [CrossRef] [PubMed]
55. Martin, W.K.; Tennant, A.H.; Conolly, R.B.; Prince, K.; Stevens, J.S.; DeMarini, D.M.; Martin, B.L.; Thompson, L.C.; Gilmour, M.I.; Cascio, W.E.; et al. High-Throughput Video Processing of Heart Rate Responses in Multiple Wild-type Embryonic Zebrafish per Imaging Field. *Sci. Rep.* **2019**, *9*, 145. [CrossRef] [PubMed]
56. Tang, J.Y.; Cheng, Y.B.; Chuang, Y.T.; Yang, K.H.; Chang, F.R.; Liu, W.; Chang, H.W. Oxidative Stress and AKT-Associated Angiogenesis in a Zebrafish Model and Its Potential Application for Withanolides. *Cells* **2022**, *11*, 961. [CrossRef] [PubMed]
57. Weis, S.M.; Cheresh, D.A. Tumor angiogenesis: Molecular pathways and therapeutic targets. *Nat. Med.* **2011**, *17*, 1359–1370. [CrossRef] [PubMed]
58. Kleeff, J.; Michalski, C.; Friess, H.; Büchler, M.W. Pancreatic cancer: From bench to 5-year survival. *Pancreas* **2006**, *33*, 111–118. [CrossRef]
59. Li, S.; Xu, H.X.; Wu, C.T.; Wang, W.Q.; Jin, W.; Gao, H.L.; Li, H.; Zhang, S.R.; Xu, J.Z.; Qi, Z.H.; et al. Angiogenesis in pancreatic cancer: Current research status and clinical implications. *Angiogenesis* **2019**, *22*, 15–36. [CrossRef]
60. Xu, Y.; Liu, P.; Zheng, D.H.; Wu, N.; Zhu, L.; Xing, C.; Zhu, J. Expression profile and prognostic value of NNMT in patients with pancreatic cancer. *Oncotarget* **2016**, *7*, 19975–19981. [CrossRef]
61. Bi, H.C.; Pan, Y.Z.; Qiu, J.X.; Krausz, K.W.; Li, F.; Johnson, C.H.; Jiang, C.T.; Gonzalez, F.J.; Yu, A.M. N-methylnicotinamide and nicotinamide N-methyltransferase are associated with microRNA-1291-altered pancreatic carcinoma cell metabolome and suppressed tumorigenesis. *Carcinogenesis* **2014**, *35*, 2264–2272. [CrossRef] [PubMed]
62. Campagna, R.; Vignini, A. NAD(+) Homeostasis and NAD(+)-Consuming Enzymes: Implications for Vascular Health. *Antioxidants* **2023**, *12*, 376. [CrossRef]
63. van Haren, M.J.; Zhang, Y.; Thijssen, V.; Buijs, N.; Gao, Y.; Mateuszuk, L.; Fedak, F.A.; Kij, A.; Campagna, R.; Sartini, D.; et al. Macrocyclic peptides as allosteric inhibitors of nicotinamide N-methyltransferase (NNMT). *RSC Chem. Biol.* **2021**, *2*, 1546–1555. [CrossRef] [PubMed]
64. van Haren, M.J.; Gao, Y.; Buijs, N.; Campagna, R.; Sartini, D.; Emanuelli, M.; Mateuszuk, L.; Kij, A.; Chlopicki, S.; Escudé Martinez de Castilla, P.; et al. Esterase-Sensitive Prodrugs of a Potent Bisubstrate Inhibitor of Nicotinamide N-Methyltransferase (NNMT) Display Cellular Activity. *Biomolecules* **2021**, *11*, 1357. [CrossRef] [PubMed]
65. Gao, Y.; van Haren, M.J.; Buijs, N.; Innocenti, P.; Zhang, Y.; Sartini, D.; Campagna, R.; Emanuelli, M.; Parsons, R.B.; Jespers, W.; et al. Potent Inhibition of Nicotinamide N-Methyltransferase by Alkene-Linked Bisubstrate Mimics Bearing Electron Deficient Aromatics. *J. Med. Chem.* **2021**, *64*, 12938–12963. [CrossRef] [PubMed]
66. Cattaneo, M.G.; Chini, B.; Vicentini, L.M. Oxytocin stimulates migration and invasion in human endothelial cells. *Br. J. Pharmacol.* **2008**, *153*, 728–736. [CrossRef] [PubMed]
67. Sumanas, S.; Lin, S. Ets1-related protein is a key regulator of vasculogenesis in zebrafish. *PLoS Biol.* **2006**, *4*, e10. [CrossRef]
68. Song, M.; Yang, H.; Yao, S.; Ma, F.; Li, Z.; Deng, Y.; Deng, H.; Zhou, Q.; Lin, S.; Wei, Y. A critical role of vascular endothelial growth factor D in zebrafish embryonic vasculogenesis and angiogenesis. *Biochem. Biophys. Res. Commun.* **2007**, *357*, 924–930. [CrossRef]

Disclaimer/Publisher's Note: The statements, opinions and data contained in all publications are solely those of the individual author(s) and contributor(s) and not of MDPI and/or the editor(s). MDPI and/or the editor(s) disclaim responsibility for any injury to people or property resulting from any ideas, methods, instructions or products referred to in the content.

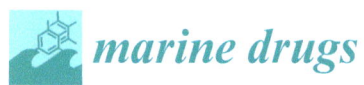

Article

Anti-Atopic Dermatitis Activity of *Epi*-Oxyzoanthamine Isolated from Zoanthid

Chieh-Chen Huang [1,2], Yuan-Hsin Lo [1,3], Yu-Jou Hsu [4], Yuan-Bin Cheng [5], Chia-Chi Kung [1,6], Cher-Wei Liang [1,7], Der-Chen Chang [8], Kang-Ling Wang [9,*] and Chi-Feng Hung [1,10,*]

1. School of Medicine, Fu Jen Catholic University, New Taipei City 242, Taiwan; m001017@ms.skh.org.tw (C.-C.H.); a00781@fjuh.fju.edu.tw (Y.-H.L.); drpainkung@gmail.com (C.-C.K.); 085027@mail.fju.edu.tw (C.-W.L.)
2. Department of Dermatology, Shin Kong Wu Ho-Su Memorial Hospital, Taipei 111, Taiwan
3. Department of Dermatology, Fu Jen Catholic University Hospital, Fu Jen Catholic University, New Taipei City 242, Taiwan
4. PhD Program in Pharmaceutical Biotechnology, Fu Jen Catholic University, New Taipei City 24205, Taiwan; 411138028@mail.fju.edu.tw
5. Department of Marine Biotechnology and Resources, National Sun Yat-Sen University, Kaohsiung 804, Taiwan; jmb@mail.nsysu.edu.tw
6. Department of Anesthesiology, Fu Jen Catholic University Hospital, Fu Jen Catholic University, New Taipei City 242, Taiwan
7. Department of Pathology, Fu Jen Catholic University Hospital, Fu Jen Catholic University, New Taipei City 242, Taiwan
8. Department of Mathematics and Statistics, Department of Computer Science, Georgetown University, Washington, DC 20057, USA; chang@georgetown.edu
9. Division of Metabolism and Endocrinology, Department of Internal Medicine, Taoyuan Armed Forces General Hospital, Taoyuan 325, Taiwan
10. School of Pharmacy, Kaohsiung Medical University, Kaohsiung 80708, Taiwan
* Correspondence: klwang@aftygh.gov.tw (K.-L.W.); skin@mail.fju.edu.tw (C.-F.H.)

Citation: Huang, C.-C.; Lo, Y.-H.; Hsu, Y.-J.; Cheng, Y.-B.; Kung, C.-C.; Liang, C.-W.; Chang, D.-C.; Wang, K.-L.; Hung, C.-F. Anti-Atopic Dermatitis Activity of *Epi*-Oxyzoanthamine Isolated from Zoanthid. *Mar. Drugs* 2023, 21, 447. https://doi.org/10.3390/md21080447

Academic Editor: Chang-Lun Shao

Received: 19 July 2023
Revised: 10 August 2023
Accepted: 10 August 2023
Published: 12 August 2023

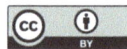

Copyright: © 2023 by the authors. Licensee MDPI, Basel, Switzerland. This article is an open access article distributed under the terms and conditions of the Creative Commons Attribution (CC BY) license (https://creativecommons.org/licenses/by/4.0/).

Abstract: Atopic dermatitis (AD, eczema) is a condition that causes dry, itchy, and inflamed skin and occurs most frequently in children but also affects adults. However, common clinical treatments provide limited relief and have some side effects. Therefore, there is a need to develop new effective therapies to treat AD. *Epi*-oxyzoanthamine is a small molecule alkaloid isolated from Formosan zoanthid. Relevant studies have shown that zoanthamine alkaloids have many pharmacological and biological activities, including anti-lymphangiogenic functions. However, there are no studies on the use of *epi*-oxyzoanthamine on the skin. In this paper, *epi*-oxyzoanthamine has been shown to have potential in the treatment of atopic dermatitis. Through in vitro studies, it was found that *epi*-oxyzoanthamine inhibited the expression of cytokines in TNF-α/IFN-γ-stimulated human keratinocyte (HaCaT) cells, and it reduced the phosphorylation of MAPK and the NF-κB signaling pathway. Atopic dermatitis-like skin inflammation was induced in a mouse model using 2,4-dinitrochlorobenzene (DNCB) in vivo. The results showed that *epi*-oxyzoanthamine significantly decreased skin barrier damage, scratching responses, and epidermal hyperplasia induced by DNCB. It significantly reduced transepidermal water loss (TEWL), erythema, ear thickness, and spleen weight, while also increasing surface skin hydration. These results indicate that *epi*-oxyzoanthamine from zoanthid has good potential as an alternative medicine for treating atopic dermatitis or other skin-related inflammatory diseases.

Keywords: atopic dermatitis; inflammation; keratinocyte; *epi*-oxyzoanthamine; zoanthid

1. Introduction

Atopic dermatitis, also known as eczema, is a chronic inflammatory relapsing skin disease. It is one of the most common skin diseases affecting infants and young children [1]. About half of children with atopic dermatitis will develop allergic rhinitis, asthma, allergic conjunctivitis, etc. [2]. Allergies or abnormal immune function are currently believed to be important factors causing atopic dermatitis, but the true, underlying cause is not yet clear [3]. Patients have skin allergic reactions to many allergens in the environment, such as dust mites and food, and elevated levels of immunoglobulin E (IgE) [4] and eosinophilic leukocytes [5] are found in the blood of many patients [3]. Notably, itching and dry skin are the main clinical symptoms [6]. Topical steroids are currently the main treatment for atopic dermatitis. However, long-term use of topical steroids can cause skin thinning and discoloration [7]. Oral antihistamines can also be used for severe itching. Yet, it should be noted that the first-generation antihistamines are prone to the side effect of drowsiness [6], limiting the overall benefit of their use. The onset of atopic dermatitis involves multiple mechanisms, and a small number of particularly severe atopic dermatitis may even require doctors to prescribe biological agents [8] or immunosuppressants for treatment. The discovery of these biological agents and oral targeted small-molecule drugs are typically very helpful to patients as they have good therapeutic effects and minimal side effects [9]. Unfortunately, the high cost of these treatments is a strong barrier and limits patient use. Therefore, it is a medical necessity to develop an atopic dermatitis treatment with few side effects at a low price.

Human beings have been using Chinese herbal medicine for thousands of years [10]. Most scientists have discovered new drugs or compound structures from land. However, with the extensive research and development by scientists, the discovery of new structural natural components in terrestrial plants has become more and more difficult. Many scientists hope to find them in the ocean [11]. The ocean area accounts for more than half of the earth's surface area. It is not only the origin of life on the earth, but also the most abundant treasure house of biological resources, including hundreds of thousands to millions of lower marine organisms and microorganisms. The ocean may also produce many chemical substances with special structures and significant biological activities depending on the geographical location, ocean currents, and depths [11,12]. In the past, many compounds have been found to have anti-cancer [13], anti-hyperlipidemia [14], anti-viral [15], pain-relieving [16], and anti-dementia effects [17]. Several of these candidates have been marketed or are in clinical trials [3].

Zoanthid is a kind of sessile marine invertebrate that is regarded as a good source of marine natural products. Zoanthenamine alkaloids are the predominant secondary metabolites of zoanthid. More than 70 of this type of compound have been identified, and the majority contain an azepane moiety [18]. These non-aromatic alkaloids demonstrate various pharmacological effects, including anti-inflammatory [19], anti-cancer [20], neuroprotective [21], antiosteoporosis [22], and antimetastatic activities [23]. However, the effect of this type of compound on atopic dermatitis is still unknown. Therefore, this article will leverage in vivo and in vitro experiments to show that *epi*-oxyzoanthamine among the zoanthamine compounds is a very good choice for atopic dermatitis.

2. Results
2.1. Effect of Epi-Oxyzoanthamine on HaCaT Cell Viability

At the beginning of the experiment, in order to prove the safety of the *epi*-oxyzoanthamine (Figure 1A), whether the toxicity of the *epi*-oxyzoanthamine is proved by cell viability test is suitable for subsequent related in vitro or in vivo studies. Thiazolyl blue tetrazolium bromide (MTT) assay was used to evaluate the cell viability. After the cells were administered for 1 h from a low dose of 1 µM to a high dose of 50 µM, we still did not find any toxicity of *epi*-oxyzoanthamine to the cells (Figure 1B). Therefore, experiments were conducted to investigate the mechanism of action of *epi*-oxyzoanthamine against atopic dermatitis in this concentration range.

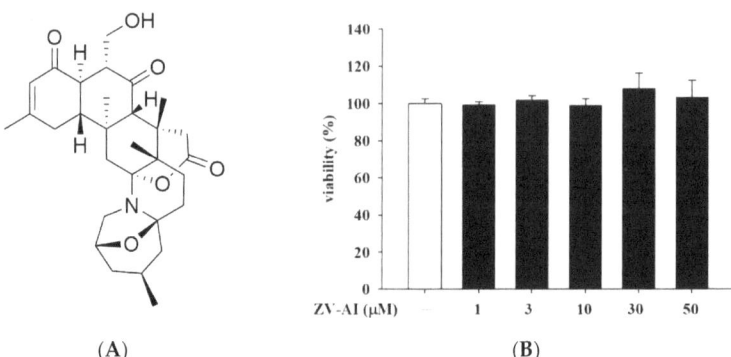

(A) (B)

Figure 1. (**A**) The chemical structure of *epi*-oxyzoanthamine. (**B**) Effects of *epi*-oxyzoanthamine (ZV-AI) on cell viabilities of keratinocytes. HaCaT cells were pretreated with different concentrations of *epi*-oxyzoanthamine for 24 h.

2.2. The Anti-Inflammatory Effect of Epi-Oxyzoanthamine in Tumor Necrosis Factor-α (TNF-α)/Interferon-γ (IFN-γ)-Induced Inflammation in HaCaT Cells

The increase of pro-inflammatory cytokines is closely related to the etiology of atopic dermatitis. Many studies have shown that IFN-γ and TNF-α stimulate keratinocytes to induce signaling pathways involved in pro-inflammatory responses. Therefore, this model is often used as an in vitro test method for skin anti-inflammatory effectiveness [24,25]. It is shown in Figure 2 that once these pro-inflammatory cytokines (TNF-α and IFN-γ) are added, the formation of intracellular cytokine mRNA is significantly increased. These cytokines include IL-1β, IL-6, and IL-8. Moreover, there was a direct relationship between the concentrations of *epi*-oxyzoanthamine (1–10 μM) and the inhibitory ability of the cytokines: as the drug concentration increased, so did the inhibitory ability (Figure 2A–C).

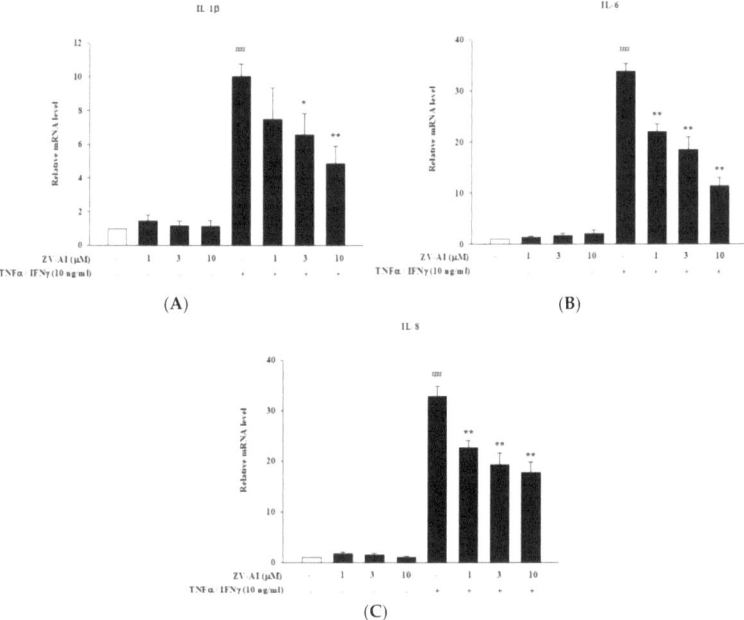

Figure 2. Effects of *epi*-oxyzoanthamine (ZV-AI) on the expression of correlated cytokines mRNA ((**A**): IL-1β, (**B**): IL-6, and (**C**): IL-8) after stimulation of TNF-α/IFN-γ. HaCaT cells were pretreated

with different concentrations of *epi*-oxyzoanthamine for 1 h, and then the cells were treated with TNF-α/IFN-γ for 1 h. ## $p < 0.01$ compared with the no-treatment group; * $p < 0.05$ and ** $p < 0.01$ compared with the TNF-α/IFN-γ-induced group.

2.3. Effects of Epi-Oxyzoanthamine on Phosphrylation of MAPK Pathway in HaCaT Cells

Many studies have shown that cytokine stimulation of skin cells activates mitogen-activated protein kinase (MAPK) pathway. Therefore, the following experiments will elucidate whether or not *epi*-oxyzoanthamine affects these pathways. First, *epi*-oxyzoanthamine demonstrated no activation or effect on the MAPK pathway (Figure 3). Next, cells were stimulated the cells with IFN-γ and TNF-α for one (or half) hour and found that the pathway to MAPK was activated and phosphorylated (Figure 4). However, the study found that if the cells were pretreated with the *epi*-oxyzoanthamine, the increased phosphorylation was indeed significantly inhibited. This phenomenon was more effective at higher concentrations (Figure 4A–C).

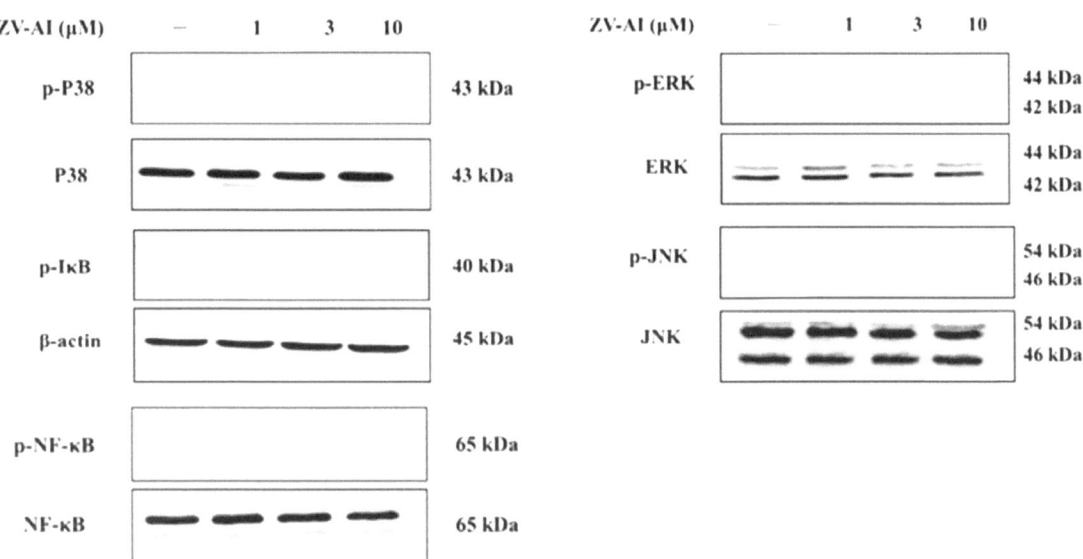

Figure 3. Effect of *epi*-oxyzoanthamine (ZV-AI) on phosphorylation of MAP kinase and transcription factor. HaCaT cells were pretreated with different concentrations of *epi*-oxyzoanthamine for 1 h.

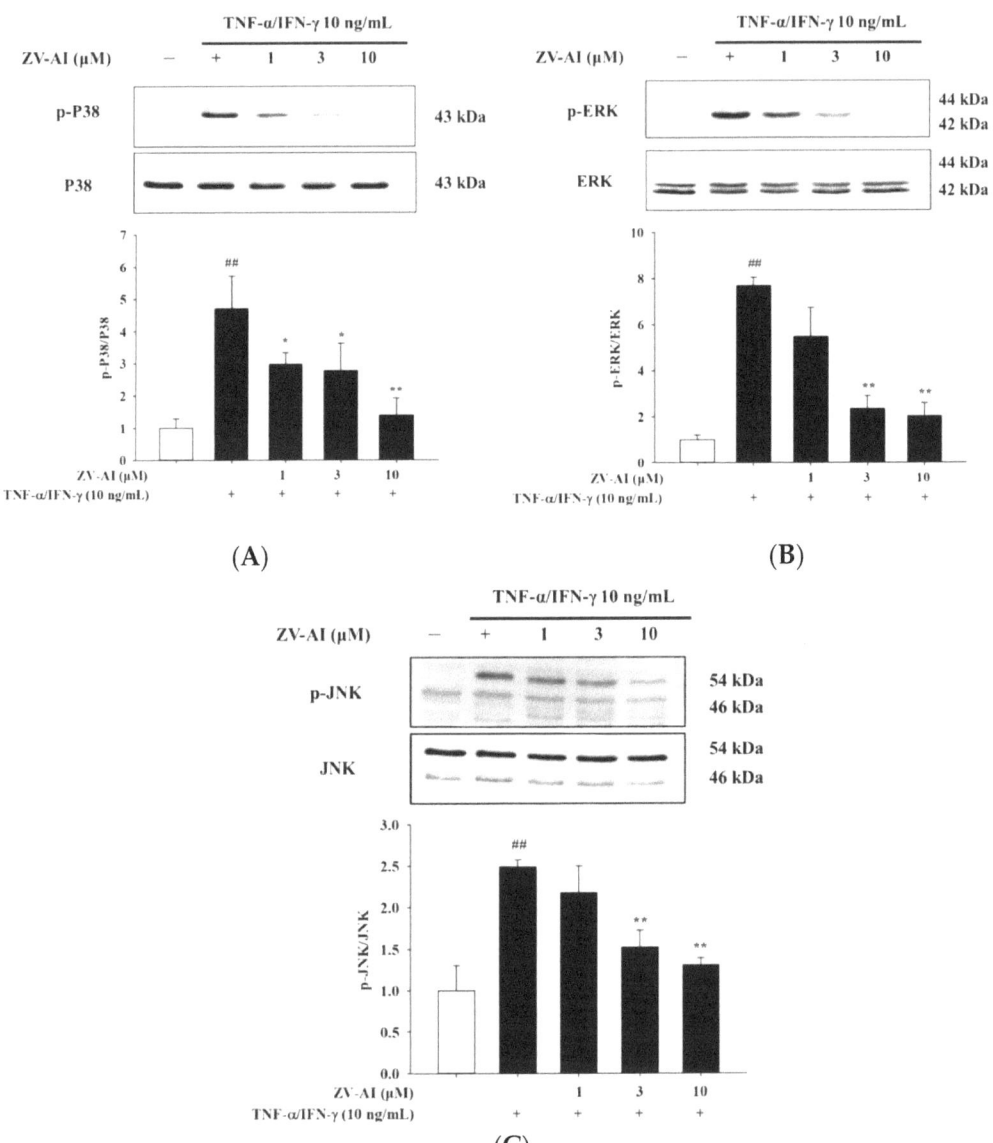

Figure 4. The effect of *epi*-oxyzoanthamine (ZV-AI) on phosphorylation of MAP kinase in TNF-α/IFN-γ-induced HaCaT cells. HaCaT cells were pretreated with different concentrations of *epi*-oxyzoanthamine for 1 h, and then the cells were treated with TNF-α/IFN-γ for 30 min (**A**,**B**) or 1 h (**C**). ## $p < 0.01$ compared with the no-treatment group; * $p < 0.05$ and ** $p < 0.01$ compared with the TNF-α/IFN-γ-induced group.

2.4. Epi-Oxyzoanthamine Reduced IκB and NF-κB Activation in TNF-α/IFN-γ-Stimulated Keratinocytes

Previous studies have cited MAP kinase as an upstream NF-κB regulatory kinase [26]. Studies have also found that IFN-γ and TNF-α also increase the phosphorylation of NF-κB and IκB. At the same time, it was found that an increase in the concentration of *epi*-

oxyzoanthamine after pretreatment caused an increase in the inhibition of phosphorylation (Figure 5).

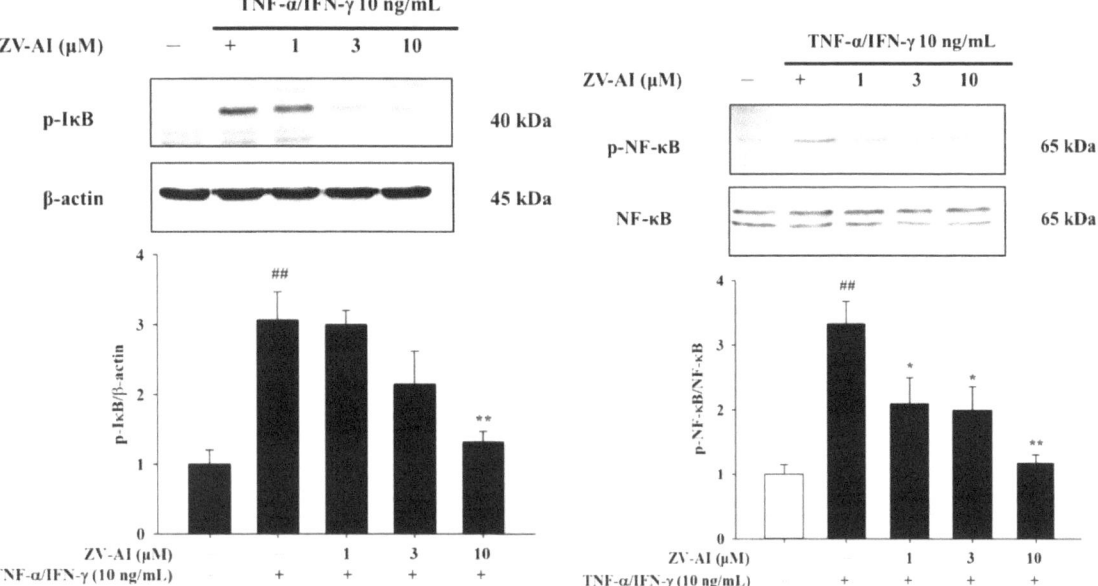

Figure 5. The effect of *epi*-oxyzoanthamine (ZV-AI) on phosphorylation of IκB (**left panel**) and NF-κB (**right panel**) in TNF-κ/IFN-γ-induced HaCaT cells. HaCaT cells were pretreated with different concentrations of *epi*-oxyzoanthamine for 1 h, and then the cells were treated with TNF-α/IFN-γ for 1 h. ## $p < 0.01$ compared with the no-treatment group; * $p < 0.05$ and ** $p < 0.01$ compared with the TNF-α/IFN-γ-induced group.

2.5. The Effect of Epi-Oxyzoanthamine on the Skin Appearance in DNCB-Induced BALB/c Mouse

After the previous in vitro studies, it was found that *epi*-oxyzoanthamine has the potential of anti-atopic dermatitis. Dinitrochlorobenzene (DNCB)-induced contact hypersensitivity (CHS) of the skin in mice is a commonly-used animal model for studying the pathogenesis of contact dermatitis [27]. Given the complexity of factors involved in the pathogenesis of AD, epidermal sensitization with stimuli such as DNCB is a common method used to identify testing drug candidates in AD [28]. When DNCB was applied to the animal's dorsal skin, it showed atopic dermatitis-like symptoms, such as desquamation and redness, epidermis thickening, skin inflammation, enlarged spleen, and the animal even had scratching behavior (Figures 6 and 7). The above pathological phenomena and symptoms after DNCB pretreatment will be alleviated with the increase of *epi*-oxyzoanthamine concentration. These same preventive effects are also commonly observed after pretreatment with dexamethasone (Figures 6 and 7).

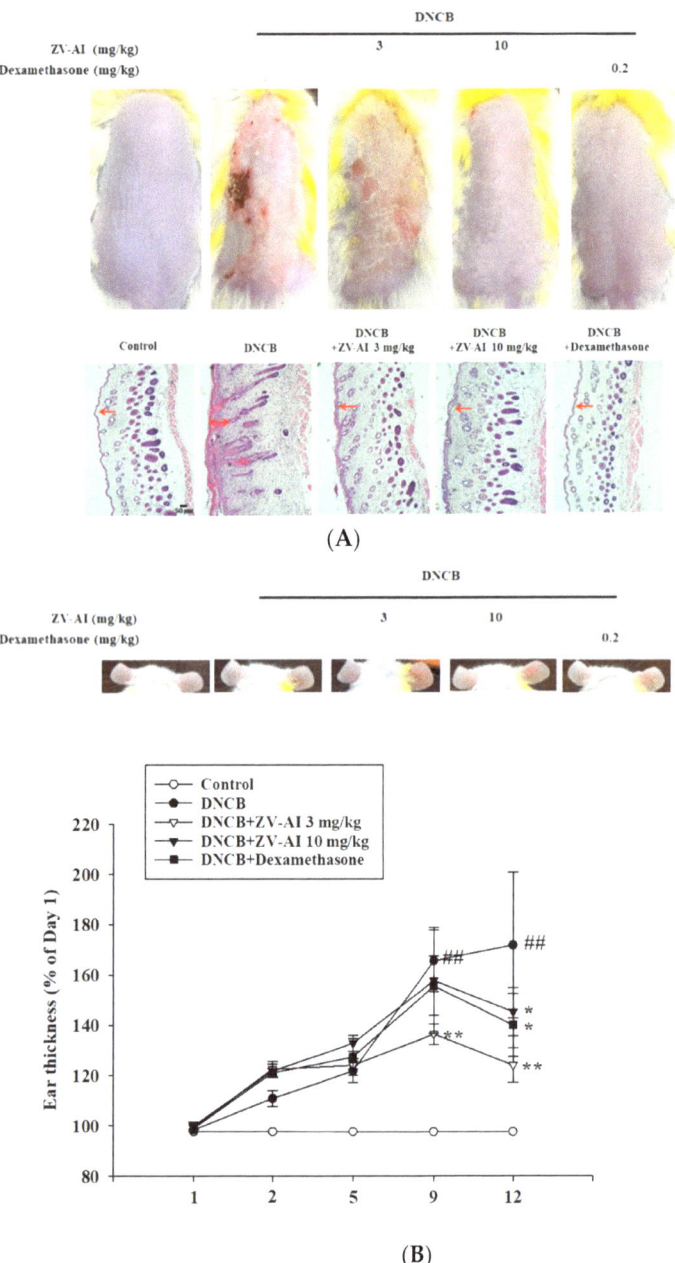

Figure 6. (**A**) Effect of *epi*-oxyzoanthamine (ZV-AI) on DNCB-induced atopic dermatitis in dorsal skin (**upper panel**). Effect of *epi*-oxyzoanthamine on DNCB-induced atopic dermatitis in ears. H and E staining of ear tissue sections. Red arrows point to the epidermis (**lower panel**). (**B**) Upper panel shows the inhibitory effect of the inflammatory response on the ear. Lower panel shows statistical results of ear inflammation thickness. ## $p < 0.01$ compared with the no-treatment group; * $p < 0.05$ and ** $p < 0.01$ compared with the DNCB-induced group.

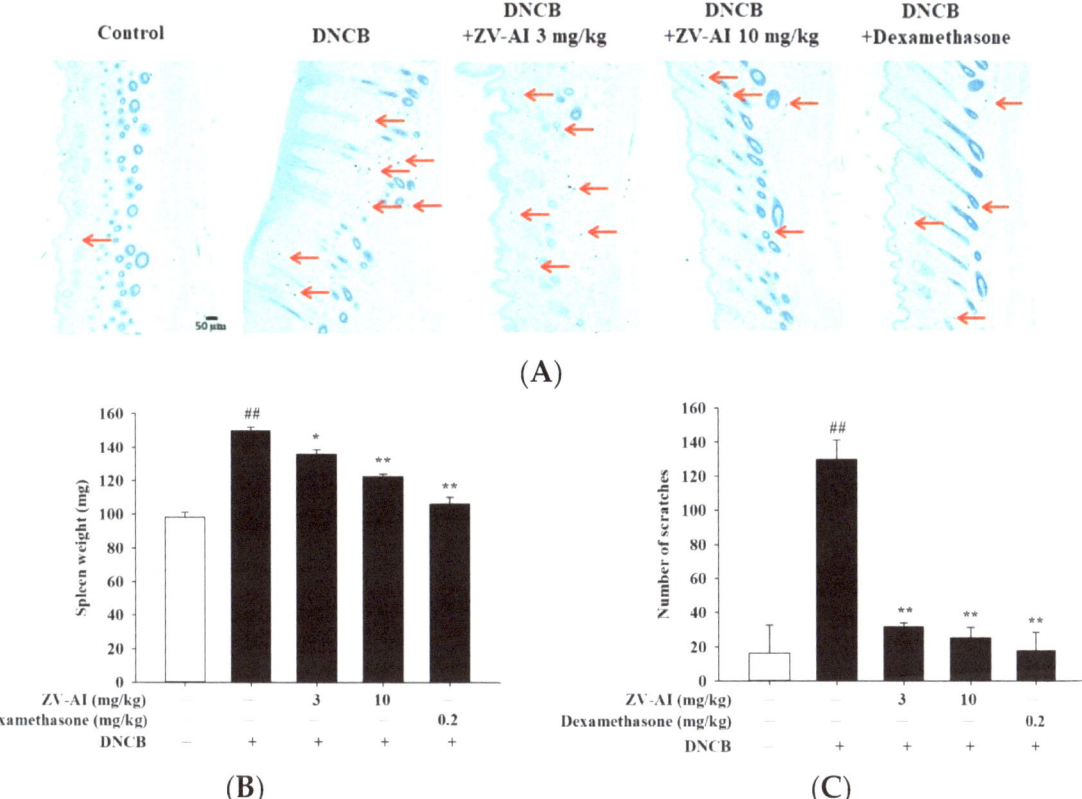

Figure 7. (**A**) Toluidine blue staining of the dorsal skin; scale bar: 50 μm (**upper panel**) and statistical analysis of the mast cells. The red arrow points to the mast cells. (**B**) Effect of *epi*-oxyzoanthamine on spleen weight. (**C**) Analysis of the effect of the change in the number of scratches in BALB/c mice with an atopic-dermatitis-like phenotype. ## $p < 0.01$ compared with the no-treatment group; * $p < 0.05$ and ** $p < 0.01$ compared with the DNCB-induced group.

2.6. Change in Physiological Functions of DNCB-Induced BALB/c Mouse Skin after Treatment with Epi-Oxyzoanthamine

From the previous pathological sections, *epi*-oxyzoanthamine does have an inhibitory effect on the inflammation caused by DNCB. The physiological values were measured to confirm the efficacy of these effects in improving physiological functions. As shown in Figure 8, improvements were found in physiological function, including transepidermal water loss, skin redness, and skin moisture content, after treatment of *epi*-oxyzoanthamine (Figure 8A–C).

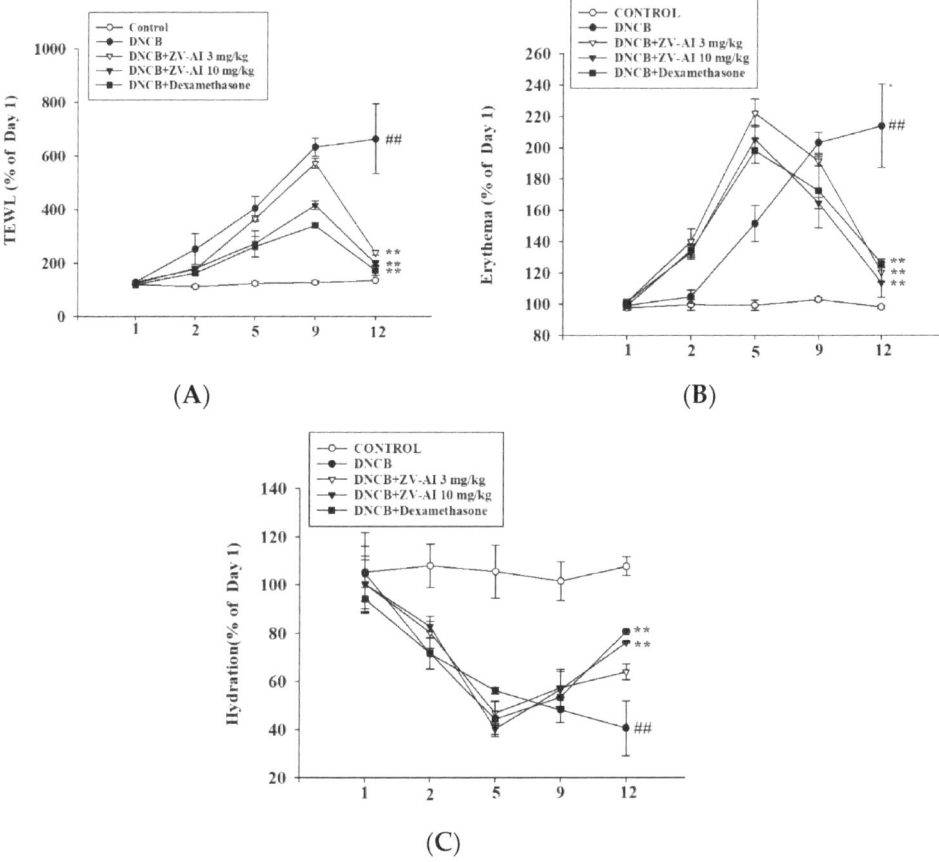

Figure 8. DNCB-induced changes in skin physiological parameters of BALB/c mice after treatment with *epi*-oxyzoanthamine (ZV-AI). Effect of changes in transepidermal water loss (TEWL, (**A**)), erythema (**B**), and hydration (**C**) in the atopic dermatitis-like phenotype of BALB/c mice. Values represent means ± SEM of at least six independent experiments. ## $p < 0.01$ compared to the no-treatment condition; ** $p < 0.01$ compared to the DNCB-induced group.

3. Discussion

Marine organisms are now a very large source of pharmaceutical resources. Scientists have also discovered many new structures of compounds here, and many structures have even been used to treat diseases. Some of them have even been used clinically or are already in clinical trials. Marine biological sources of these compounds typically include algae, bacteria, fungi, sponges, corals, and other marine animals [29]. Most of their discovered physiological activities are anti-bacterial, anti-viral, anti-tumor, or anti-inflammatory. Among them, the biological activities of sponges, algae, and bacteria have been studied the most, and have shown anti-tumor and anti-bacterial effects [29,30]. There are relatively few drugs from corals [31]. Therefore, our study demonstrates that *epi*-oxyzoanthamine isolated from zoanthid has good anti-dermatological potential, especially in the treatment of atopic dermatitis. These results will open up the application of related compounds produced by corals in the treatment of skin diseases, especially in the treatment of atopic dermatitis.

In previous studies on marine organisms against atopic dermatitis, some studies reported that the red algae—*Pyropia yezoensis*-extract inhibited the production of pro-inflammatory chemokines induced by IFN-γ and TNF-α in HaCaT cells by down-regulating NF-κB [32]. Down-regulation of NF-κB and STAT1 pathways by *Polyopes affinis* suppresses IFN-γ and TNF-α-induced inflammation in human keratinocytes [33]. Red algae—*Sarcodia suiae* sp. ethanol extract has anti-inflammatory effects, alleviates AD symptoms, suppresses inflammatory responses in skin tissue, and restores barrier function in DNCB-induced AD mice [34]. Polysaccharide of brown seaweed—laminarin-topical administration has a protective effect on oxazolone-induced atopic dermatitis-like lesions. Topical application of laminarin can alleviate the overproduction of IgE, mast cell infiltration, and expression of pro-inflammatory cytokines oxazolone-induced atopic dermatitis [35]. Trifuhalol A, a phlorotannin isolated from brown seaweed—*Agarum cribrosum*, inhibited the activations of immune cells and the biosynthesis of cytokines in differentiated B cells and keratinocytes, respectively. Trifuhalol A alleviated pruritus in the Compound 48/80-induced systemic anaphylaxis model and improved symptoms in house dust mite (HDM)-induced AD mice [36]. *Sargassum* polyphenol extract alleviates DNCB-induced atopic dermatitis in NC/Nga mice by restoring skin barrier function [37]. Based on these findings, the effects of marine drugs against atopic dermatitis are attributed to the immunomodulation and regulations of the skin barrier. As shown by the results of this study, *epi*-oxyzoanthamine reduced the cytokines-induced expression of pro-inflammatory cytokines. The mechanisms of action could regulate the map kinase and reduce the action of transcription factor (NF-κB). Therefore, *epi*-oxyzoanthamine could decrease the production of cytokines including IL1β, IL6, and IL8. The appearance of dysfunction of skin barrier is a major symptom in atopic dermatitis patients. Trans-epidermal water loss is an indicator of the skin barrier. Using in vivo studies, it was found that the increase of TEWL-induced DNCB was decreased after treatment of *epi*-oxyzoanthamine. On the other hand, the hydration of the epidermal is increased after the treatment of *epi*-oxyzoanthamine (Figure 8). The erythema and hyperplasia of dorsal skin are the appearance of inflammatory skin. The anti-inflammatory activity of *epi*-oxyzoanthamine was shown in Figures 7 and 8. It was also found that the infiltration of mast cells and the weight of the spleen after treatment of DNCB were decreased after pretreatment with *epi*-oxyzoanthamine. These effects indicate that dysregulation of the immune system could modulate by pretreatment with *epi*-oxyzoanthamine.

Soft corals are an indispensable source of metabolites with medicinal properties [38]. In the past, many studies have discovered many new compounds with anti-cancer, antibacterial, and anti-viral properties in soft corals [39–42]. Compounds found in soft corals have also been recently reported by many studies for their anti-inflammatory effects. Because inflammation plays an increasingly important role in many clinical diseases [43,44], these compounds are also of particular interest in the application of inflammatory diseases [45–48]. In recent years, the incidence of diverse chronic inflammatory skin diseases has been increasing, especially atopic dermatitis. Therefore, the discovery of a potent and potential chemical structure of zoanthenamine from zoanthid can be applied to inflammatory skin diseases. In the past, scholars only found that zoanthamines have anti-inflammatory, anti-bacterial, anti-platelet, anti-lymphangiogenesis neuroprotective effects [19,21,49,50]. However, no scholars have proposed the effect on inflammatory dermatitis. Therefore, this is the first to suggest that zoanthamines have anti-inflammatory dermatitis effects. Zoanthamine alkaloids are specific secondary metabolites of marine zoanthids. Importantly, these results show that its ability to resist atopic dermatitis is not inferior to that of components isolated from land plants. Moreover, their mechanism of action is very similar [24,25,51]. Future work will look to identify any unique mechanisms that are used by zoanthamine alkaloids to promote anti-inflammatory dermatitis effects.

4. Materials and Methods

4.1. Isolation of Epi-Oxyzoanthamine

The lyophilized specimens of *Zoanthus vietnamensis* (1.1 kg) were exhaustively extracted with 95% EtOH to afford 248.2 g of crude extract. An alkaloid-enriched portion of the extract (22.4 g) was subjected to a silica gel column eluted with a stepped hexanes/EtOAc/MeOH (3/1/0 to 0/4/1) to give nine fractions (S1–S9). Fraction S5 (4.9 g) was fractionated by a silica gel column (hexanes/CH$_2$Cl$_2$/MeOH, 25/10/1 to 0/5/1) to yield six fractions (S5-1 to S5-6). Fraction S5-2 (2.8 g) was applied on a silica gel column (hexanes/acetone, 3/2 to 0/1) to obtain six fractions (S5-2-1 to S5-2-6). Fraction S5-2-3 (491.0 mg) was separated by a silica column (hexanes/acetone, 2/1 to 0/1) to get *epi*-oxyzoanthamine (110.2 mg) [23]. The structure of *epi*-oxyzoanthamine was confirmed by comparing its NMR and MS data with the literature data [52]. The specimens of *Zoanthus vietnamensis* were collected in the northern coastal area of Taiwan, in April 2017. The animal material was identified by Yuan-Bin Cheng [53].

4.2. Culture of Human Keratinocyte

The human epidermal keratinocyte line (HaCaT) was used for this study. The HaCaT cell line was provided by Dr. Nan-Lin Wu, Department of Dermatology, Mackay Memorial Hospital, Taiwan. HaCaT was cultured in a 75T flask containing 10% fetal bovine serum (fetal bovine serum, FBS) and Dulbecco's Modified Eagle Medium (DMEM) with 1% antibiotics (Grand Island, NY, USA). The cells were placed in an incubator at 37 °C and 5% CO$_2$, and the cells were allowed to grow to about 80–90% saturation, and then the cells were subcultured.

4.3. Western Blotting

Western blots were used to analyze changes in various proteins in cells. Related methods are described in more depth in a previously published paper [24]. HaCaT cells were seeded in 3.5 cm culture dishes. HaCaT cells were seeded in 3.5 cm dishes. After cells reached 90% confluence and were starved for 24 h, they were pretreated with *epi*-oxyzoanthamine for 1 h and then stimulated with TNF-α/IFN-γ for 1 h, respectively. After scraping, cells were crushed by sonication and centrifuged (13,200 rpm, 10 min, 4 °C). After centrifugation, the supernatant was taken, and protein was quantified using the Pierce Protein Assay Kit (Pierce, Rockford, IL, USA). Approximately 20–40 μg of protein was electrophoresed on a 10% SDS-polyacrylamide gel, followed by electroporation with PVDF membranes. After the transfer, the PVDF membrane was placed in a TBS-T solution (Tris-buffered salt/0.05% tween 20) containing 5% nonfat dry milk for 1 h with continuous shaking to avoid nonspecific binding. Then, the PVDF membrane was washed 3 times with TBS-T (30 min in total). After that, the primary antibody was added (diluted 1:1000). PVDF membranes were left overnight at 4 °C and then washed 3 times with TBS-T for 10 min each. Finally, after adding the secondary antibody for 1 h (diluted to 1:1000), the PVDF membrane was washed 3 times with TBS-T, then the developing solution was added, and the membrane was put into the chemiluminescence extraction system (Biostep GmbH Chemiluminescence Imager CELVIN; Type CELVIN®S420 FL, Calibre Scientific, LA, USA) for photography.

4.4. Real-Time Quantitative Reverse Transcription Polymerase Chain Reaction (RT-qPCR)

HaCaT cells were seeded in 3.5 cm Petri dishes. Cells can reach 90% confluency after 24 h. Cells were pretreated with *epi*-oxyzoanthamine for 1 h and stimulated with TNF-α/IFN-γ for 1 h. Cells were scraped and centrifuged (16,000× *g*, 10 min, 4 °C) and the supernatant was removed. RNA was purified using a total RNA isolation kit (GeneDireX®, Vegas, NV, USA) according to the operating procedure of iScript™ cDNA Synthesis Kit (BIO-RAD, Hercules, CA, USA), reagents were added one by one and specified conditions were followed closely to convert RNA into cDNA. Additionally, PowerUp™ SYBR™ Green Master Mix (Applied Biosystems™, Waltham, MA, USA) was used. 7.5 μL ddH$_2$O, 2 μL cDNA, 0.25 μL forward and reverse primers, and 10 μL SYBR GREEN were added and mixed well. The relevant primer sequences are listed in Table 1. Finally, RNA was quantified using the ABI StepOnePlus™ Real-Time PCR System (Applied Biosystems™, Waltham, MA, USA).

Table 1. Primers used for RT-qPCR.

Name	Forward Primer Sequence (5′–3′)	Reverse Primer Sequence (5′–3′)
IL-1β	CTC TCA CCT CTC CTA CTC ACT	ATC AGA ATG TGG GAG CGA AT
IL-6	ATC AGA ATG TGG GAG CGA AT	GGA CCG AAG GCG CTT GTG GAG
IL-8	ACT GAG AGT GAT TGA GAG TGG AC	AAC CCT CTG CAC CCA GTT TTC
GAPDH	CTG CTC CTG TTC GAC AGT	CCG TTG ACT CCG ACC TTC AC

4.5. Animal Model of DNCB-Induced Atopic Dermatitis-like Skin Inflammation

Male mice (BALB/c, 8 weeks old) were purchased from Taiwan National Laboratory Animal Center. The mice were kept in a temperature-controlled and humidity-controlled animal room (controlled at 21 ± 2 °C and 50 ± 20%, respectively). Mice were housed at the Animal Center of Fu Jen Catholic University in Taiwan with controlled laminar filtered airflow and a 12-h light/dark cycle. This experiment was performed after review by the Institutional Animal Care and Use Committee of Fu Jen Catholic University, Taiwan (approval number A10964).

The mice were first divided into four groups: control group, DNCB group, *epi*-oxyzoanthamine (3 and 10 mg/kg) plus DNCB group, and 0.2 mg/kg dexamethasone plus DNCB group. For in vivo experiments, *epi*-oxyzoanthamine was dissolved in dimethylsulfoxide (DMSO), while DNCB was dissolved in 75% ethanol. The former was administered by intraperitoneal injection, while the latter was applied to the skin of the back and right ear in 100 µL and 20 µL, respectively. During the first three days, mice were anesthetized and had their dorsal hair removed. A small magnet (1 mm in diameter and 3 mm in length) was embedded in each mouse's hind paw. Three days later, the behavior of the mice was observed, and it was ensured that mice were in good physical condition and the skin in the depilated area on the back was normal before starting the experiment. Skin-related physiological values including transepidermal water loss (TEWL), erythema, skin moisture, ear thickness, and number of scratches were measured before the experiment. Photographs were also taken to document changes in the appearance of the skin and ears. The whole experimental process was carried out in a room with constant temperature and humidity. The first phase (days 1–4) is the allergic atopic dermatitis phase. After measuring the physiological value of the mice, 1% DNCB was evenly applied to the skin of the dorsal and right ear. On the fifth day, intraperitoneal injection of *epi*-oxyzoanthamine began. The second phase (days 5 to 14) involved reinduction of atopic dermatitis. We then evenly applied 0.5% DNCB on the back and right ear skin of mice in four experimental groups. The next day, the physiological values of the skin were tested and recorded and photographed. After completing all tests on day 15, mice were euthanized with carbon dioxide (CO_2) and dorsal skin tissue and spleens were removed for subsequent experimental analysis.

4.6. Data and Statistical Analysis

Sigma-Plot software (version 10.0) was used for all statistical analyses of the data. All data are presented as mean ± SEM. Statistical significance was assessed by unpaired two-tailed Student's *t*-test. $p < 0.05$ was considered significant (* $p < 0.05$, ## and ** $p < 0.01$).

5. Conclusions

The results showed that *epi*-oxyzoanthamine significantly decreased skin barrier damage, scratching responses, and epidermal hyperplasia induced by DNCB. It significantly reduced transepidermal water loss (TEWL), erythema, ear thickness, and spleen weight, while also increasing surface skin hydration. These results indicate that *epi*-oxyzoanthamine from zoanthid has good potential as an alternative medicine for treating atopic dermatitis or other skin-related inflammatory diseases.

Author Contributions: Conceptualization, C.-C.H., Y.-H.L., K.-L.W. and C.-F.H.; Data curation, Y.-J.H.; Funding acquisition, C.-C.H., Y.-H.L. and K.-L.W.; Investigation, C.-C.H., C.-C.K. and C.-F.H.; Methodology, Y.-H.L., Y.-J.H. and Y.-B.C.; Resources, C.-C.H., C.-C.K., C.-W.L., K.-L.W. and C.-F.H.; Validation, Y.-J.H.; Writing—original draft, Y.-B.C., D.-C.C. and C.-F.H.; Writing—review and editing, D.-C.C., K.-L.W. and C.-F.H. All authors have read and agreed to the published version of the manuscript.

Funding: This work was supported by grants from the National Science and Technology Council, Fu Jen Catholic University Hospital, Shin Kong Wu Ho-Su Memorial Hospital, and Taoyuan Armed Force General Hospital (numbers 110-2320-B-030-004-MY3, 110-FJUH-04, 106-SKH-FJU-05, and TYAFGH-A-112017) in Taiwan.

Institutional Review Board Statement: Not applicable.

Data Availability Statement: Not applicable.

Acknowledgments: We thank Yun-Di Wu and Ting-Hsuan Chao for their participation in this study.

Conflicts of Interest: The authors declare no conflict of interest.

References

1. Salimian, J.; Salehi, Z.; Ahmadi, A.; Emamvirdizadeh, A.; Davoudi, S.M.; Karimi, M.; Korani, M.; Azimzadeh Jamalkandi, S. Atopic dermatitis: Molecular, cellular, and clinical aspects. *Mol. Biol. Rep.* **2022**, *49*, 3333–3348. [CrossRef]
2. Maiello, N.; Comberiati, P.; Giannetti, A.; Ricci, G.; Carello, R.; Galli, E. New Directions in Understanding Atopic March Starting from Atopic Dermatitis. *Children* **2022**, *9*, 450. [CrossRef]
3. Li, W.; Man, X.Y. Immunotherapy in atopic dermatitis. *Immunotherapy* **2022**, *14*, 1149–1164. [CrossRef]
4. Weidinger, S.; Novak, N. Atopic dermatitis. *Lancet* **2016**, *387*, 1109–1122. [CrossRef]
5. Gandhi, N.A.; Pirozzi, G.; Graham, N.M.H. Commonality of the IL-4/IL-13 pathway in atopic diseases. *Expert Rev. Clin. Immunol.* **2017**, *13*, 425–437. [CrossRef]
6. Eichenfield, L.F.; Tom, W.L.; Berger, T.G.; Krol, A.; Paller, A.S.; Schwarzenberger, K.; Bergman, J.N.; Chamlin, S.L.; Cohen, D.E.; Cooper, K.D.; et al. Guidelines of care for the management of atopic dermatitis: Section 2. Management and treatment of atopic dermatitis with topical therapies. *J. Am. Acad. Derm.* **2014**, *71*, 116–132. [CrossRef]
7. Saeki, H.; Ohya, Y.; Furuta, J.; Arakawa, H.; Ichiyama, S.; Katsunuma, T.; Katoh, N.; Tanaka, A.; Tsunemi, Y.; Nakahara, T.; et al. English Version of Clinical Practice Guidelines for the Management of Atopic Dermatitis 2021. *J. Derm.* **2022**, *49*, e315–e375. [CrossRef]
8. Chovatiya, R.; Paller, A.S. JAK inhibitors in the treatment of atopic dermatitis. *J. Allergy Clin. Immunol.* **2021**, *148*, 927–940. [CrossRef]
9. Fishbein, A.B.; Silverberg, J.I.; Wilson, E.J.; Ong, P.Y. Update on Atopic Dermatitis: Diagnosis, Severity Assessment, and Treatment Selection. *J. Allergy Clin. Immunol. Pr.* **2020**, *8*, 91–101. [CrossRef]
10. Zhou, X.; Li, C.-G.; Chang, D.; Bensoussan, A. Current Status and Major Challenges to the Safety and Efficacy Presented by Chinese Herbal Medicine. *Medicines* **2019**, *6*, 14. [CrossRef]
11. Lindequist, U. Marine-Derived Pharmaceuticals—Challenges and Opportunities. *Biomol. Ther.* **2016**, *24*, 561–571. [CrossRef]
12. Haque, N.; Parveen, S.; Tang, T.; Wei, J.; Huang, Z. Marine Natural Products in Clinical Use. *Mar. Drugs* **2022**, *20*, 528. [CrossRef]
13. Murphy, T.; Yee, K.W.L. Cytarabine and daunorubicin for the treatment of acute myeloid leukemia. *Expert Opin. Pharm.* **2017**, *18*, 1765–1780. [CrossRef]
14. Kammoun, I.; Ben Salah, H.; Ben Saad, H.; Cherif, B.; Droguet, M.; Magné, C.; Kallel, C.; Boudawara, O.; Hakim, A.; Gharsallah, N.; et al. Hypolipidemic and cardioprotective effects of *Ulva lactuca* ethanolic extract in hypercholesterolemic mice. *Arch. Physiol. Biochem.* **2018**, *124*, 313–325. [CrossRef]
15. Perera, R.; Herath, K.; Sanjeewa, K.K.A.; Jayawardena, T.U. Recent Reports on Bioactive Compounds from Marine Cyanobacteria in Relation to Human Health Applications. *Life* **2023**, *13*, 1411. [CrossRef]
16. Ardizzone, A.; Mannino, D.; Capra, A.P.; Repici, A.; Filippone, A.; Esposito, E.; Campolo, M. New Insights into the Mechanism of *Ulva pertusa* on Colitis in Mice: Modulation of the Pain and Immune System. *Mar. Drugs* **2023**, *21*, 298. [CrossRef]
17. Buijs, Y.; Bech, P.K.; Vazquez-Albacete, D.; Bentzon-Tilia, M.; Sonnenschein, E.C.; Gram, L.; Zhang, S.D. Marine Proteobacteria as a source of natural products: Advances in molecular tools and strategies. *Nat. Prod. Rep.* **2019**, *36*, 1333–1350. [CrossRef]
18. Guillen, P.O.; Jaramillo, K.B.; Genta-Jouve, G.; Thomas, O.P. Marine natural products from zoantharians: Bioactivity, biosynthesis, systematics, and ecological roles. *Nat. Prod. Rep.* **2020**, *37*, 515–540. [CrossRef]
19. Hsu, Y.-M.; Chang, F.-R.; Lo, I.W.; Lai, K.-H.; El-Shazly, M.; Wu, T.-Y.; Du, Y.-C.; Hwang, T.-L.; Cheng, Y.-B.; Wu, Y.-C. Zoanthamine-Type Alkaloids from the Zoanthid *Zoanthus kuroshio* Collected in Taiwan and Their Effects on Inflammation. *J. Nat. Prod.* **2016**, *79*, 2674–2680. [CrossRef]
20. Cheng, Y.-B.; Lo, I.W.; Shyur, L.-F.; Yang, C.-C.; Hsu, Y.-M.; Su, J.-H.; Lu, M.-C.; Chiou, S.-F.; Lan, C.-C.; Wu, Y.-C.; et al. New alkaloids from Formosan zoanthid *Zoanthus kuroshio*. *Tetrahedron* **2015**, *71*, 8601–8606. [CrossRef]

21. Chen, S.-R.; Wang, S.-W.; Lin, Y.-C.; Yu, C.-L.; Yen, J.-Y.; Chen, Y.-F.; Cheng, Y.-B. Additional alkaloids from *Zoanthus vietnamensis* with neuroprotective and anti-angiogenic effects. *Bioorg. Chem.* **2021**, *109*, 104700. [CrossRef] [PubMed]
22. Yamaguchi, K.; Yada, M.; Tsuji, T.; Kuramoto, M.; Uemura, D. Suppressive effect of norzoanthamine hydrochloride on experimental osteoporosis in ovariectomized mice. *Biol. Pharm. Bull.* **1999**, *22*, 920–924. [CrossRef] [PubMed]
23. Chen, S.-R.; Wang, S.-W.; Sheu, J.-H.; Chang, T.-H.; Cheng, Y.-B. Zoanthamine Alkaloid Derivatives from the Zoantharian *Zoanthus vietnamensis* with Antimetastatic Activity. *J. Org. Chem.* **2020**, *85*, 12553–12560. [CrossRef]
24. Wang, C.-C.; Hsiao, C.-Y.; Hsu, Y.-J.; Ko, H.-H.; Chang, D.-C.; Hung, C.-F. Anti-Inflammatory Effects of Cycloheterophyllin on Dinitrochlorobenzene-Induced Atopic Dermatitis in HaCaT Cells and BALB/c Mice. *Molecules* **2022**, *27*, 2610. [CrossRef]
25. Tsai, Y.-C.; Chang, H.-H.; Chou, S.-C.; Chu, T.W.; Hsu, Y.-J.; Hsiao, C.-Y.; Lo, Y.-H.; Wu, N.-L.; Chang, D.-C.; Hung, C.-F. Evaluation of the Anti-Atopic Dermatitis Effects of α-Boswellic Acid on Tnf-α/Ifn-γ-Stimulated HaCat Cells and DNCB-Induced BALB/c Mice. *Int. J. Mol. Sci.* **2022**, *23*, 9863. [CrossRef]
26. Saha, R.N.; Jana, M.; Pahan, K. MAPK p38 regulates transcriptional activity of NF-kappaB in primary human astrocytes via acetylation of p65. *J. Immunol.* **2007**, *179*, 7101–7109. [CrossRef] [PubMed]
27. Garrigue, J.L.; Nicolas, J.F.; Fraginals, R.; Benezra, C.; Bour, H.; Schmitt, D. Optimization of the mouse ear swelling test for in vivo and in vitro studies of weak contact sensitizers. *Contact Dermat.* **1994**, *30*, 231–237. [CrossRef]
28. Jin, H.; He, R.; Oyoshi, M.; Geha, R.S. Animal models of atopic dermatitis. *J. Investig. Derm.* **2009**, *129*, 31–40. [CrossRef]
29. Carroll, A.R.; Copp, B.R.; Davis, R.A.; Keyzers, R.A.; Prinsep, M.R. Marine natural products. *Nat. Prod. Rep.* **2023**, *40*, 275–325. [CrossRef]
30. Chung, Y.; Jeong, S.; Lee, I.-K.; Yun, B.-S.; Lee, J.S.; Ro, S.; Park, J.K. Regulation of p53 Activity by (+)-Epiloliolide Isolated from *Ulva lactuca*. *Mar. Drugs* **2021**, *19*, 450. [CrossRef]
31. Negm, W.A.; Ezzat, S.M.; Zayed, A. Marine organisms as potential sources of natural products for the prevention and treatment of malaria. *RSC Adv.* **2023**, *13*, 4436–4475. [CrossRef] [PubMed]
32. Ha, Y.; Lee, W.H.; Jeong, J.; Park, M.; Ko, J.Y.; Kwon, O.W.; Lee, J.; Kim, Y.J. Pyropia yezoensis Extract Suppresses IFN-Gamma- and TNF-Alpha-Induced Proinflammatory Chemokine Production in HaCaT Cells via the Down-Regulation of NF-κB. *Nutrients* **2020**, *12*, 1238. [CrossRef] [PubMed]
33. Ha, Y.; Lee, W.H.; Kim, J.K.; Jeon, H.K.; Lee, J.; Kim, Y.J. Polyopes affinis Suppressed IFN-γ- and TNF-α-Induced Inflammation in Human Keratinocytes via Down-Regulation of the NF-κB and STAT1 Pathways. *Molecules* **2022**, *27*, 1836. [CrossRef] [PubMed]
34. Chen, P.C.; Lo, Y.H.; Huang, S.Y.; Liu, H.L.; Yao, Z.K.; Chang, C.I.; Wen, Z.H. The anti-inflammatory properties of ethyl acetate fraction in ethanol extract from *Sarcodia suiae* sp. alleviates atopic dermatitis-like lesion in mice. *Biosci. Biotechnol. Biochem.* **2022**, *86*, 646–654. [CrossRef]
35. Lee, T.K.; Kim, D.W.; Ahn, J.H.; Lee, C.H.; Lee, J.C.; Lim, S.S.; Kang, I.J.; Hong, S.; Choi, S.Y.; Won, M.H.; et al. Protective Effects of Topical Administration of Laminarin in Oxazolone-Induced Atopic Dermatitis-like Skin Lesions. *Mar. Drugs* **2022**, *20*, 669. [CrossRef]
36. Bong, S.K.; Park, N.J.; Lee, S.H.; Lee, J.W.; Kim, A.T.; Liu, X.; Kim, S.M.; Yang, M.H.; Kim, Y.K.; Kim, S.N. Trifuhalol A Suppresses Allergic Inflammation through Dual Inhibition of TAK1 and MK2 Mediated by IgE and IL-33. *Int. J. Mol. Sci.* **2022**, *23*, 10163. [CrossRef]
37. Mihindukulasooriya, S.P.; Dinh, D.T.T.; Herath, K.; Kim, H.J.; Han, E.J.; Cho, J.; Ko, M.O.; Jeon, Y.J.; Ahn, G.; Jee, Y. *Sargassum horneri* extract containing polyphenol alleviates DNCB-induced atopic dermatitis in NC/Nga mice through restoring skin barrier function. *Histol. Histopathol.* **2022**, *37*, 839–852. [CrossRef]
38. Du, Y.Q.; Liang, L.F.; Guo, Y.W. Cladiella Octocorals: Enormous Sources of Secondary Metabolites with Diverse Structural and Biological Properties. *Chem. Amp; Biodivers.* **2023**, *20*, e202201065. [CrossRef]
39. Chen, Z.H.; Lu, S.Q.; Han, G.Y.; Li, X.W.; Guo, Y.W. Sinuhirtone A, An Uncommon 17,19-Dinorxeniaphyllanoid, and Nine Related New Terpenoids from the Hainan Soft Coral *Sinularia hirta*. *Mar. Drugs* **2022**, *20*, 113088. [CrossRef]
40. Liu, J.; Xia, F.; Ouyang, H.; Wang, W.; Li, T.; Shi, Y.; Yan, X.; Yan, X.; He, S. Nardosinane-related antimicrobial terpenoids from *Lemnalia* sp. soft coral. *Phytochemistry* **2022**, *196*, 113088. [CrossRef]
41. Liu, M.; Li, P.; Tang, X.; Luo, X.; Liu, K.; Zhang, Y.; Wang, Q.; Li, G. Lemnardosinanes A-I: New Bioactive Sesquiterpenoids from Soft Coral *Lemnalia* sp. *J. Org. Chem.* **2021**, *86*, 970–979. [CrossRef]
42. Yan, X.; Ouyang, H.; Wang, W.; Liu, J.; Li, T.; Wu, B.; Yan, X.; He, S. Antimicrobial Terpenoids from South China Sea Soft Coral *Lemnalia* sp. *Mar. Drugs* **2021**, *19*, 294. [CrossRef] [PubMed]
43. Matar, D.Y.; Ng, B.; Darwish, O.; Wu, M.; Orgill, D.P.; Panayi, A.C. Skin Inflammation with a Focus on Wound Healing. *Adv. Wound Care* **2022**, *12*, 269–287. [CrossRef] [PubMed]
44. Zhang, H.; Wang, M.; Xu, Y. Understanding the mechanisms underlying obesity in remodeling the breast tumor immune microenvironment: From the perspective of inflammation. *Cancer Biol. Med.* **2023**, *20*, 268–286. [CrossRef] [PubMed]
45. Tai, C.J.; Su, J.H.; Huang, C.Y.; Huang, M.S.; Wen, Z.H.; Dai, C.F.; Sheu, J.H. Cytotoxic and anti-inflammatory eunicellin-based diterpenoids from the soft coral *Cladiella krempfi*. *Mar. Drugs* **2013**, *11*, 788–799. [CrossRef]
46. Zeng, Z.R.; Li, W.S.; Nay, B.; Hu, P.; Zhang, H.Y.; Wang, H.; Li, X.W.; Guo, Y.W. Sinunanolobatone A, an Anti-inflammatory Diterpenoid with Bicyclo[13.1.0]pentadecane Carbon Scaffold, and Related Casbanes from the Sanya Soft Coral *Sinularia nanolobata*. *Org. Lett.* **2021**, *23*, 7575–7579. [CrossRef]

47. Wang, C.; Zhang, J.; Shi, X.; Li, K.; Li, F.; Tang, X.; Li, G.; Li, P. Sarcoeleganolides C-G, Five New Cembranes from the South China Sea Soft Coral *Sarcophyton elegans*. *Mar. Drugs* **2022**, *20*, 574. [CrossRef]
48. Huynh, T.H.; Liu, C.J.; Liu, Y.H.; Chien, S.Y.; Wen, Z.H.; Fang, L.S.; Chen, J.J.; Wu, Y.C.; Su, J.H.; Sung, P.J. Briavioids E-G, Newly Isolated Briarane-Diterpenoids from a Cultured Octocoral *Briareum violaceum*. *Mar. Drugs* **2023**, *21*, 124. [CrossRef]
49. Behenna, D.C.; Stockdill, J.L.; Stoltz, B.M. The Biology and Chemistry of the Zoanthamine Alkaloids. *Angew. Chem. Int. Ed.* **2008**, *47*, 2365–2386. [CrossRef]
50. Chen, S.-R.; Wang, S.-W.; Su, C.-J.; Hu, H.-C.; Yang, Y.-L.; Hsieh, C.-T.; Peng, C.-C.; Chang, F.-R.; Cheng, Y.-B. Anti-Lymphangiogenesis Components from Zoanthid *Palythoa tuberculosa*. *Mar. Drugs* **2018**, *16*, 47. [CrossRef]
51. Yang, C.-C.; Hung, Y.-L.; Ko, W.-C.; Tsai, Y.-J.; Chang, J.-F.; Liang, C.-W.; Chang, D.-C.; Hung, C.-F. Effect of Neferine on DNCB-Induced Atopic Dermatitis in HaCaT Cells and BALB/c Mice. *Int. J. Mol. Sci.* **2021**, *22*, 8237. [CrossRef] [PubMed]
52. Daranas, A.H.; Fernández, J.; Gavín, J.; Norte, M. Epioxyzoanthamine, a new zoanthamine-type alkaloid and the unusual deuterium exchange in this series. *Tetrahedron* **1998**, *54*, 7891–7896. [CrossRef]
53. Chen, S.R.; Wang, S.W.; Chang, F.R.; Cheng, Y.B. Anti-Lymphangiogenic Alkaloids from the Zoanthid *Zoanthus vietnamensis* Collected in Taiwan. *J. Nat. Prod.* **2019**, *82*, 2790–2799. [CrossRef] [PubMed]

Disclaimer/Publisher's Note: The statements, opinions and data contained in all publications are solely those of the individual author(s) and contributor(s) and not of MDPI and/or the editor(s). MDPI and/or the editor(s) disclaim responsibility for any injury to people or property resulting from any ideas, methods, instructions or products referred to in the content.

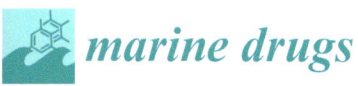

Review

Marine Microorganism Molecules as Potential Anti-Inflammatory Therapeutics

Malia Lasalo [1], Thierry Jauffrais [2], Philippe Georgel [3] and Mariko Matsui [1,*]

[1] Group Bioactivities of Natural Compounds and Derivatives (BIONA), Institut Pasteur of New Caledonia, Member of the Pasteur Network, Noumea 98845, New Caledonia; mlasalo@pasteur.nc

[2] Ifremer, Institut de Recherche pour le Développement (IRD), Centre Nationale de la Recherche Scientifique (CNRS), Université de la Réunion, Université de la Nouvelle-Calédonie, UMR 9220 ENTROPIE, 101 Promenade Roger Laroque, Noumea 98897, New Caledonia; thierry.jauffrais@ifremer.fr

[3] Team Neuroimmunology and Peptide Therapy, Biotechnologie et Signalisation Cellulaire, UMR 7242, University of Strasbourg, 67085 Strasbourg, France; pgeorgel@unistra.fr

* Correspondence: mmatsui@pasteur.nc; Tel.: +687-272666

Abstract: The marine environment represents a formidable source of biodiversity, is still largely unexplored, and has high pharmacological potential. Indeed, several bioactive marine natural products (MNPs), including immunomodulators, have been identified in the past decades. Here, we review how this reservoir of bioactive molecules could be mobilized to develop novel anti-inflammatory compounds specially produced by or derived from marine microorganisms. After a detailed description of the MNPs exerting immunomodulatory potential and their biological target, we will briefly discuss the challenges associated with discovering anti-inflammatory compounds from marine microorganisms.

Keywords: anti-inflammatory; inflammation; microorganisms; MNPs

1. Introduction

Chronic inflammatory diseases (CIDs) have emerged as a significant global concern, with a prevalence of 5 to 7% of Western society in 2010 [1]. These illnesses, such as psoriasis, rheumatoid arthritis (RA), inflammatory bowel disease (IBD), Crohn's disease (CD), or ulcerative colitis (UC), can be debilitating, leading to a reduced quality of life and, in the most severe cases, premature death [2].

Conventional treatments based on corticoids and non-steroidal anti-inflammatory drugs (NSAIDs) often lead to severe side effects, including gastrointestinal ulceration and bleeding, osteoporosis, hypertension, and glaucoma. Drug development more recently has focused on monoclonal antibodies targeting inflammatory cytokines such as tumor necrosis factor-α (TNF-α) or interleukins (e.g., IL-6) [3], or inhibitors of pathways activated by inflammatory cytokines, such as Janus Kinase inhibitors (Jakinibs) [4]. Although these therapies have shown considerable clinical efficacy, many patients remain unresponsive, and others may develop resistance to monoclonal antibody treatment. Furthermore, the use of such immunomodulatory molecules carries a limited but notable risk of developing opportunistic infections, such as Herpes Zoster Virus [5].

As life expectancy increases, there is an increased likelihood of developing CIDs, and therefore, managing these diseases has become more challenging. Hence, continuing to explore innovative treatment exploration and improving their response to these debilitating diseases is crucial. In this regard, the discovery of bioactive molecules from marine microorganisms represents a groundbreaking pharmaceutical development that could promote the identification of novel therapeutic compounds to treat CIDs.

Here, we aim to review marine microorganisms that produce molecules with potential pharmaceutical relevance, categorizing them based on producing genus and species, compounds' molecular structures, and their mechanism of action on immune signaling pathways. Additionally, we will provide a brief overview of the difficulties related to identifying anti-inflammatory compounds derived from marine microorganisms.

While previous reviews have primarily centered on symbiotic bacteria, to the best of our knowledge, none have yet highlighted the anti-inflammatory properties of these microorganisms. For this review, we selected 208 articles published from 2000 to 2024. One anterior reference was retained for the historical aspect of a specific molecule. The search engines Google Scholar, Science Direct, PubMed, and MarinLit databases were used with the keywords "marine natural products" combined with "anti-inflammatory", "macro-organisms", "microorganisms", "clinical pipeline", "clinical use", and "bioactivities." The database Worms (https://www.marinespecies.org/, accessed on 17 January 2024) was used to identify the species of marine organisms.

2. The Link between the Inflammation and CIDs

Harmful stimuli such as pathogens, toxic compounds, injuries, or irradiation induce cell damage and trigger an inflammatory response, a crucial component of our innate immune system [6]. This process involves the detection of danger signals that are recognized by dedicated immune receptors [7], enabling the elimination of such unwanted signals and the initiation of the healing process, thereby maintaining tissue homeostasis and a healthy condition. However, this process requires strict control and must be initiated locally and temporarily. In fact, systemic and chronic inflammations are associated with most human diseases and mortality [2]. Although some features of inflammatory responses may vary depending on the initial stimulus and its location in the body, they are characterized by dedicated signaling pathways and transcriptional signatures.

2.1. Inflammatory Pathways

Deciphering the regulatory pathways and mediators involved in inflammation is crucial for developing effective treatments against various diseases. A central player in inflammation is the NF-κB transcription factor, which controls the production of pro-inflammatory cytokines and, subsequently, the recruitment of immune cells. The nuclear translocation of NF-κB is regulated by IκB, which, once phosphorylated by upstream kinases in response to innate immune receptor engagement, is degraded by the proteasome (reviewed in [8]). In the case of IBD, the overactivation of this pathway directly causes an increase in the production of pro-inflammatory cytokines such as TNF-α, IL-1, and IL-6, consequently fueling chronic inflammation [9].

Similarly, Mitogen-activated Protein Kinases (MAPKs) are a family of protein kinases that respond to various stimuli, including inflammatory cytokines. They influence cell proliferation, differentiation, survival, and apoptosis. The activation of MAPKs leads to the phosphorylation and activation of p38 transcription factors, which also activate inflammatory response genes [10]. In the joint tissue of RA patients, the mentioned pathway regulates the production of pro-inflammatory cytokines. Also, it has a crucial role in the signaling cascade downstream of interleukin (IL-1), IL-17, and TNF-α, leading to cartilage destruction [11].

The JAK-STAT pathway is another highly conserved signaling mechanism significantly regulating inflammatory gene expression. Upon ligands (which are primarily cytokines, such as interferons) binding to their cognate receptors, intracellular receptor-associated Janus-activated kinases (JAKs) phosphorylate each other and dimerize, creating docking sites for Signal Transducers and Activators of Transcription (STATs), which are latent, cytoplasmic transcription factors. The cytoplasmic STATs undergo phosphorylation and subsequent dimerization, enabling their translocation to the nucleus, where they modulate immune-related gene expression [12]. Under normal conditions, this pathway is governed by negative regulators of JAK/STAT, including the suppressor of cytokine signaling and protein inhibitor of activated STAT. However, in the context of rheumatoid arthritis (RA), the malfunction of these regulators leads to joint damage commonly observed in affected patients [13].

Finally, inflammasome (among which is the NOD-like receptor family, the pyrin domain containing three signaling, or NLRP3 is the best described) signaling is also activated during many inflammatory responses. Inflammasomes require a sensor, an adaptor, and a pro-caspase that, following puncta formation, leads to IL-1β secretion, an important player in several (auto) inflammatory disorders, such as gouty arthritis [14].

Because dysregulation of NF-κB, MAPKs, JAK-STAT, or inflammasomes activity is often associated with inflammatory, autoimmune, or metabolic diseases, a thorough investigation of the corresponding pathways offers tremendous opportunities to develop more effective treatments for these diseases and improve patient outcomes.

2.2. Therapeutic Strategies to Target Inflammation

Until the end of the 20th century, CIDs therapeutics relied essentially on glucocorticoids and other small chemicals (non-steroidal) based on their anti-inflammatory, immunomodulatory, or anti-proliferative properties. Over the past 20 years, the management of patients who have rheumatoid arthritis (RA), one of the most frequent CIDs, witnessed significant improvements with the development and marketing of biologic and targeted-synthetic disease-modifying antirheumatic drugs (b/tsDMARDs). These molecules are designed to target and neutralize cytokines (such as TNF-α) and their receptors, to deplete specific cell populations (such as B lymphocytes with the anti-CD20 antibody), to modulate T cells activation (using the CTLA4-Ig) or to impact signaling pathways (with JAK inhibitors for instance) [15].

In this regard, TNF-α inhibitors completely changed the therapeutic strategy of RA patients, moving from relieving their symptoms to complete remission, which is the goal of the current therapy.

However, despite that considerable progress, many unmet clinical needs persist for CID patients. Indeed, even in the case of RA, a significant proportion of patients remain refractory to available therapies, and others develop resistance to effective drugs (as can be observed following anti-TNF-α treatment) [16]. For IBD patients, ~10% to 30% of patients resist the anti-TNF-α agent (primary non-responder), and 20% to 50% of responding patients (secondary loss of response) develop a resistance to the treatment within one year [17]. In addition, many chronic inflammatory syndromes (like scleroderma or Sjögren syndrome) are still without any reference treatment [18]. Therefore, the search for alternative therapeutic options remains current.

Table 1. MNPs with anti-inflammatory activity. ?: no species identified.

Organisms	Macro-Organisms				Target/Mode of Action	Ref(s).
	Classification (Phylum)	Species	Type of Molecules	Molecules		
Sponge	Porifera	*Fasciospongia cavernosa*	Terpene lactone	Cavernolide	TNF-α, NO, and PGE2 inhibition in RAW 264.7 cells	[19]
Sponge	Porifera	*Dysidea* spp.	Sesquiterpene	Dysidotronic acid	TNF-α, IL-1, NO, PGE2 inhibition in RAW 264.7 cells	[20]
Sponge	Porifera	*Plakortis* spp.	α-exomethylene-γ-lactone	Plakolide A	iNOS inhibition in RAW 264.7 cells	[21]
Sponge	Porifera	*Luffariella variabilis*	Sesterterpene	Manoalide	Eicosanoids synthesis inhibition in human polymorphonuclear leukocytes	[22]
Caribbean sponge	Porifera	*Cacospongia linteiformis*	Sesterterpene	Cyclolinteinone	iNOS and COX-2 inhibition in LPS-stimulated J774 macrophages	[23]
Sponge	Porifera	*Dysidea* sp. and *Petrosaspongia nigra*	Merosesquiterpene & Sesterterpene	Bolinaquinone and petrosaspongiolide M	Protection against TNBS-induced colitis in BALB/c mice	[24]
Sponge	Porifera	*Petrosia* spp.	Polyacetylenes	Petrocortyne D, Petrocortyne E, Petrocortyne F, Petrocortyne G, Petrocortyne H	Inhibition of PLA2 activity in K-562 cell line	[25]
Sponge	Porifera	*Petrosia* spp.	Polyacetylenic alcohol	Petrocortyne A	TNF-α inhibition in LPS-activated RAW 264.7 and PMA/LPS-treated U937 cells and NO inhibition in LPS- or IFNγ-treated RAW 264.7 cells	[26]
Sponge	Porifera	*Theonella swinhoe*	Steroid	Solomonsterol A	Reduction in arthritic score in anti-type II collagen antibody-induced arthritis murine model	[27]
Sponge	Porifera	*Geodia barretti*	Alpha amino acids and derivatives	Barettin	TNF-α and IL-1β inhibition in LPS-stimulated THP-1 cells	[28]

Table 1. Cont.

Organisms	Macro-Organisms					
	Classification (Phylum)	Species	Type of Molecules	Molecules	Target/Mode of Action	Ref(s).
Sponge	Porifera	*Geodia berretti*	Alkaloids	6-bromoindole derivatives geobarettin B, 6-bromoindole derivatives geobarettin C, 6-bromoindole alkaloids 6-bromoconicamin, barettin	IL-12 p40 inhibition and IL-10 increasing in dendritic cells	[29]
Sponge	Porifera	*Halichondria okadai*	Alkaloid	Halichlorine	VCAM-1, ICAM-1, and E-selectin inhibition in LPS-stimulated aortic endothelial cells, inhibition of macrophage adhesion to cultured cell monolayers, an anti-inflammatory effect associated with NF-κB pathway	[30]
Sponge	Porifera	*Stylissa*	Alkaloid	Pyrrole alkaloid (10Z)-debromohymenialdisine	IL-1β, IL-6, TNF-α, iNOS, COX-2, NO and PGE2 inhibition in co-cultures of LPS-stimulated Caco-2 and THP-1 cells	[31]
Sponge	Porifera	*Stylissa flabellata*	Alkaloids	Stylissadine A, Stylissadine B	Antagonistic effect on P2X7 receptors in THP-1 cells	[32]
Soft coral	Cnidaria	*Sinularia dissecta*	Diterpene	Seco-sethukarailin	Inhibition of pro-inflammatory cytokines in bone marrow-derived dendritic cells	[33]
Soft coral	Cnidaria	*Pseudopterogorgia elisabethae*	Diterpenes	Pseudopterosin E, Pseudopterosin A	Reduction of PMA-induced mouse ear edema; PGE2 and LCT4 inhibition in zymosan-stimulated murine peritoneal macrophages	[34]
Soft coral	Cnidaria	*Sinularia gibberosa*	Steroid	Gibberoketosterol	Inhibition of pro-inflammatory iNOS and COX-2 proteins in LPS-stimulated RAW264.7 cells	[35]
Okinawan soft coral	Cnidaria	*Sinularia* spp.	Diterpenes	Norcembranolide and sinuleptolide	TNF-α and NO inhibition in LPS-stimulated RAW 264.7 cells	[36]

Table 1. *Cont.*

Organisms	Macro-Organisms					
	Classification (Phylum)	Species	Type of Molecules	Molecules	Target/Mode of Action	Ref(s).
Soft coral	Cnidaria	*Sinularia lochmodes*	Sesquiterpene	Lochmolins A, Lochmolins B	Inhibition of COX-2 expression in LPS-activated RAW 264.7 cells	[37]
				Lochmolins C	Inhibition of COX-2 expression in LPS-activated RAW 264.7 cells	[38]
				Lochmolins D	Inhibition of COX-2 expression in LPS-activated RAW 264.7 cells	[37]
Soft coral	Cnidaria	*Lemnalia cervicorni*	Sesquiterpene	Lemnalol	Inhibition of iNOS and COX-2 expression in LPS-activated RAW 264.7 cells; inhibition of iNOS and COX-2 expression in carrageenan-activated rat paws	[39]
Soft coral	Cnidaria	*Lemnalia flava*	Sesquiterpene	Flavalin A	iNOS and COX-2 inhibition in RAW 264.7 cells	[40]
Soft coral	Cnidaria	*Lobophytum crassum*	Diterpenes	Crassumol E 1R,4R,2E,7E,11E-cembra-2,7,11-trien-4-ol	Inhibition of NF-κB activation in TNF-α-activated HepG2 cells	[41]
Soft coral	Cnidaria		Diterpenes	Lobocrasol A, Lobocrasol B	Inhibition of NF-κB activation in TNF-α-activated HepG2 cells	[42]
Soft coral	Cnidaria	*Scleronephthya gracillimum*	Steroid	Sclerosteroid J	Inhibition of iNOS and COX-2 expression in LPS-activated RAW 264.7 cells	[43]
Octocoral	Cnidaria	*Pseudopterogorgia acerosa*	Diterpene	Pseudopterane	Inhibition of NO, TNF-α, IL-1β and IFNγ-induced protein production in LPS-activated peritoneal macrophages	[44]

Table 1. Cont.

		Macro-Organisms				
Organisms	Classification (Phylum)	Species	Type of Molecules	Molecules	Target/Mode of Action	Ref(s).
Coral	Cnidaria	Rumphella antipathies (classification rhumpaella antipathes Linnaeus 1758)	Sesquiterpene	Clovane compound 1	Inhibition of superoxide anions generation and elastase release	[45]
			Sesquiterpene	Clovane compound 2	Inhibition of elastase release in fMLP/CB-activated human neutrophils	[45]
			Sesquiterpene	Rumphellaone C	Inhibition of superoxide anion generation and elastase release in human neutrophils	[46]
			Sesquiterpene	Rumphellol A	Inhibition of superoxide generation and elastase release in human neutrophils	[47]
			Sesquiterpene	Rumphelloll B		
Coral	Cnidaria	Briareum excavatum	Diterpene	Excavatolide B	Inhibition of iNOS expression in carrageenan-activated rat paws	[48]
Coral	Cnidaria	Briareum excacatum	Diterpene	Excavatolide B	Inhibition of 12-O-tetradecanoylphorbol-13-acetate (TPA)-induced vascular permeability; inhibition of TPA-induced matrix metalloproteinase-9 expression in mouse skin; inhibition of IL-6 expression of LPS-activated mouse bone marrow-derived dendritic cells	[49]
Anemone	Cnidaria	Zoanthus kuroshio	Alkaloid	5α-iodozoanthenamine	Anti-inflammatory effect on—neutrophils, reduction of superoxide anion generation, and elastase by cells	[50]
Anemone	Cnidaria	Zoanthus vulchellus	Alkaloids	3-hydroxinorzoanthamine Norzoanthine Roanthamine	ROS and NO inhibition in LPS-stimulated BV-2 cells	[51]
Starfish	Echinodermata	Marthasterias glacialis	Steroid	Ergosta-7,22-dien-3-ol	Inhibition of iNOS protein level in LPS-activated RAW 264.7 cells	[52]
Starfish	Echinodermata	Astropecten polycanthus	Steroid	Steroid compound 5	Inhibition of IL-12 p40, IL-6, and TNF-α production in LPS-activated mice bone marrow-derived dendritic cells	[53]

Table 1. *Cont.*

Organisms	Macro-Organisms					
	Classification (Phylum)	Species	Type of Molecules	Molecules	Target/Mode of Action	Ref(s).
Starfish	Echinodermata	*Asterias amurensis*	Fatty acid	Fatty acids	Inhibition of the expression of inflammatory genes via NF-κB and MAPK pathways in LPS-stimulated RAW 264.7 cells	[54]
Starfish	Echinodermata	*Marthasterias glacialis*	Fatty acid	Cis 11-eicosenoic and cis 11,14 eicosadienoic acids	Inhibition of iNOS, COX-2, IκBα, and NF-κB gene expression in LPS-stimulated RAW 264.7 cells	[52]
Starfish	Echinodermata	*Protoreaster nodosus*	Steroid	Oxygenated steroid derivatives	IL-12 p40, IL-6, and TNF-α inhibition in bone marrow-derived dendritic cells	[55]
Starfish	Echinodermata	*Protoreaster lincki*	Steroids	Protolinckioside A, Protolinckioside B, Protolinckioside C, Protolinckioside D	Reduction of ROS formation and NO production in LPS-stimulated RAW 264.7 cells	[56]
Starfish	Echinodermata	*Anthenea aspera*	Steroid	Anthenoside O		[57]
Starfish	Echinodermata	*Pentaceraster regulus*	Steroid	Pentareguloside C, Pentareguloside D, Pentareguloside E	Reduction of ROS formation and NO production in LPS-stimulated RAW 264.7 cells	[58]
Starfish	Echinodermata	*Acanthaster planci*	Pyrrole oligoglycoside	Plancipyrroside A, Plancipyrroside B	Reduction of ROS formation and NO production in LPS-stimulated RAW 264.7 cells	[59]
Starfish	Echinodermata	*Asterina batheri*	Pyrrole oligoglycoside	Astebatherioside B, Astebatherioside C, Astebatherioside D	IL-12 p40 inhibition in LPS-stimulated bone marrow-derived dendritic cells	[60]
Sea cucumber	Echinodermata	*Holothuria grisea*	Protein	Lectin	Inhibition of neutrophil migration to the peritoneal cavity in carrageenan-activated rats; reduction of myeloperoxidase activity in carrageenan-activated rats	[61]

Table 1. Cont.

Organisms	Macro-Organisms					
	Classification (Phylum)	Species	Type of Molecules	Molecules	Target/Mode of Action	Ref(s).
Sea cucumber	Echinodermata	*Apostichopus japonicus* and *Stichopus chloronotus*	Sulfated polysaccharide	Fucosylated chondroitin sulfate	Reduction of neutrophil migration, inhibition of paw edema in carrageenan-induced paw edema in rats	[62]
Sea cucumber	Echinodermata	*Isostichopus badionotus*	Sulfated polysaccharide	Fucosylated chondroitin sulfate	Suppression of TPA-mediated up-regulation of TNF-α, IL-6, NF-κB, iNOS, IL-10, IL-11, COX-2 and STAT3 genes in mouse ear tissue	[63]
Sea cucumber	Echinodermata	*Isostichopus badionotus*	Sulfated polysaccharide	Fucoidan	Regulation of serum inflammatory cytokines (TNF-α, CRP, MIP-1, IL-1β, IL-6, and IL-10) and their mRNA expression, inactivation of JNK and IκB/NF-κB pathways	[64]
Sea cucumber	Echinodermata	*Holothuria albiventer* and *Cucumaria frondosa*	Sulfated polysaccharide	Sulfated fucan/FCS	Suppression of TNF-α and IL-6 production	[65]
Sea cucumber	Echinodermata	*Holothuria tomasi*	Triterpenes glycoside		Inhibition of IL-6, TNF-α levels in STZ-induced diabetic rats	[66]
Sea cucumber	Echinodermata	*Pearsonothuria graeffei*	Triterpenes glycoside	Holothurin A and Echinoside A	Inhibition of IL-1β, TNF-α, IL-6 and infiltration of macrophages in obese mice via p-ERK/cPLA2/COX-1 pathway and reduction of the PGE2 levels	[67]
Sea cucumber	Echinodermata	*Apostichopus japonicus* and *Acaudina 'eucoprocta*	Peptide	Oligopeptides	Downregulation of pro-inflammatory cytokines transcription, upregulation of anti-inflammatory cytokines, and inhibition of TLR4/MyD88/NF-κB signaling pathway	[68]
Sea cucumber	Echinodermata	*Cucumaria frondosa*	Fatty acid	Eicosapentaenoic acid	Inhibition of TNF-α, IL-6, and MCP1 expression, attenuation of macrophage infiltration in the liver in mice, attenuation of the phosphorylation of NF-κB in RAW 264.7 cells	[69]

Table 1. Cont.

Organisms	Classification (Phylum)	Species	Type of Molecules	Molecules	Target/Mode of Action	Ref(s).
			Macro-Organisms			
Sea cucumber	Echinodermata	Cucumaria frondosa	Lipid	Frondanol	Reduction of inflammation-associated changes in the colon in mice, reduction of cytokine content at the protein and mRNA level	[70]
Sea cucumber	Echinodermata	Cucumaria frondosa	Lipid	Sphingolipids	Inhibition of pro-inflammatory cytokines IL-1β, IL-6 TNF-α and increasing anti-inflammatory IL-10 via inhibition of phosphorylation of JNK and translocation of NF-κB	[71]
Sea cucumber	Echinodermata	Cucumaria frondosa	Lipid	Frondaol A5	Attenuation of circulating inflammatory cytokines and suppression of mRNA expression of inflammatory markers such as 5-LOX and FLAP	[72]
Sea urchins	Echinodermata	Scaphechinus mirabilis	Dark red pigment	EchA	Attenuation of macrophage activation and infiltration (neutrophils), inhibition of TNF-α and IFNγ in bleomycin-induced scleroderma mouse model	[73]
Sea urchins	Echinodermata	?	Dark red pigment	EchA	Decreasing DIA, improvement of colon length and suppression of tissue damage, suppression of macrophage activation	[74]
Sea urchins	Echinodermata	?	Dark red pigment	EchA	TNF-α and NF-κB inhibition in Lewis rats	[75]
Sea urchins	Echinodermata	Paracentrotus lividus	Dark red pigment	EchA	Potent stabilizing effect on the human red blood cells, suppression of the production of IL-6 and TNF-α in septic rats	[76]
Sea urchins	Echinodermata	Scaphechinus mirabilis	Pigment	Spinochrome A	Reduction of chronic inflammation in cotton-pellet granuloma rat model	[77]
Sea urchins	Echinodermata	Scaphechinus mirabilis	Pigment	Spinochrome B		[77]

Table 1. Cont.

Organisms	Macro-Organisms					
	Classification (Phylum)	Species	Type of Molecules	Molecules	Target/Mode of Action	Ref(s).
Sea urchins	Echinodermata	Echinometra mathaei, diadema savignyi, tripneustes gratilla and Toxopneustes pileolus	Pigment	Spinochromes	TNF-α inhibition in J774 macrophages	[78]
Sea urchins	Echinodermata	Echinometra mathaei, diadema savignyi, tripneustes gratilla and Toxopneustes pileolus	Pigment	EchA	IL-12 p40, IL-6, IL-1β and TNF-α inhibition in THP-1 cells	[79,80]
Sea urchins	Echinodermata	Strongylocentrotus droebachiensis	Peptide	Centrocin 1 (CEN1HC-Br)	COX-2 and 5-LOX inhibition by using the 2,7-dichlorofluorescein method	[81]
Sea urchins	Echinodermata	Salmacis bicolor	Isochroman derived polyketide	Salmachroman	COX-1, COX-2, and 5-LOX inhibition by the 2,7-dichlorofluorescein method	[82]
Sea urchins	Echinodermata	Salmacis bicolor	Polyoxygenated furanocembranoid derivatives	Salmacembrane A Salmacembrane B	Inhibition of 5-LOX, COX-1 and COX-2 inhibition by the 2,7-dichlorofluorescein method	[83]
Sea urchins	Echinodermata	Stomopmeustes variolaris	Cembrane type of diterpene	4-hydroxy-1-(16methoxyprop-16-en-15-yl)-8-methyl-21,22-dioxatricyclo[11.3.1.15,8]octadecane-3,19-dione	COX-2, 5-LOX, iNOS inhibition in RAW 264.7 cells	[84]
Sea urchins	Echinodermata	Stomopmeustes variolaris	Macrocyclic lactone	Stomopneulactones D	Inhibition of proinflammatory cytokines by the inactivation of JNK/p38 MAPK and NF-kB pathways	[85]
Sea urchins	Echinodermata	Brisaster latifrons	Sulfonic acid	(Z)-4-methylundeca-1,9-diene-6-sulfonic acid	Inhibition of iNOS, COX-2, and cytokines, downregulation of the NF-κB and JNK/P38 MAPK signaling pathway	[86]
Sea urchins	Echinodermata	Hemicentrotus pulcherrimus and Diadema setosum	Lipid	Hp-s1 ganglioside		

Table 1. Cont.

Organisms	Classification (Phylum)	Species	Type of Molecules	Molecules	Target/Mode of Action	Ref(s).
			Macro-Organisms			
Ascidian	Chordata	*Aplidium orthium*	Alkaloids	Alkaloid tubastrine, Orthidine A, Orthidine B, Orthidine C, Orthidine E, Orthidine F	Reduction of the superoxide synthesis in PMA-stimulated neutrophils in vitro and in vivo models	[87]
Ascidian	Chordata	*Aplidium* spp.	Alkaloids	Ascidiathiazone A, Ascidiathiazone B	Reduction of the superoxide production by PMA-stimulated neutrophils in vitro and in vivo in murine gout model	[88]
Ascidian	Chordata	*Pycnoclavella kottae*	Alkaloid	Kottamide D	Reduction of superoxide synthesis by PMA and N-formylmethionyl-leucyl-phenylalanine (fMLP)-activated neutrophils *in vitro*	[89]
Red algae	Rhodophyta	*Gracilaria opuntia*	Alkaloid	Azocinyl morpholinone	Inhibition of the carrageenan-induced paw edema	[90]
Green algae	Chlorophyta	*Enteromorpha prolifera*	Chlorophyll	Pheophytin	Suppression of the production of superoxide anion in mouse macrophages	[91]
Green algae	Chlorophyta	*Ulva lactuca*	Sterol	3-0-B-D-glucopyranosil-stigmata-5,25,-dien sterol	Topical anti-inflammatory activity in mouse edema	[92]
Green algae	Chlorophyta	*Caulerpa racemosa*	Alkaloid	Caulerpin / Sulfated polysaccharides	Inhibition of capsaicin-induced ear edema model and significant reduction of the number of recruited cells; reduction in neutrophil counts in the peritoneal cavity and paws of carrageenan-treated rats; reduction of edema volume in carrageenan and dextran-activated mouse paws	[93,94]

Table 1. Cont.

Macro-Organisms						
Organisms	Classification (Phylum)	Species	Type of Molecules	Molecules	Target/Mode of Action	Ref(s).
Green algae	Chlorophyta	Enteromorpha prolifera	Chlorophyll	Pheophytin A	Significant suppression of TPA-induced inflammatory reactions such as edema formation in BALB/c mouse ears	[91]
Green algae	Chlorophyta	Caulerpa mexicana	Sulfated polysaccharides	Sulfated polysaccharides	Reduction of edema volume and neutrophilic infiltration in carrageenan-activated raw paws; Reduction of edema volume in dextran and histamine-activated rat paws	[95]
Green algae	Chlorophyta	Caulerpa cupressoids	Protein	Lectin	Reduction of leukocyte counts and myeloperoxidase activity in rat temporomandibular joint synovial lavage fluid in zymosan-activated rats	[96]
Brown algae	Heterokontophyta	Ecklonia cava	Pholorotannin	Dieckol	Inhibition of NO, PGE2, and the expression of iNOS production in murine BV2 microglia	[97]
Brown algae	Heterokontophyta	Undaria pinnatifida	Fatty acid	Ω-3 polyunsaturated fatty acids	Inhibition of the mouse ear inflammation induced by PMA	[98]
Brown algae	Heterokontophyta	Laminaria japonica	Sulfated polysaccharide	Fucoidan	NO and IL-6 inhibition in Caco-2 cells	[99]
Brown algae	Heterokontophyta	Fucus vesiculosus	Sulfated polysaccharide	Fucoidan	Reduction of NO, PGE2, TNF-α and IL-1β production in RAW 264.7 cells	[100]

Microorganisms						
Organisms	Classification (Phylum)	Species	Type of Molecules	Molecules	Target/Mode of Action	Ref(s).
Dinoflagellate (microalgae)	Dinoflagellata	Symbiodinium spp.	Amphoteric iminium	6,6,6-tricyclic iminium ring and aryl sulfate moiety	Inhibition of the COX-2 activity in RAW 264.7 cells	[101]
Haptophyte (microalgae)	Haptophyta	Isochrysis galbana	Galactolipids	Monogalactosyldiacylglycerol, Digalactosyldiacylglycerol	Inhibition of the synthesis of TNF-α, IL-1β, IL-6, IL-17 in THP-1 cells	[102]

Table 1. Cont.

Organisms	Classification (Phylum)	Species	Type of Molecules	Molecules	Target/Mode of Action	Ref(s).
Microorganisms						
Green microalgae	Chlorophyta	Chlorella vulgaris	Polyunsaturated fatty acid	Linoleic acid and α-linolenic	Inhibition of TNF-α, IL-6, PGE2, and NO production in RAW 264.7 cells	[103]
Red microalgae	Rhodophyta	Porphyridium cruentum	Fatty acids	Fatty acids	Inhibition of superoxide anion production by peritoneal leukocytes primed with PMA	[104]
Red microalgae	Rhodophyta	Porphyridium cruentum	Exopolysaccharide (EPS)	EPS	Inhibition of 77% of COX-2 in human keratinocytes and murine fibroblasts Balb/c-3T3	[105]
			Pigment	Phycoerythrin	Inhibition of COX-2 in human keratinocytes and murine fibroblasts Balb/c-3T3	[105]
Cyanobacteria	Cyanobacteria	Spirulina subsalsa	Lipids (glycophospholipids, phospholipids)	Sulfoquinovosyl diacylglycerols, monogalactosylodiglycerides, cerebrosides; ceramides, phosphatidylcholines, phosphatidylethanolamines	Inhibitory effects on platelet-activating factor and thrombin-induced platelet aggregation	[106]
Cyanobacteria	Cyanobacteria	Lyngbya majuscula	Malyngamide	Malyngamide F acetate	Inhibition of the NO production in RAW 264.7 cells	[107]
Cyanobacteria	Cyanobacteria	Caldora sp.	Azirine	Dysidazirine carboxylic acid	Inhibition of the NO production by almost 50% at 50 µM in RAW 264.7 cells	[108]
Fungi	Ascomycota	Chaetomium globosum QEN-14	Alkaloid	Chaetoglobosin Fex	Inhibition of TNF-α and IL-6 production in LPS-activated RAW 264.7 cells	[109]

Table 1. Cont.

Organisms	Microorganisms					Ref(s).
	Classification (Phylum)	Species	Type of Molecules	Molecules	Target/Mode of Action	
Fungi	Ascomycota	*Stachybotrys* sp. HH1 ZSDS1F1-2 (isolated from a sponge from Xisha Island, China, in April 2012)	Xanthonne	Xanthone derivatives 3 (others), Xanthone derivatives 4 (others), Xanthone derivatives 11 (others)	Inhibition of COX-2	[110]
Fungi	Ascomycota	*Aspergillus* spp.	Diketopiperazine alkaloids	5-prenyl-dihydrovariecolorin F	Inhibition of iNOS and COX-2 activity, reduction of NO and PGE2 levels in LPS-stimulated RAW 264.7 and BV2 cells	[111]
Fungi	Ascomycota	*Aspergillus* spp.	Diketopiperazine alkaloids	5-prenyl-dihydrorubrumazine A		
Fungi	Ascomycota	*Aspergillus* sp. SF-6354	Polyketide	TMC-256C1	NO and PGE2 inhibition in LPS-activated BV2 cells	[112]
Fungi	Ascomycota	*Aspergillus* sp. SCSIO Ind09F01	Polyketides	Diorcinol, Cordyol C, 3,7-dihydroxy-1,9-dimethyldibenzofuran	Inhibition of COX-2 (IC$_{50}$ = 2.4–10.6 µM)	[113]
Fungi	Ascomycota	*Aspergillus* sp. SF-5974 and *Aspergillus* sp. SF-5976	Polyketides	Cladosporin 8-O-α-ribofuranoside, Cladosporin, Asperentin 6-O-methyl ether Cladosporin 8-O-methyl ether, 4′-hydroxyasperentin, 5′-hydroxyasperentin	Inhibition of NO and PGE2 expression, (IC$_{50}$ = 20–65 µM) in LPS-activated microglial cells	[114]
Fungi	Ascomycota	*Aspergillus* sp. SF-5044	Polyketide	Asperlin	Inhibition of NO and PGE2 expression in LPS-activated murine macrophages	[115]

Table 1. Cont.

Organisms	Classification (Phylum)	Species	Type of Molecules	Molecules	Target/Mode of Action	Ref(s).
				Microorganisms		
Fungi	Ascomycota	Aspergillus sp.	Peptide	Aurantiamide acetate	Inhibition of NO and PGE2 expression in LPS-activated BV2 cells	[116]
Fungi	Ascomycota	A.europaeus WZXY-SX-4-1	Polyketides	Eurobenzophenone B, Euroxanthone A, 3-de-O-methylsulochrin, Yicathin B, Dermolutein, Methylemodin	Inhibition of NF-κB activation and NO expression in LPS-activated SW480 cells	[117]
Fungi	Ascomycota	Aspergillus sp. ZLO-1b14	Terpenes	Aspertetranone A, Aspertetranone B, Aspertetranone C, Aspertetranone D	Inhibition of IL-6 expression in LPS-activated RAW 264.7 cells	[118]
Fungi	Ascomycota	A.sydowii J05B-7F-4	Polyketide	Violaceol II, Cordyol E	Inhibition of NO (IC$_{50}$ = 73 μM) expression in LPS-activated RAW 264.7 cells	[119]
Fungi	Ascomycota	A.niger SCSIO Jcsw6F30	Polyketides	Aurasperone F, Aurasperone C, Asperpyrone A	Inhibition of COX-2 expression (IC$_{50}$ = 11.1, 4.2, and 6.4 μM for F, C, and A, respectively) in LPS-activated RAW 264.7 cells	[120]
Fungi	Ascomycota	A. flocculosus 16D-1	Alkaloids	Preussin C, Preussin D, Preussin E, Preussin F, Preussin G, Preussin H, Preussin I, Preussin J, Preussin K	Inhibition of IL-6 expression in LPS-activated THP-1 cells	[121]

Table 1. Cont.

Organisms	Microorganisms					
	Classification (Phylum)	Species	Type of Molecules	Molecules	Target/Mode of Action	Ref(s).
Fungi	Ascomycota	A.versicolor	Alkaloids	Asperversiamide B, Asperversiamide C, Asperversiamide F, Asperversiamide G	Inhibition of iNOS expression in LPS-activated RAW 264.7 cells	[122]
Fungi	Ascomycota	A.terreus	Alkaloid	Luteoride E	Inhibition of NO in LPS-activated RAW 264.7 cells	[123]
Fungi	Ascomycota	A.terreus	Terpene	Lovastatin	Inhibition of NO production in LPS-activated RAW 264.7 cells	[123]
Fungi	Ascomycota	A.terreus CFCC 81836	Terpene	Brasilanone A	Inhibition NO production in LPS-activated RAW 264.7 cells	[124]
Fungi	Ascomycota	A.terreus CFCC 81836	Terpene	Brasilanone E		[124]
Fungi	Ascomycota (phylum)	A.terreus	Polyketide	Versicolactone G	Inhibition of NO production (IC$_{50}$ = 15.72 and 29.34 μM for G and A, respectively) in LPS-activated RAW 264.7 cells	[123]
Fungi	Ascomycota	A.terreus	Polyketide	Territrem A		
Fungi	Ascomycota	A.terreus	Peptide	Methyl 3,4,5-trimethoxy-2-(2-(nicotinamido)benzamido)benzoate	Inhibition of NO production in LPS-activated RAW 264.7 cells	[123]
Fungi	Ascomycota	A. terreus (isolated from the coral Sarcophyton subviride)	Aliphatic alcohol	(3E,7E)-4,8-dimethyl-undecane-3,7-diene-1,11-diol, 14α-hydroxyergosta-4,7,22-triene-3,6-dione	Inhibition of NO expression in LPS-activated RAW 264.7 cells	[123]
Fungi	Ascomycota	Aspergillus sp. SCSIOW2	Terpenes	Dihydrobipolaroxins B-D Dihydrobipolaroxin	NO inhibition in RAW 264.7 cells	[125]
Fungi	Ascomycota	Eurotium sp., SF-5989	Alkaloid	Neoechinulin B	Inhibition of NO production in amyloid-β 1-42-activated BV-2 cells	[126]
Fungi	Ascomycota	Eurotium sp SF-5989	Polyketide	Flavoglaucin Isotecrahydroauroglaucin	Inhibition of NO and PGE2 expression in LPS-activated RAW 264.7 cells	[127]

Table 1. Cont.

Organisms	Microorganisms				Target/Mode of Action	Ref(s).
	Classification (Phylum)	Species	Type of Molecules	Molecules		
Fungi	Ascomycota	*Eurotium* spp.	Indolic alkaloid	Neoechinulin A	Reduction of NO and PGE2 production by inhibiting iNOS and COX-2 expression and reduced the production of IL-1β, TNF-α in LPS-stimulated RAW 264.7 cells	[126]
Fungi	Ascomycota	*Eurotium* sp. SF-5989	Alkaloid	Neoechinulin A	Inhibition of NO and PGE2 in LPS-stimulated RAW 264.7 macrophages	[126]
Fungi	Ascomycota	*E.amstelodami*	Polyketide	Asperflavin	Inhibition of 4.6% and 55.9% of NO and PGE2 expression, respectively, in LPS-activated RAW 264.7 cells	[128]
Fungi	Ascomycota	*E.amstelodami*	Polyketide	Questinol	Inhibition of 73% and 43.5% of NO and PGE2 expression, respectively, in LPS-stimulated RAW 264.7 cells	[129]
Fungi	Ascomycota	*Penicillium* sp. SF-5859 (isolated from a sponge)	Polyketides	Curvularin, (11R,15S)-11-hydroxycurvularin, (11S,15S)-11-hydroxycurvularin, (11R,15S)-11-methoxycurvularin, (11S,15S)-11-methoxycurvularin, (10E,15S)-10,11-dehydrocurvularin, (10Z,15S)-10,11-dehydrocurvularin	Inhibition of NO and PGE2 expression (IC_{50} values ranging from 1.9 to 18.7 μM) in LPS-stimulated RAW 264.7 cells	[130]
Fungi	Ascomycota	*Graphostroma* sp. MCCC 3A00421	Terpene	Graphostromane F	Inhibition of NO in LPS-activated RAW 264.7 cells	[131]
Fungi	Ascomycota	*Graphostroma* sp. MCCC 3A00421	Terpene	Khusinol B	Inhibition of NO expression in LPS-activated RAW 264.7 cells	[132]

Table 1. Cont.

	Microorganisms					
Organisms	Classification (Phylum)	Species	Type of Molecules	Molecules	Target/Mode of Action	Ref(s).
Fungi	Ascomycota	*P.chrysogenum* SCSIO41901	Alkaloid	Chrysamide C	Inhibition of IL-17 expression in mice T-cells	[133]
Fungi	Ascomycota	*Penicillium* sp. SF-5295	Alkaloid	Viridicatol	Inhibition of NO and PGE2 expression in LPS-activated RAW 264.7 and in LPS-activated BV2 cells	[134]
Fungi	Ascomycota	*Penicillium* sp.	Alkaloids	Brevicompanine E, Brevicompanine H	Inhibition of NO production in LPS-activated RAW 264.7 cells	[135]
Fungi	Ascomycota	*Penicillium* sp. SF-5995	Alkaloid	Methylpenicinoline	Inhibition of NO, PGE2, iNOS and COX-2 expression in LPS-induced RAW 264.7 cells and BV2 microglia	[136]
Fungi	Ascomycota	*Penicillium* sp. SF-5497	Terpenes	7-acetoxydehydroaustinol, Austinolide, 7-acetoxydehydroaustin, 11-hydroxyisoaustinone, 11-acetoxyisoaustinone	Inhibition of NO expression in LPS-activated BV-2 cells	[137]
Fungi	Ascomycota	*Penicillium* sp. SF 6013	Terpenes	2E,4Z-tanzawaic acid D, Tanzawaicaids A, Tanzawaicaids E	Inhibition of NO expression in LPS-activated RAW 264.7 cells	[138]
Fungi	Ascomycota	*Penicillium* sp. SF-5629	Polyketide	Citrinin H1	Inhibition of NO and prostaglandin E2 expression (IC$_{50}$ = 8.1 and 8.0 μM) in LPS-activated BV2 cells	[139]
Fungi	Ascomycota	*Penicillium* sp SF-5292	Polyketide	Penicillospirone	Inhibition of NO and PGE2 expression (with IC$_{50}$ values of 21.9–27.6 μM) in LPS-activated RAW 264.7 and BV2 cells	[134]
Fungi	Ascomycota	*Penicillium* sp. SF-5292	Polyketide	Penicillinolide A	Inhibition of NO, PGE2, TNF-α, IL-1β, and IL-6 expression (IC$_{50}$ = 20.47, 17.54, 8.63, 11.32, and 20.92 μM, respectively) in LPS-activated RAW 264.7 and BV2 cells	[140]

Table 1. Cont.

Organisms	Classification (Phylum)	Microorganisms Species	Type of Molecules	Molecules	Target/Mode of Action	Ref(s).
Fungi	Ascomycota	*Penicillium* sp. J05B-3-F-1	Hexylitaconic acid derivatives	Methyl 8-hydroxy-3-methoxycarbonyl-2-methylenenonanoate, (3S)-Methyl 9-hydroxy-3-methoxycarbonyl-2-methylenenonanoate	Inhibition of pro-inflammatory cytokines and NO expression in LPS-activated RAW 264.7 cells	[141]
Fungi	Ascomycota	*P. atrovenetum*	Terpene	Citreohybridonol	Anti-neuroinflammatory activity	[142]
Fungi	Ascomycota	*P. steckii 108YD142*	Terpenes	Tanzawaic acid Q, Tanzawaic acid A, Tanzawaic acid C, Tanzawaic acid D, Tanzawaic acid K	Inhibition of NO expression in LPS-activated RAW 264.7 cells	[143]
Fungi	Ascomycota	*P. paxilili*	Polyketide	Pyrenocine A	Inhibition of TNF-α and PGE2 expression in LPS-activated RAW 264.7 cells	[144]
Fungi	Ascomycota	*P. thomii KMM 4667*	Terpene	Thomimarine E	Inhibition of 22.5% of NO production in LPS-activated RAW 264.7 cells	[145]
Fungi	Ascomycota	*P. thomii KMM 4667*	Polyketide	Guaiadiol A, 4,10,11 trihydroxyguaiane	Inhibition of 24.1% and 36.6% of NO production at 10 μM in LPS-activated RAW 264.7 cells	[145]
Fungi	Ascomycota	*P. citrinum SYP-F-2720*	Peptide	(S)-2-(2-hydroxypropanamido) benzoic acid	Reduction of the inflammation in xylene-induced mouse ear edema model	[146]
Fungi	Ascomycota	*Hypocreales* sp. HLS-104	Terpene	1R,6R,7R,10S-10-hydroxy-4(5)-cadinen-3-one	Inhibition of NO expression in LPS-activated RAW 264.7 cells with Emax value of 26.46% at 1 μM	[147]
Fungi	Ascomycota	*Hypocreales* sp. HLS-104	Polyketide	(R)-5,6-dihydro-6-pentyl-2H-pyran-2-one		[147]
Fungi	Ascomycota	*F. heterosporum CNC-477*	Sesterpene polyol	Mangicol A	Inhibition of PMA-induced mouse ear edema assay	[148]
Fungi	Ascomycota	*F. heterosporum CNC-477*	Sesterpene polyol	Mangicol B		

Table 1. Cont.

Organisms	Microorganisms					
	Classification (Phylum)	Species	Type of Molecules	Molecules	Target/Mode of Action	Ref(s).
Fungi	Basidiomycota	Chondrostereum sp. NTOU4196	Sesquiterpenes	Chondroterpene A, Chondroterpene B, Chondroterpene H, Hirsutanol A, Chondrosterin A, Chondrosterin B	Inhibition of NO expression in LPS-activated BV-2 cells	[149]
Fungi	Ascomycota	Pleosporales sp.	Terpenes	Pleosporallin A, Pleosporallin B, Pleosporallin C	Inhibition of IL-6 expression in LPS-activated RAW 264.7 cells	[150]
Fungi	Ascomycota	Phoma sp. NTOU4195	Polyketide	Phomaketides A–C, FR-111142	Inhibition of NO expression (IC_{50} values ranging from 8.8 to 19.3 μM) in LPS-activated RAW 264.7 cells	[151]
Fungi	Ascomycota	Stachybotrys chartarum 952	Terpenes	Stachybotrysin C, Stachybonoid F, Stachybotylactone	Inhibition of NO expression in LPS-activated RAW 264.7 cells	[152]
Fungi	Ascomycota	Leptosphaerulina chartarum 3608	Polyketide	(4R,10S,4'S)-leptothalenone B	Inhibition of NO in LPS-activated RAW 264.7 cells (IC_{50} = 44.5 μM)	[153]
Fungi	Ascomycota	Glimcstix sp. ZSD51-F11	Polyketides	Expansol A, Expansol B, Expansol C, Expansol D, Expansol E, Expansol F	Inhibition of COX-1 (IC_{50} = 5.3, 16.2, 30.2, 41 and 56.8 μM, for A, B, C, E, F respectively) and COX-2 (IC_{50} = 3.1, 5.6, 3, 5.1, 3.2 and 3.7 μM, for A, B, C, D, E, F, respectively)	[154]
Fungi	Ascomycota	Diaporthe sp. HLY-1	Polyketide	Mycoepoxydiene	Inhibition of NO and TNF-α, IL-6, and IL-1β expression in LPS-activated macrophages	[155]
Fungi	Ascomycota	Aspergillus violaceofuscus	Peptides	Violaceotide A, diketopiperazine dimer	Inhibition of IL-10 expression in LPS-activated THP1 cells	[156]

Table 1. Cont.

Organisms	Microorganisms					
	Classification (Phylum)	Species	Type of Molecules	Molecules	Target/Mode of Action	Ref(s).
Fungi	Ascomycota	*Acremonium* sp.	Peptide	Oxepinamide A	Inhibition of RTX-activated mouse ear edema assay	[157]
Fungi	Ascomycota	*Alternaria* sp.	Peptide	Alternaramide	Inhibition NO and PGE2 expression in LPS-activated RAW 264.7 and BV2 cells	[158]
Fungi	Ascomycota	*Trichoderma citrinoviride* (isolated from green alga *Cladophora*)	Sorbicillinoid	Trichodermanone C	Inhibitory effect on nitrite levels in LPS-activated J774A.1 macrophages	[159]
Fungi	Ascomycota	*Paraconiothyrium* sp. VK-13	Polyketide	1-(2,5-dihydroxyphenyl)-3-hydroxybutan-1-one, 1-(2,5-dihydroxyphenyl)-2-buten-1-one	Inhibition of NO and PGE2 expression in LPS-activated RAW 264.7 cells (IC_{50} = 3.9–12.5 μM).	[160]
Fungi	Basidiomycota	*Cystobasidium larynges* IV17-028	Phenazine derivatives	6-[1-(2-aminobenzoyloxy)ethyl]-1-phenazinecarboxylic acid, Saphenol, (R)-saphenic acid, Phenazine-1-carboxylic acid, 6-(1-hydroxyethyl) phenazine-1-carboxylic acid, 6-acetyl-phenazine-1-carboxylic acid	Inhibition of NO production in RAW 264.7 cells	[161]
Fungi	Ascomycota	*Penicillium sp JF-55* (polyketide)	Phenylpropanoid	Penstyrylpyrone	Inhibition of NO, PGE2, TNF-α, IL-1β in LPS-activated murine peritoneal macrophages	[162]
Bacteria	Actinobacteria	*Streptomyces* spp.	Alkaloid	Actinoquinoline A Actinoquinoline B	Inhibition of COX-1 and COX-2	[163]

Table 1. *Cont.*

Organisms	Microorganisms				Type of Molecules	Molecules	Target/Mode of Action	Ref(s).
	Classification (Phylum)	Species						
Bacteria	Actinobacteria	*Streptomyces caniferus*			Macrolide	Caniferolide A	Inhibition of NF-κB p65 translocation and pro-inflammatory cytokines expression in BV2 microglial cells	[164]
Bacteria	Actinobacteria	*Nocardiopsis* sp.			Macrolide	Fijiolide A	Reduction of TNF-α-induced NF-κB in human embryonic kidney cells 293 (IC_{50} = 0.57 μM)	[165]
Bacteria	Actinobacteria	*Kocuria* sp. strain AG5			Exopolysaccharide	EPS5	Inhibition of LOX-5 and COX-2 (IC_{50} = 15.39 ± 0.82 μg/mL and 28.06 ± 1.1 μg/mL, respectively)	[166]
Bacteria	Bacillota	*Bacillus subtilis* B5			Macrolactin derivative	7,13-epoxyl-macrolactin A; 7-O-2′E-butenoyl macrolactin A	Inhibition of inducible nitric oxide synthase (iNOS), interleukin-1β (IL-1β), and interleukin-6 (IL-6) expression in LPS-stimulated RAW 264.7 macrophages	[167]

3. Marine Microorganisms vs. Macro-Organisms: Who Are the Actual Producers of Metabolites?

Oceans are a vast and unexplored world, teeming with life and diversity. Recent advancements in bioprospecting and molecular technologies foster the identification of new marine organisms, from macroscopic to microscopic biota, in this fascinating ecosystem [168]. However, the number of unknown marine species is estimated between 60,000 and 1,950,000, depending on the literature [169]. In the early days, bioprospecting campaigns focused on larger species like cnidarians, sponges, or soft corals due to technical limitations [170]. Between the 1990s and the 2010s, marine invertebrates have been found to produce almost 10,000 new marine natural products (MNPs) [171]. These discoveries have revealed the immense potential of marine organisms for developing innovative compounds for therapeutic and industrial applications. Many metabolites produced by marine macro-organisms have shown promising biological properties, such as anti-inflammatory activity for 43.7% of compounds (Figure 1a). These metabolites belong to different classes of molecules like terpenes (26%), alkaloids (20%), lipids (20%), pigments (8%), polysaccharides (6%) as shown in Figure 1b. Among macro-organisms, those belonging to the phylum Echinodermata produce the most anti-inflammatory molecules (Table 1), inhibiting pro-inflammatory cytokines and the NF-κB pathway but also reducing inflammation in vivo (Table 1). Since then, the possibility of further exploring and leveraging marine ecosystems has been genuinely exciting as it could unlock countless benefits for human health.

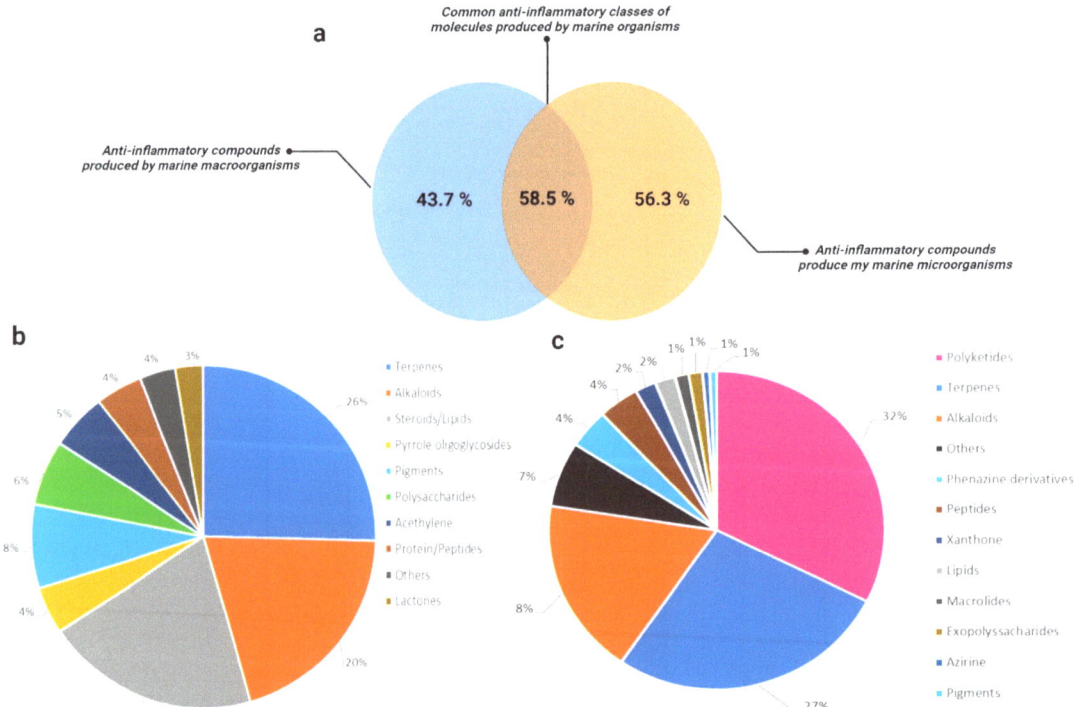

Figure 1. Chemical classification of MNPs with anti-inflammatory activity as reported between 2000 and 2024. Percentage of known anti-inflammatory compounds produced by marine organisms (**a**), by marine macro-organisms (**b**), and microorganisms (**c**) according to the structure type.

An ongoing exploration of marine ecosystems has extended to extreme environments such as deep ocean trenches, geographical poles, or hydrothermal vents; furthermore, technological improvement of microorganisms conservation during collects prompted bioprospecting campaigns to focus on microorganisms such as microalgae, marine fungi, cyanobacteria, and other groups of marine microorganisms. These microscopic life forms represent over 90% of the marine biomass and play a critical role in geochemical processes necessary for terrestrial life [172]. They are also remarkable for their ability to thrive, even in the harshest environments, producing rare and unique compounds that cannot be found in terrestrial biotopes. Furthermore, marine microorganisms are highly metabolically efficient, producing large amounts of metabolites while consuming limited energy [173]. Over the past year, MNPs obtained from marine bacteria, fungi, and cyanobacteria increased by 22%, 85%, and 61%, respectively, between 2018 and 2020, underscoring the impact of marine microorganisms on scientific research [174]. Yet, macro-organisms such as sponges and cnidarians have also been shown to produce MNPs [175]. The identification of these sources has led to inquiries and discussions about the actual producers of these metabolites.

Recent studies have uncovered that certain compounds previously thought to be specifically produced by marine macro-organisms are actually the metabolic byproducts of associated microorganisms [176], as illustrated by bryostatin, which has been confirmed to originate from microbes. The discovery of this metabolite has been made through the identification of polyketide synthase genes involved in its biosynthesis and found in the genome of the bryozoan bacterial symbiont *Candidatus Endobugula sertula* [177]. Another striking example is the fungus *Penicilium canescens* found in the ascidian *Styela plicata*, which exhibited anti-inflammatory activity. Furthermore, the findings presented in Figure 1a indicate that 58.3% of common anti-inflammatory classes of molecules are produced by both marine macro-organisms and microorganisms. This suggests that microorganisms may play a crucial role in producing these compounds, as many microorganisms live in symbiosis with macro-organisms.

In comparison with macro-organisms, microorganisms represent a significant source of anti-inflammatory molecules, contributing a noteworthy 56% of these compounds (Figure 1a). Moreover, the diversity of their metabolites is astounding, including terpenes (27%), alkaloids (18%), peptides (4%), lipids (2%), and pigments (1%) as indicated in Figure 1C. However, the most intriguing aspect is the specific type of molecules, such as polyketides (32%) and phenazine derivatives (4%) produced by marine fungi that target pro-inflammatory cytokines like TNF-α or IL-6, as well as inflammatory markers like NO (Table 1, Figure 2). Given that these mediators are produced upon activation of the NF-kB pathway or are involved in the activation of the JAK-STAT pathway, it is plausible that the MNPs derived from fungi may inhibit these pathways. Additionally, marine microorganisms, particularly bacteria, can produce specific compounds that are not found in macro-organisms. These compounds, such as exopolysaccharides, macrolides, and azirine, can target inflammatory mediators such as cyclooxygenases, NO, TNF-α, and the NF-κB pathway (Table 1, Figure 2). It is worth noting that among microorganisms, most of the compounds are produced by fungi, particularly those belonging to the Ascomycota phylum (Table 1). In addition, they are the major producers of polyketides, one of the specific molecules mentioned above. Furthermore, although most specific molecules targeted the NF-κB pathway (Table 1), their structural characteristics prompt consideration of whether their modes of action could reveal new pathways and targets for modulating inflammation, thus extending our understanding of the interplay between marine compounds and the inflammatory process. These results suggest that fungi could potentially serve as valuable sources of anti-inflammatory molecules.

Considering the vast potential of microorganisms in the production of anti-inflammatory compounds, further research must be conducted to unlock their full potential and develop new treatments for inflammatory diseases.

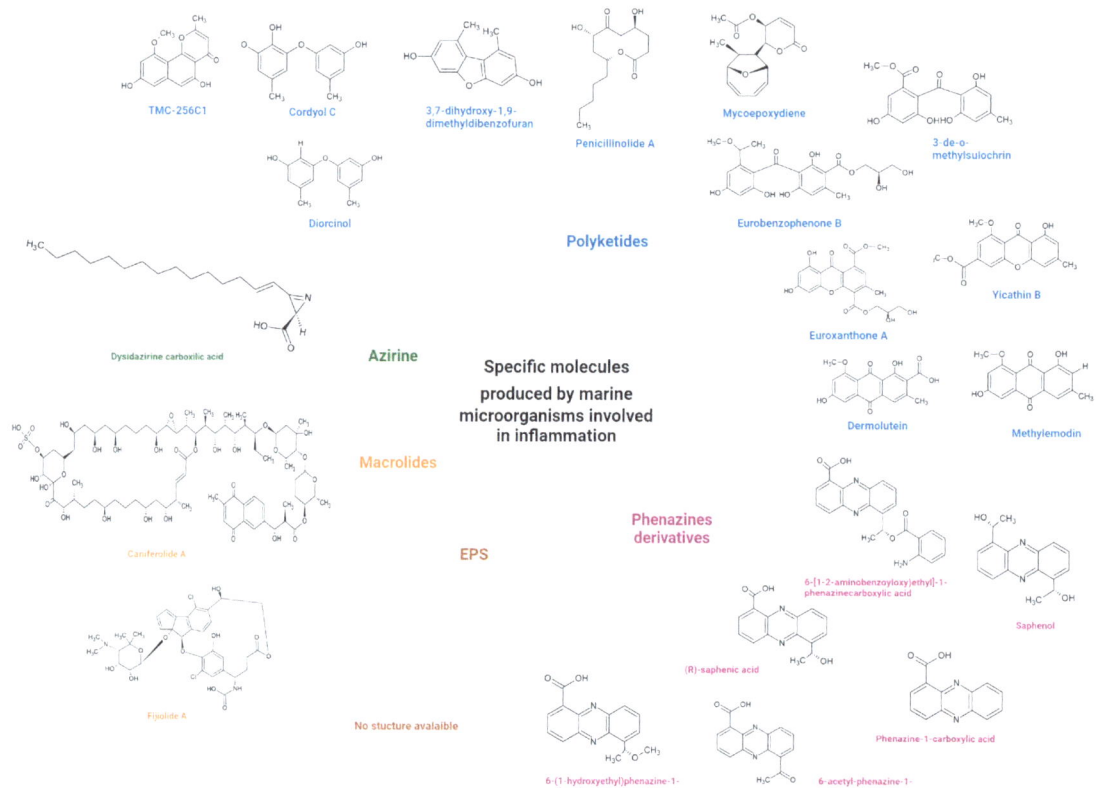

Figure 2. Chemical structure of specific molecules produced by marine microorganisms according to their classification. Regarding polyketides, only a few molecules were presented for each specific target involved in inflammation.

4. Challenges and Future Directions

Exploring the potential of marine microorganisms as anti-inflammatory agents presents a myriad of challenges and promising future opportunities. One significant challenge lies in the development of anti-inflammatory drugs derived from marine sources, which may encounter barriers impacting the speed and efficiency of the process. Additionally, regulatory hurdles could potentially impede the approval and commercialization of marine-derived pharmaceuticals for anti-inflammatory purposes. Scaling up the production of bioactive compounds from marine microorganisms to meet demand poses a significant challenge, while ensuring the cost-effectiveness of extracting and utilizing these compounds for anti-inflammatory therapies is a critical consideration. The intricate complexity of marine ecosystems and the vast diversity of microorganisms further address the challenges in identifying and isolating effective anti-inflammatory compounds.

Looking towards the future, the quest for potent and effective anti-inflammatory natural products from marine organisms requires ongoing and rigorous research. It is essential to explore innovative approaches in marine drug discovery to uncover new and promising anti-inflammatory compounds. In the future, efforts should be focused on optimizing the drug development process from marine sources to enhance its efficacy and speed. Collaboration among researchers, industry members, and regulatory bodies is crucial for advancing marine-based anti-inflammatory therapies. Furthermore, emphasizing sustainable harvesting practices for marine microorganisms intended for anti-inflammatory purposes is vital for ensuring long-term viability.

By addressing these challenges and focusing on future directions, we can unlock marine microorganisms' full potential as valuable sources of anti-inflammatory agents, leading to significant advancements in healthcare and therapeutic treatments.

5. Conclusions

The inter-relations between microorganisms and macro-organisms are complex, ranging from parasitic to symbiotic systems. In this regard, metagenomic analysis offers major insights to decipher the complexity of a micro-environment comprising a macro-organism and its hosts without providing any clues as to which among the various interacting, living species is actually responsible for the synthesis of the bioactive metabolites (Figure 3). On the other hand, microbiota identification and microbial isolation from a macro-organism is an attractive alternative, enabling the isolation and identification of specific bacterial species, their culture, and, ultimately, the demonstration of their ability to produce compounds of pharmaceutical interest. Indeed, microorganisms have emerged as a promising avenue for drug discovery, offering a solution to the challenges posed by low quantities of secondary metabolites and the difficulty of obtaining sufficient biomass necessary for pharmaceutical companies to perform clinical trials. Bacterial or microalgal cultures can provide a continuous source of biomass production within a subsequent purification of bioactive metabolites. These steps could revolutionize drug discovery by making it also more environmentally friendly by reducing the exploitation of marine resources.

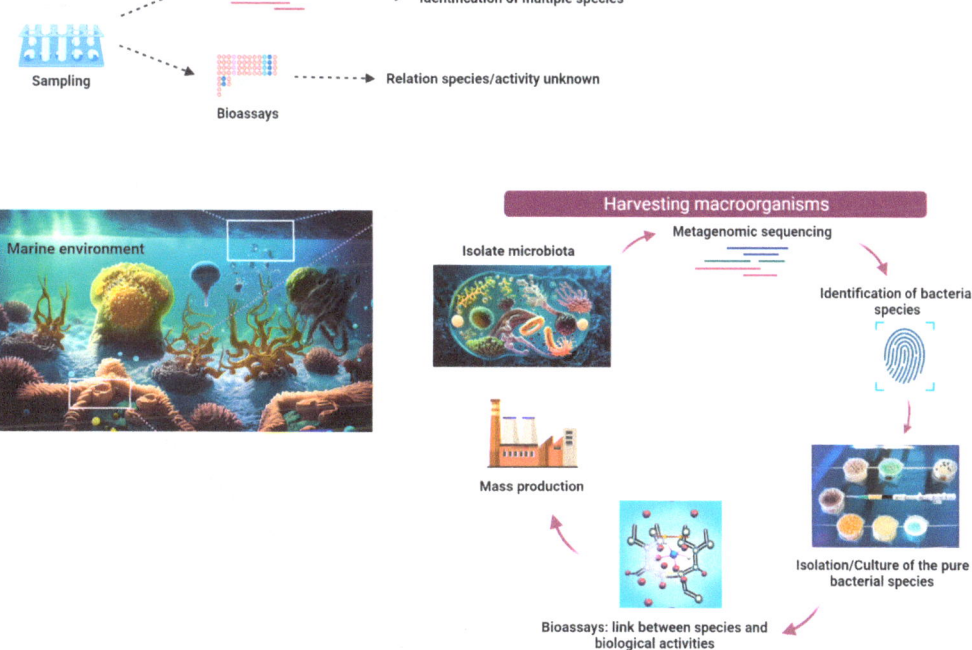

Figure 3. Metagenomic approach to discover the metabolites produced by the microbiota of marine macro-organisms. Two strategies are illustrated. In the top figure, whole metagenomics sequencing enables the identification of most species present in a microenvironment without driving the determination of a species/activity relationship. In the bottom part, microbiota isolation from the environment or macro-organisms leads to bacterial identification, specific culture, and a possible link between a metabolite and bioactivity.

Author Contributions: Conceptualization, M.L., P.G. and M.M.; writing—original draft preparation, M.L.; writing—review and editing, M.L., P.G., T.J. and M.M; supervision, M.M. All authors have read and agreed to the published version of the manuscript.

Funding: This study is supported by the French National Research Agency (ANR; project CHARM N°ANR-21-CE43-0015-01). ML and MM positions are financed by the ANR and by the Government of New Caledonia, respectively.

Data Availability Statement: All data in this review are openly available without any restrictions.

Acknowledgments: We are thankful to Catherine Vonthron-Sénéchau and to Cyril Antheaume (University of Strasbourg) for a critical reading of the first version of the manuscript.

Conflicts of Interest: The authors declare no conflicts of interest.

References

1. El-Gabalawy, H.; Guenther, L.C.; Bernstein, C.N. Epidemiology of immune-mediated inflammatory diseases: Incidence, prevalence, natural history, and comorbidities. *J. Rheumatol. Suppl.* **2010**, *85*, 2–10. [CrossRef] [PubMed]
2. Furman, D.; Campisi, J.; Verdin, E.; Carrera-Bastos, P.; Targ, S.; Franceschi, C.; Ferrucci, L.; Gilroy, D.W.; Fasano, A.; Miller, G.W.; et al. Chronic inflammation in the etiology of disease across the life span. *Nat. Med.* **2019**, *25*, 1822–1832. [CrossRef]
3. Castelli, M.S.; McGonigle, P.; Hornby, P.J. The pharmacology and therapeutic applications of monoclonal antibodies. *Pharmacol. Res. Perspect.* **2019**, *7*, e00535. [CrossRef]
4. Alexander, M.; Luo, Y.; Raimondi, G.; O'shea, J.J.; Gadina, M. Jakinibs of All Trades: Inhibiting Cytokine Signaling in Immune-Mediated Pathologies. *Pharmaceuticals* **2021**, *15*, 48. [CrossRef] [PubMed]
5. Choi, S.R.; Shin, A.; Ha, Y.J.; Lee, Y.J.; Lee, E.B.; Kang, E.H. Comparative risk of infections between JAK inhibitors versus TNF inhibitors among patients with rheumatoid arthritis: A cohort study. *Arthritis Res. Ther.* **2023**, *25*, 129. [CrossRef]
6. Medzhitov, R. The spectrum of inflammatory responses. *Science* **2021**, *374*, 1070–1075. [CrossRef] [PubMed]
7. Gong, T.; Liu, L.; Jiang, W.; Zhou, R. DAMP-sensing receptors in sterile inflammation and inflammatory diseases. *Nat. Rev. Immunol.* **2020**, *20*, 95–112. [CrossRef]
8. Liu, T.; Zhang, L.; Joo, D.; Sun, S.C. NF-κB signaling in inflammation. *Signal Transduct. Target. Ther.* **2017**, *2*, 17023. [CrossRef]
9. Laurindo, L.F.; Santos, A.R.D.O.D.; Carvalho, A.C.A.D.; Bechara, M.D.; Guiguer, E.L.; Goulart, R.D.A.; Vargas Sinatora, R.; Araújo, A.C.; Barbalho, S.M. Phytochemicals and Regulation of NF-kB in Inflammatory Bowel Diseases: An Overview of In Vitro and In Vivo Effects. *Metabolites* **2023**, *13*, 96. [CrossRef]
10. Awasthi, A.; Raju, M.B.; Rahman, M.A. Current Insights of Inhibitors of p38 Mitogen-Activated Protein Kinase in Inflammation. *Med. Chem.* **2021**, *17*, 555–575. [CrossRef] [PubMed]
11. Liu, S.; Ma, H.; Zhang, H.; Deng, C.; Xin, P. Recent advances on signaling pathways and their inhibitors in rheumatoid arthritis. *Clin. Immunol.* **2021**, *230*, 108793. [CrossRef] [PubMed]
12. Philips, R.L.; Wang, Y.; Cheon, H.; Kanno, Y.; Gadina, M.; Sartorelli, V.; Horvath, C.M.; Darnell, J.E.; Stark, G.R.; O'shea, J.J. The JAK-STAT pathway at 30: Much learned, much more to do. *Cell* **2022**, *185*, 3857–3876. [CrossRef] [PubMed]
13. Malemud, C.J. The role of the JAK/STAT signal pathway in rheumatoid arthritis. *Ther. Adv. Musculoskelet. Dis.* **2018**, *10*, 117–127. [CrossRef] [PubMed]
14. Prakash, A.V.; Park, I.-H.; Park, J.W.; Bae, J.P.; Lee, G.S.; Kang, T.J. NLRP3 Inflammasome as Therapeutic Targets in Inflammatory Diseases. *Biomol. Ther.* **2023**, *31*, 395–401. [CrossRef] [PubMed]
15. Sparks, J.A.; Harrold, L.R.; Simon, T.A.; Wittstock, K.; Kelly, S.; Lozenski, K.; Khaychuk, V.; Michaud, K. Comparative effectiveness of treatments for rheumatoid arthritis in clinical practice: A systematic review. *Semin. Arthritis Rheum.* **2023**, *62*, 152249. [CrossRef] [PubMed]
16. Cush, J.J. Rheumatoid Arthritis: Early Diagnosis and Treatment. *Rheum. Dis. Clin. N. Am.* **2022**, *48*, 537–547. [CrossRef] [PubMed]
17. Kim, K.U.; Kim, J.; Kim, W.-H.; Min, H.; Choi, C.H. Treatments of inflammatory bowel disease toward personalized medicine. *Arch. Pharm. Res.* **2021**, *44*, 293–309. [CrossRef] [PubMed]
18. Longhino, S.; Chatzis, L.G.; Dal Pozzolo, R.; Peretti, S.; Fulvio, G.; La Rocca, G.; Navarro Garcia, I.C.; Orlandi, M.; Quartuccio, L.; Baldini, C. Sjögren's syndrome: One year in review 2023. *Clin. Exp. Rheumatol.* **2023**, *41*, 2343–2356. [CrossRef] [PubMed]
19. Posadas, I.; Terencio, M.C.; De Rosa, S.; Payá, M. Cavernolide: A new inhibitor of huma, sPLA2 sharing unusual chemical features. *Life Sci.* **2000**, *67*, 3007–3014. [CrossRef]
20. Posadas, I.; Terencio, M.C.; Giannini, C.; D'Auria, M.V.; Payá, M. Dysidotronic acid, a new sesquiterpenoid, inhibits cytokine production and the expression of nitric oxide synthase. *Eur. J. Pharmacol.* **2001**, *415*, 285–292. [CrossRef]
21. Gunasekera, S.P.; Isbrucker, R.A.; Longley, R.E.; Wright, A.E.; Pomponi, S.A.; Reed, J.K. Plakolide a, a new gamma-lactone from the marine sponge *Plakortis* sp. *J. Nat. Prod.* **2004**, *67*, 110–111. [CrossRef]
22. Cabré, F.; Carabaza, A.; Suesa, N.; García, A.M.; Rotllan, E.; Gómez, M.; Tost, D.; Mauleón, D.; Carganico, G. Effect of manoalide on human 5-lipoxygenase activity. *Inflamm. Res.* **1996**, *45*, 218–223. [CrossRef]

23. D'Acquisto, F.; Lanzotti, V.; Carnuccio, R. Cyclolinteinone, a sesterterpene from sponge Cacospongia linteiformis, prevents inducible nitric oxide synthase and inducible cyclo-oxygenase protein expression by blocking nuclear factor-kappaB activation in J774 macrophages. *Biochem. J.* **2000**, *346 Pt 3*, 793–798. [CrossRef] [PubMed]
24. Busserolles, J.; Payá, M.; D'Auria, M.V.; Gomez-Paloma, L.; Alcaraz, M.J. Protection against 2,4,6-trinitrobenzenesulphonic acid-induced colonic inflammation in mice by the marine products bolinaquinone and petrosaspongiolide M. *Biochem. Pharmacol.* **2005**, *69*, 1433–1440. [CrossRef]
25. Shin, J.; Seo, Y.; Cho, K.W. Five new polyacetylenes from a sponge of the genus petrosia. *J. Nat. Prod.* **1998**, *61*, 1268–1273. [CrossRef]
26. Hong, S.; Kim, S.H.; Rhee, M.H.; Kim, A.R.; Jung, J.H.; Chun, T.; Yoo, E.S.; Cho, J.Y. In vitro anti-inflammatory and pro-aggregative effects of a lipid compound, petrocortyne A, from marine sponges. *Naunyn Schmiedebergs Arch. Pharmacol.* **2003**, *368*, 448–456. [CrossRef]
27. Mencarelli, A.; D'Amore, C.; Renga, B.; Cipriani, S.; Carino, A.; Sepe, V.; Perissutti, E.; D'Auria, M.V.; Zampella, A.; Distrutti, E.; et al. Solomonsterol A, a marine pregnane-X-receptor agonist, attenuates inflammation and immune dysfunction in a mouse model of arthritis. *Mar. Drugs* **2013**, *12*, 36–53. [CrossRef] [PubMed]
28. Lind, K.F.; Hansen, E.; Østerud, B.; Eilertsen, K.-E.; Bayer, A.; Engqvist, M.; Leszczak, K.; Jørgensen, T.; Andersen, J.H. Antioxidant and anti-inflammatory activities of barettin. *Mar. Drugs* **2013**, *11*, 2655–2666. [CrossRef] [PubMed]
29. Di, X.; Rouger, C.; Hardardottir, I.; Freysdottir, J.; Molinski, T.F.; Tasdemir, D.; Omarsdottir, S. 6-Bromoindole Derivatives from the Icelandic Marine Sponge Geodia barretti: Isolation and Anti-Inflammatory Activity. *Mar. Drugs* **2018**, *16*, 437. [CrossRef]
30. Tsubosaka, Y.; Murata, T.; Yamada, K.; Uemura, D.; Hori, M.; Ozaki, H. Halichlorine reduces monocyte adhesion to endothelium through the suppression of nuclear factor-kappaB activation. *J. Pharmacol. Sci.* **2010**, *113*, 208–213. [CrossRef]
31. Lee, S.M.; Kim, N.H.; Lee, S.; Kim, Y.N.; Heo, J.D.; Rho, J.R.; Jeong, E.J. (10Z)-Debromohymenialdisine from Marine Sponge *Stylissa* sp. Regulates Intestinal Inflammatory Responses in Co-Culture Model of Epithelial Caco-2 Cells and THP-1 Macrophage Cells. *Molecules* **2019**, *24*, 3394. [CrossRef] [PubMed]
32. Buchanan, M.S.; Carroll, A.R.; Addepalli, R.; Avery, V.M.; Hooper, J.N.; Quinn, R.J. Natural products, stylissadines A and B, specific antagonists of the P2X7 receptor, an important inflammatory target. *J. Org. Chem.* **2007**, *72*, 2309–2317. [CrossRef] [PubMed]
33. Nguyen, P.T.; Nguyen, H.N.; Nguyen, X.C.; Bui, H.T.; Tran, H.Q.; Nguyen, T.T.N.; Bui, T.T.L.; Yang, S.Y.; Choi, C.H.; Kim, S.; et al. Steroidal Constituents from the Soft Coral Sinularia dissecta and Their Inhibitory Effects on Lipopolysaccharide-Stimulated Production of Pro-inflammatory Cytokines in Bone Marrow-Derived Dendritic Cells. *Bull. Korean Chem. Soc.* **2013**, *34*, 949–952. [CrossRef]
34. Mayer, A.M.; Jacobson, P.B.; Fenical, W.; Jacobs, R.S.; Glaser, K.B. Pharmacological characterization of the pseudopterosins: Novel anti-inflammatory natural products isolated from the Caribbean soft coral, *Pseudopterogorgia elisabethae*. *Life Sci.* **1998**, *62*, Pl401–Pl407. [CrossRef]
35. Ahmed, A.F.; Hsieh, Y.-T.; Wen, Z.-H.; Wu, Y.-C.; Sheu, J.-H. Polyoxygenated sterols from the Formosan soft coral *Sinularia gibberosa*. *J. Nat. Prod.* **2006**, *69*, 1275–1279. [CrossRef] [PubMed]
36. Takaki, H.; Koganemaru, R.; Iwakawa, Y.; Higuchi, R.; Miyamoto, T. Inhibitory Effect of Norditerpenes on LPS-Induced TNF-α Production from the Okinawan Soft Coral, *Sinularia* sp. *Biol. Pharm. Bull.* **2003**, *26*, 380–382.
37. Tseng, Y.J.; Shen, K.P.; Lin, H.L.; Huang, C.Y.; Dai, C.F.; Sheu, J.H. Lochmolins A-G, new sesquiterpenoids from the soft coral *Sinularia lochmodes*. *Mar. Drugs* **2012**, *10*, 1572–1581. [CrossRef]
38. Chen, K.J.; Tseng, C.-K.; Chang, F.-R.; Yang, J.-I.; Yeh, C.-C.; Chen, W.-C.; Wu, S.-F.; Chang, H.-W.; Lee, J.-C. Aqueous extract of the edible *Gracilaria tenuistipitata* inhibits hepatitis C viral replication via cyclooxygenase-2 suppression and reduces virus-induced inflammation. *PLoS ONE* **2013**, *8*, e57704. [CrossRef]
39. Lee, H.P.; Huang, S.-Y.; Lin, Y.-Y.; Wang, H.-M.; Jean, Y.-H.; Wu, S.-F.; Duh, C.-Y.; Wen, Z.-H. Soft coral-derived lemnalol alleviates monosodium urate-induced gouty arthritis in rats by inhibiting leukocyte infiltration and iNOS, COX-2 and c-Fos protein expression. *Mar. Drugs* **2013**, *11*, 99–113. [CrossRef]
40. Lu, Y.; Li, P.-J.; Hung, W.-Y.; Su, J.-H.; Wen, Z.-H.; Hsu, C.-H.; Dai, C.-F.; Chiang, M.Y.; Sheu, J.-H. Nardosinane sesquiterpenoids from the Formosan soft coral *Lemnalia flava*. *J. Nat. Prod.* **2011**, *74*, 169–174. [CrossRef] [PubMed]
41. Cuong, N.X.; Thao, N.P.; Luyen, B.T.T.; Ngan, N.T.T.; Thuy, D.T.T.; Song, S.B.; Nam, N.H.; Van Kiem, P.; Kim, Y.H.; Van Minh, C. Cembranoid diterpenes from the soft coral *Lobophytum crassum* and their anti-inflammatory activities. *Chem. Pharm. Bull.* **2014**, *62*, 203–208. [CrossRef]
42. Thao, N.P.; Luyen, B.T.T.; Ngan, N.T.T.; Song, S.B.; Cuong, N.X.; Nam, N.H.; Van Kiem, P.; Kim, Y.H.; Van Minh, C. New anti-inflammatory cembranoid diterpenoids from the Vietnamese soft coral *Lobophytum crassum*. *Bioorg. Med. Chem. Lett.* **2014**, *24*, 228–232. [CrossRef]
43. Fang, H.Y.; Hsu, C.-H.; Chao, C.-H.; Wen, Z.-H.; Wu, Y.-C.; Dai, C.-F.; Sheu, J.-H. Cytotoxic and anti-inflammatory metabolites from the soft coral *Scleronephthya gracillimum*. *Mar. Drugs* **2013**, *11*, 1853–1865. [CrossRef] [PubMed]
44. Gonzalez, Y.; Doens, D.; Santamaría, R.; Ramos, M.; Restrepo, C.M.; de Arruda, L.B.; Lleonart, R.; Gutiérrez, M.; Fernández, P.L. A pseudopterane diterpene isolated from the octocoral *Pseudopterogorgia acerosa* inhibits the inflammatory response mediated by TLR-ligands and TNF-alpha in macrophages. *PLoS ONE* **2013**, *8*, e84107. [CrossRef]

45. Chung, H.M.; Wang, W.-H.; Hwang, T.-L.; Wu, Y.-C.; Sung, P.-J. Natural clovanes from the gorgonian coral *Rumphella antipathies*. *Nat. Prod. Commun.* **2013**, *8*, 1037–1040. [CrossRef]
46. Chung, H.M.; Wang, W.H.; Hwang, T.L.; Li, J.J.; Fang, L.S.; Wu, Y.C.; Sung, P.J. Rumphellaones B and C, new 4,5-seco-caryophyllane sesquiterpenoids from *Rumphellan antipathies*. *Molecules* **2014**, *19*, 12320–12327. [CrossRef]
47. Chung, H.M.; Wang, W.-H.; Hwang, T.-L.; Chen, J.-J.; Fang, L.-S.; Wen, Z.-H.; Wang, Y.-B.; Wu, Y.-C.; Sung, P.-J. Rumphellols A and B, new caryophyllene sesquiterpenoids from a Formosan gorgonian coral, *Rumphella antipathies*. *Int. J. Mol. Sci.* **2014**, *15*, 15679–15688. [CrossRef] [PubMed]
48. Lin, Y.Y.; Lin, S.-C.; Feng, C.-W.; Chen, P.-C.; Su, Y.-D.; Li, C.-M.; Yang, S.-N.; Jean, Y.-H.; Sung, P.-J.; Duh, C.-Y.; et al. Anti-Inflammatory and Analgesic Effects of the Marine-Derived Compound Excavatolide B Isolated from the Culture-Type Formosan Gorgonian *Briareum excavatum*. *Mar. Drugs* **2015**, *13*, 2559–2579. [CrossRef]
49. Wei, W.C.; Lin, S.-Y.; Chen, Y.-J.; Wen, C.-C.; Huang, C.-Y.; Palanisamy, A.; Yang, N.-S.; Sheu, J.-H. Topical application of marine briarane-type diterpenes effectively inhibits 12-O-tetradecanoylphorbol-13-acetate-induced inflammation and dermatitis in murine skin. *J. Biomed. Sci.* **2011**, *18*, 94. [CrossRef] [PubMed]
50. Hsu, Y.M.; Chang, F.R.; Lo, I.W.; Lai, K.H.; El-Shazly, M.; Wu, T.Y.; Du, Y.C.; Hwang, T.L.; Cheng, Y.B.; Wu, Y.C. Zoanthamine-Type Alkaloids from the Zoanthid *Zoanthus kuroshio* Collected in Taiwan and Their Effects on Inflammation. *J. Nat. Prod.* **2016**, *79*, 2674–2680. [CrossRef]
51. Guillen, P.O.; Gegunde, S.; Jaramillo, K.B.; Alfonso, A.; Calabro, K.; Alonso, E.; Rodriguez, J.; Botana, L.M.; Thomas, O.P. Zoanthamine Alkaloids from the Zoantharian *Zoanthus* cf. *pulchellus* and Their Effects in Neuroinflammation. *Mar. Drugs* **2018**, *16*, 242. [CrossRef] [PubMed]
52. Pereira, D.M.; Correia-da-Silva, G.; Valentão, P.; Teixeira, N.; Andrade, P.B. Anti-inflammatory effect of unsaturated fatty acids and Ergosta-7,22-dien-3-ol from Marthasterias glacialis: Prevention of CHOP-mediated ER-stress and NF-kappaB activation. *PLoS ONE* **2014**, *9*, e88341. [CrossRef]
53. Thao, N.P.; Cuong, N.X.; Luyen, B.T.T.; Van Thanh, N.; Nhiem, N.X.; Koh, Y.-S.; Ly, B.M.; Nam, N.H.; Van Kiem, P.; Van Minh, C.; et al. Anti-inflammatory asterosaponins from the starfish *Astropecten monacanthus*. *J. Nat. Prod.* **2013**, *76*, 1764–1770. [CrossRef]
54. Monmai, C.; Go, S.H.; Shin, I.S.; You, S.; Kim, D.O.; Kang, S.; Park, W.J. Anti-Inflammatory Effect of Asterias amurensis Fatty Acids through NF-kappaB and MAPK Pathways against LPS-Stimulated RAW264.7 Cells. *J. Microbiol. Biotechnol.* **2018**, *28*, 1635–1644. [CrossRef]
55. Thao, N.P.; Luyen, B.T.T.; Koo, J.E.; Kim, S.; Koh, Y.S.; Cuong, N.X.; Nam, N.H.; Van Kiem, P.; Kim, Y.H.; Van Minh, C. Anti-inflammatory components of the Vietnamese starfish *Protoreaster nodosus*. *Biol. Res.* **2015**, *48*, 12. [CrossRef]
56. Malyarenko, T.V.; Kicha, A.A.; Kalinovsky, A.I.; Ivanchina, N.V.; Popov, R.S.; Pislyagin, E.A.; Menchinskaya, E.S.; Padmakumar, K.P.; Stonik, V.A. Four New Steroidal Glycosides, Protolinckiosides A-D, from the Starfish *Protoreaster lincki*. *Chem. Biodivers.* **2016**, *13*, 998–1007. [CrossRef]
57. Malyarenko, T.V.; Kharchenko, S.D.; Kicha, A.A.; Ivanchina, N.V.; Dmitrenok, P.S.; Chingizova, E.A.; Pislyagin, E.A.; Evtushenko, E.V.; Antokhina, T.I.; Minh, C.V.; et al. Anthenosides L-U, Steroidal Glycosides with Unusual Structural Features from the Starfish *Anthenea aspera*. *J. Nat. Prod.* **2016**, *79*, 3047–3056. [CrossRef] [PubMed]
58. Kicha, A.A.; Kalinovsky, A.I.; Ivanchina, N.V.; Malyarenko, T.V.; Dmitrenok, P.S.; Kuzmich, A.S.; Sokolova, E.V.; Stonik, V.A. Furostane Series Asterosaponins and Other Unusual Steroid Oligoglycosides from the Tropical Starfish *Pentaceraster regulus*. *J. Nat. Prod.* **2017**, *80*, 2761–2770. [CrossRef]
59. Vien, L.T.; Hanh, T.T.H.; Huong, P.T.T.; Dang, N.H.; Van Thanh, N.; Lyakhova, E.; Cuong, N.X.; Nam, N.H.; Van Kiem, P.; Kicha, A.; et al. Pyrrole Oligoglycosides from the Starfish *Acanthaster planci* Suppress Lipopolysaccharide-Induced Nitric Oxide Production in RAW264.7 Macrophages. *Chem. Pharm. Bull.* **2016**, *64*, 1654–1657. [CrossRef]
60. Thao, N.P.; Dat, L.D.; Ngoc, N.T.; Tu, V.A.; Hanh, T.T.H.; Huong, P.T.T.; Nhiem, N.X.; Tai, B.H.; Cuong, N.X.; Nam, N.H.; et al. Pyrrole and furan oligoglycosides from the starfish *Asterina batheri* and their inhibitory effect on the production of pro-inflammatory cytokines in lipopolysaccharide-stimulated bone marrow-derived dendritic cells. *Bioorg. Med. Chem. Lett.* **2013**, *23*, 1823–1827. [CrossRef] [PubMed]
61. Moura Rda, M.; Aragão, K.S.; de Melo, A.A.; Carneiro, R.F.; Osório, C.B.; Luz, P.B.; de Queiroz, A.F.; Dos Santos, E.A.; de Alencar, N.M.; Cavada, B.S. Holothuria grisea agglutinin (HGA): The first invertebrate lectin with anti-inflammatory effects. *Fundam. Clin. Pharmacol.* **2013**, *27*, 656–668. [CrossRef] [PubMed]
62. Mou, J.; Li, Q.; Qi, X.; Yang, J. Structural comparison, antioxidant and anti-inflammatory properties of fucosylated chondroitin sulfate of three edible sea cucumbers. *Carbohydr. Polym.* **2018**, *185*, 41–47. [CrossRef]
63. Olivera-Castillo, L.; Grant, G.; Kantún-Moreno, N.; Barrera-Pérez, H.A.; Montero, J.; Olvera-Novoa, M.A.; Carrillo-Cocom, L.M.; Acevedo, J.J.; Puerto-Castillo, C.; Solís, V.M.; et al. A Glycosaminoglycan-Rich Fraction from Sea Cucumber *Isostichopus badionotus* Has Potent Anti-Inflammatory Properties In Vitro and In Vivo. *Nutrients* **2020**, *12*, 1698. [CrossRef] [PubMed]
64. Wang, J.; Hu, S.; Jiang, W.; Song, W.; Cai, L.; Wang, J. Fucoidan from sea cucumber may improve hepatic inflammatory response and insulin resistance in mice. *Int. Immunopharmacol.* **2016**, *31*, 15–23. [CrossRef] [PubMed]
65. Zhu, Q.; Lin, L.; Zhao, M. Sulfated fucan/fucosylated chondroitin sulfate-dominated polysaccharide fraction from low-edible-value sea cucumber ameliorates type 2 diabetes in rats: New prospects for sea cucumber polysaccharide based-hypoglycemic functional food. *Int. J. Biol. Macromol.* **2020**, *159*, 34–45. [CrossRef]

66. El Barky, A.R.; Hussein, S.A.; Alm-Eldeen, A.A.; Hafez, Y.A.; Mohamed, T.M. Anti-diabetic activity of *Holothuria thomasi* saponin. *Biomed. Pharmacother.* **2016**, *84*, 1472–1487. [CrossRef]
67. Chen, C.; Han, X.; Dong, P.; Li, Z.; Yanagita, T.; Xue, C.; Zhang, T.; Wang, Y. Sea cucumber saponin liposomes ameliorate obesity-induced inflammation and insulin resistance in high-fat-diet-fed mice. *Food Funct.* **2018**, *9*, 861–870. [CrossRef] [PubMed]
68. Wan, H.; Han, J.; Tang, S.; Bao, W.; Lu, C.; Zhou, J.; Ming, T.; Li, Y.; Su, X. Comparisons of protective effects between two sea cucumber hydrolysates against diet induced hyperuricemia and renal inflammation in mice. *Food Funct.* **2020**, *11*, 1074–1086. [CrossRef]
69. Tian, Y.; Liu, Y.; Xue, C.; Wang, J.; Wang, Y.; Xu, J.; Li, Z. The exogenous natural phospholipids, EPA-PC and EPA-PE, contribute to ameliorate inflammation and promote macrophage polarization. *Food Funct.* **2020**, *11*, 6542–6551. [CrossRef]
70. Subramanya, S.B.; Chandran, S.; Almarzooqi, S.; Raj, V.; Al Zahmi, A.S.; Al Katheeri, R.A.; Al Zadjali, S.A.; Collin, P.D.; Adrian, T.E. Frondanol, a Nutraceutical Extract from *Cucumaria frondosa*, Attenuates Colonic Inflammation in a DSS-Induced Colitis Model in Mice. *Mar. Drugs* **2018**, *16*, 148. [CrossRef]
71. Hu, S.; Wang, J.; Wang, J.; Xue, C.; Wang, Y. Long-chain bases from sea cucumber mitigate endoplasmic reticulum stress and inflammation in obesity mice. *J. Food Drug Anal.* **2017**, *25*, 628–636. [CrossRef] [PubMed]
72. Janakiram, N.B.; Mohammed, A.; Bryant, T.; Lightfoot, S.; Collin, P.D.; Steele, V.E.; Rao, C.V. Improved innate immune responses by Frondanol A5, a sea cucumber extract, prevent intestinal tumorigenesis. *Cancer Prev. Res.* **2015**, *8*, 327–337. [CrossRef] [PubMed]
73. Park, G.T.; Yoon, J.-W.; Yoo, S.-B.; Song, Y.-C.; Song, P.; Kim, H.-K.; Han, J.; Bae, S.-J.; Ha, K.-T.; Mishchenko, N.P.; et al. Echinochrome A Treatment Alleviates Fibrosis and Inflammation in Bleomycin-Induced Scleroderma. *Mar. Drugs* **2021**, *19*, 237. [CrossRef]
74. Oh, S.J.; Seo, Y.; Ahn, J.-S.; Shin, Y.Y.; Yang, J.W.; Kim, H.K.; Han, J.; Mishchenko, N.P.; Fedoreyev, S.A.; Stonik, V.A.; et al. Echinochrome A Reduces Colitis in Mice and Induces In Vitro Generation of Regulatory Immune Cells. *Mar. Drugs* **2019**, *17*, 622. [CrossRef] [PubMed]
75. Lennikov, A.; Kitaichi, N.; Noda, K.; Mizuuchi, K.; Ando, R.; Dong, Z.; Fukuhara, J.; Kinoshita, S.; Namba, K.; Ohno, S.; et al. Amelioration of endotoxin-induced uveitis treated with the sea urchin pigment echinochrome in rats. *Mol. Vis.* **2014**, *20*, 171–177.
76. Sadek, S.A.; Hassanein, S.S.; Mohamed, A.S.; Soliman, A.M.; Fahmy, S.R. Echinochrome pigment extracted from sea urchin suppress the bacterial activity, inflammation, nociception, and oxidative stress resulted in the inhibition of renal injury in septic rats. *J. Food Biochem.* **2022**, *46*, e13729. [CrossRef] [PubMed]
77. Hou, Y.; Carne, A.; McConnell, M.; Bekhit, A.A.; Mros, S.; Amagase, K.; Bekhit, A.E.-D.A. In vitro antioxidant and antimicrobial activities, and in vivo anti-inflammatory activity of crude and fractionated PHNQs from sea urchin (*Evechinus chloroticus*). *Food Chem.* **2020**, *316*, 126339. [CrossRef]
78. Brasseur, L.; Hennebert, E.; Fievez, L.; Caulier, G.; Bureau, F.; Tafforeau, L.; Flammang, P.; Gerbaux, P.; Eeckhaut, I. The Roles of Spinochromes in Four Shallow Water Tropical Sea Urchins and Their Potential as Bioactive Pharmacological Agents. *Mar. Drugs* **2017**, *15*, 179. [CrossRef]
79. Han, R.; Blencke, H.-M.; Cheng, H.; Li, C. The antimicrobial effect of CEN1HC-Br against Propionibacterium acnes and its therapeutic and anti-inflammatory effects on acne vulgaris. *Peptides* **2018**, *99*, 36–43. [CrossRef]
80. Björn, C.; Håkansson, J.; Myhrman, E.; Sjöstrand, V.; Haug, T.; Lindgren, K.; Blencke, H.-M.; Stensvåg, K.; Mahlapuu, M. Anti-infectious and anti-inflammatory effects of peptide fragments sequentially derived from the antimicrobial peptide centrocin 1 isolated from the green sea urchin, Strongylocentrotus droebachiensis. *AMB Express* **2012**, *2*, 67. [CrossRef]
81. Francis, P.; Chakraborty, K. An anti-inflammatory salmachroman from the sea urchin Salmacis bicolor. A prospective duel inhibitor of cyclooxygenase-2 and 5-lipoxygenase. *Nat. Prod. Res.* **2021**, *35*, 5102–5111. [CrossRef] [PubMed]
82. Francis, P.; Chakraborty, K. Anti-inflammatory polyoxygenated furanocembranoids, salmacembranes A B from the sea urchin Salmacis bicolor attenuate pro-inflammatory cyclooxygenases and lipoxygenase. *Med. Chem. Res.* **2020**, *29*, 2066–2076. [CrossRef]
83. Francis, P.; Chakraborty, K. Antioxidant and anti-inflammatory cembrane-type diterpenoid from Echinoidea sea urchin *Stomopneustes variolaris* attenuates pro-inflammatory 5-lipoxygenase. *Med. Chem. Res.* **2020**, *29*, 656–664. [CrossRef]
84. Chakraborty, K.; Francis, P. Stomopneulactone D from long-spined sea urchin *Stomopneustes variolaris*: Anti-inflammatory macrocylic lactone attenuates cyclooxygenase-2 expression in lipopolysaccharide-activated macrophages. *Bioorg. Chem.* **2020**, *103*, 104140. [CrossRef]
85. Lee, D.S.; Cui, X.; Ko, W.; Kim, K.S.; Kim, I.C.; Yim, J.H.; An, R.B.; Kim, Y.C.; Oh, H. A new sulfonic acid derivative, (Z)-4-methylundeca-1,9-diene-6-sulfonic acid, isolated from the cold water sea urchin inhibits inflammatory responses through JNK/p38 MAPK and NF-kappaB inactivation in RAW 264.7. *Arch. Pharm. Res.* **2014**, *37*, 983–991. [CrossRef] [PubMed]
86. Shih, J.H.; Tsai, Y.F.; Li, I.H.; Chen, M.H.; Huang, Y.S. Hp-s1 Ganglioside Suppresses Proinflammatory Responses by Inhibiting MyD88-Dependent NF-kappaB and JNK/p38 MAPK Pathways in Lipopolysaccharide-Stimulated Microglial Cells. *Mar. Drugs* **2020**, *18*, 496. [CrossRef] [PubMed]
87. Pearce, A.N.; Chia, E.W.; Berridge, M.V.; Maas, E.W.; Page, M.J.; Harper, J.L.; Webb, V.L.; Copp, B.R. Orthidines A–E, tubastrine, 3,4-dimethoxyphenethyl-β-guanidine, and 1,14-sperminedihomovanillamide: Potential anti-inflammatory alkaloids isolated from the New Zealand ascidian *Aplidium orthium* that act as inhibitors of neutrophil respiratory burst. *Tetrahedron* **2008**, *64*, 5748–5755. [CrossRef]

88. Pearce, A.N.; Chia, E.W.; Berridge, M.V.; Clark, G.R.; Harper, J.L.; Larsen, L.; Maas, E.W.; Page, M.J.; Perry, N.B.; Webb, V.L.; et al. Anti-inflammatory thiazine alkaloids isolated from the New Zealand ascidian *Aplidium* sp.: Inhibitors of the neutrophil respiratory burst in a model of gouty arthritis. *J. Nat. Prod.* **2007**, *70*, 936–940. [CrossRef]
89. Appleton, D.R.; Page, M.J.; Lambert, G.; Berridge, M.V.; Copp, B.R. Kottamides A-D: Novel bioactive imidazolone-containing alkaloids from the New Zealand ascidian *Pycnoclavella kottae*. *J. Org. Chem.* **2002**, *67*, 5402–5404. [CrossRef]
90. Makkar, F.; Chakraborty, K. Previously undescribed antioxidative azocinyl morpholinone alkaloid from red seaweed *Gracilaria opuntia* with anti-cyclooxygenase and lipoxygenase properties. *Nat. Prod. Res.* **2018**, *32*, 1150–1160. [CrossRef]
91. Okai, Y.; Higashi-Okai, K. Potent anti-inflammatory activity of pheophytin a derived from edible green alga, *Enteromorpha prolifera* (Sujiao-nori). *Int. J. Immunopharmacol.* **1997**, *19*, 355–358. [CrossRef] [PubMed]
92. Awad, N.E. Biologically active steroid from the green alga *Ulva lactuca*. *Phytother. Res.* **2000**, *14*, 641–643. [CrossRef] [PubMed]
93. de Souza, E.T.; de Lira, D.P.; de Queiroz, A.C.; Silva, D.J.C.D.; de Aquino, A.B.; Campessato Mella, E.A.; Lorenzo, V.P.; De Miranda, G.E.C.; de Araujo-Junior, J.X.; de Oliveira Chaves, M.C.; et al. The antinociceptive and anti-inflammatory activities of caulerpin, a bisindole alkaloid isolated from seaweeds of the genus *Caulerpa*. *Mar. Drugs* **2009**, *7*, 689–704. [CrossRef] [PubMed]
94. Ribeiro, N.A.; Abreu, T.M.; Chaves, H.V.; Bezerra, M.M.; Monteiro, H.S.A.; Jorge, R.J.B.; Benevides, N.M.B. Sulfated polysaccharides isolated from the green seaweed *Caulerpa racemosa* plays antinociceptive and anti-inflammatory activities in a way dependent on HO-1 pathway activation. *Inflamm. Res.* **2014**, *63*, 569–580. [CrossRef]
95. Carneiro, J.G.; Rodrigues, J.A.G.; Vanderlei, E.d.S.O.; Souza, R.B.; Quinderé, A.L.G.; Coura, C.O.; de Araújo, I.W.F.; Chaves, H.V.; Bezerra, M.M.; Benevides, N.M.B. Peripheral antinociception and anti-inflammatory effects of sulphated polysaccharides from the alga *Caulerpa mexicana*. *Basic Clin. Pharmacol. Toxicol.* **2014**, *115*, 335–342. [CrossRef]
96. da Conceicao Rivanor, R.L.; Chaves, H.V.; Val, D.R.D.; de Freitas, A.R.; Lemos, J.C.; Rodrigues, J.A.G.; Pereira, K.M.A.; de Araújo, I.W.F.; Bezerra, M.M.; Benevides, N.M.B. A lectin from the green seaweed *Caulerpa cupressoides* reduces mechanical hyper-nociception and inflammation in the rat temporomandibular joint during zymosan-induced arthritis. *Int. Immunopharmacol.* **2014**, *21*, 34–43. [CrossRef] [PubMed]
97. Lee, J.-B.; Koizumi, S.; Hayashi, K.; Hayashi, T. Structure of rhamnan sulfate from the green alga *Monostroma nitidum* and its anti-herpetic effect. *Carbohydr. Polym.* **2010**, *81*, 572–577. [CrossRef]
98. Khan, M.N.; Cho, J.-Y.; Lee, M.-C.; Kang, J.-Y.; Park, N.G.; Fujii, H.; Hong, Y.-K. Isolation of two anti-inflammatory and one pro-inflammatory polyunsaturated fatty acids from the brown seaweed *Undaria pinnatifida*. *J. Agric. Food Chem.* **2007**, *55*, 6984–6988. [CrossRef]
99. Yang, H.S.; Haj, F.G.; Lee, M.; Kang, I.; Zhang, G.; Lee, Y. Laminaria japonica Extract Enhances Intestinal Barrier Function by Altering Inflammatory Response and Tight Junction-Related Protein in Lipopolysaccharide-Stimulated Caco-2 Cells. *Nutrients* **2019**, *11*, 1001. [CrossRef] [PubMed]
100. Jeong, J.-W.; Hwang, S.J.; Han, M.H.; Lee, D.-S.; Yoo, J.S.; Choi, I.-W.; Cha, H.-J.; Kim, S.; Kim, H.-S.; Kim, G.-Y.; et al. Fucoidan inhibits lipopolysaccharide-induced inflammatory responses in RAW 264.7 macrophages and zebrafish larvae. *Mol. Cell. Toxicol.* **2017**, *13*, 405–417. [CrossRef]
101. Kita, M.; Ohishi, N.; Washida, K.; Kondo, M.; Koyama, T.; Yamada, K.; Uemura, D. Symbioimine and neosymbioimine, amphoteric iminium metabolites from the symbiotic marine dinoflagellate *Symbiodinium* sp. *Bioorg. Med. Chem.* **2005**, *13*, 5253–5258. [CrossRef] [PubMed]
102. de Los Reyes, C.; Ortega, M.J.; Rodríguez-Luna, A.; Talero, E.; Motilva, V.; Zubía, E. Molecular Characterization and Anti-inflammatory Activity of Galactosylglycerides and Galactosylceramides from the Microalga *Isochrysis galbana*. *J. Agric. Food Chem.* **2016**, *64*, 8783–8794. [CrossRef]
103. Sibi, G.; Rabina, S. Inhibition of Pro-inflammatory Mediators and Cytokines by Chlorella Vulgaris Extracts. *Pharmacogn. Res.* **2016**, *8*, 118–122. [CrossRef]
104. Bergé, J.P.; Debiton, E.; Dumay, J.; Durand, P.; Barthomeuf, C. In vitro anti-inflammatory and anti-proliferative activity of sulfolipids from the red alga *Porphyridium cruentum*. *J. Agric. Food Chem.* **2002**, *50*, 6227–6232. [CrossRef]
105. Liberti, D.; Imbimbo, P.; Giustino, E.; D'elia, L.; Silva, M.; Barreira, L.; Monti, D.M. Shedding Light on the Hidden Benefit of *Porphyridium cruentum* Culture. *Antioxidants* **2023**, *12*, 337. [CrossRef] [PubMed]
106. Shiels, K.; Tsoupras, A.; Lordan, R.; Zabetakis, I.; Murray, P.; Saha, S.K. Anti-inflammatory and antithrombotic properties of polar lipid extracts, rich in unsaturated fatty acids, from the Irish marine cyanobacterium *Spirulina subsalsa*. *J. Funct. Foods* **2022**, *94*, 105124. [CrossRef]
107. Villa, F.A.; Lieske, K.; Gerwick, L. Selective MyD88-dependent pathway inhibition by the cyanobacterial natural product malyngamide F acetate. *Eur. J. Pharmacol.* **2010**, *629*, 140–146. [CrossRef]
108. Gunasekera, S.P.; Kokkaliari, S.; Ratnayake, R.; Sauvage, T.; Dos Santos, L.A.; Luesch, H.; Paul, V.J. Anti-Inflammatory Dysidazirine Carboxylic Acid from the Marine Cyanobacterium *Caldora* sp. Collected from the Reefs of Fort Lauderdale, Florida. *Molecules* **2022**, *27*, 1717. [CrossRef]
109. Dou, H.; Song, Y.; Liu, X.; Gong, W.; Li, E.; Tan, R.; Hou, Y. Chaetoglobosin Fex from the marine-derived endophytic fungus inhibits induction of inflammatory mediators via Toll-like receptor 4 signaling in macrophages. *Biol. Pharm. Bull.* **2011**, *34*, 1864–1873. [CrossRef] [PubMed]
110. Qin, C.; Lin, X.; Lu, X.; Wan, J.; Zhou, X.; Liao, S.; Tu, Z.; Xu, S.; Liu, Y. Sesquiterpenoids and xanthones derivatives produced by sponge-derived fungus *Stachybotry* sp. HH1 ZSDS1F1-2. *J. Antibiot.* **2015**, *68*, 121–125. [CrossRef] [PubMed]

111. Kwon, J.; Lee, H.; Ko, W.; Kim, D.-C.; Kim, K.-W.; Kwon, H.C.; Guo, Y.; Sohn, J.H.; Yim, J.H.; Kim, Y.-C.; et al. Chemical constituents isolated from Antarctic marine-derived *Aspergillus* sp. SF-5976 and their anti-inflammatory effects in LPS-stimulated RAW 264.7 and BV2 cells. *Tetrahedron* **2017**, *73*, 3905–3912. [CrossRef]
112. Kim, D.C.; Cho, K.H.; Ko, W.; Yoon, C.S.; Sohn, J.H.; Yim, J.H.; Kim, Y.C.; Oh, H. Anti-Inflammatory and Cytoprotective Effects of TMC-256C1 from Marine-Derived Fungus *Aspergillus* sp. SF-6354 via up-Regulation of Heme Oxygenase-1 in Murine Hippocampal and Microglial Cell Lines. *Int. J. Mol. Sci.* **2016**, *17*, 529. [CrossRef]
113. Tian, Y.; Qin, X.; Lin, X.; Kaliyaperumal, K.; Zhou, X.; Liu, J.; Ju, Z.; Tu, Z.; Liu, Y. Sydoxanthone C and acremolin B produced by deep-sea-derived fungus *Aspergillus* sp. SCSIO Ind09F01. *J. Antibiot.* **2015**, *68*, 703–706. [CrossRef] [PubMed]
114. Kim, D.C.; Quang, T.H.; Ngan, N.T.T.; Yoon, C.S.; Sohn, J.H.; Yim, J.H.; Feng, Y.; Che, Y.; Kim, Y.C.; Oh, H. Dihydroisocoumarin Derivatives from Marine-Derived Fungal Isolates and Their Anti-inflammatory Effects in Lipopolysaccharide-Induced BV2 Microglia. *J. Nat. Prod.* **2015**, *78*, 2948–2955. [CrossRef]
115. Lee, D.S.; Jeong, G.-S.; Li, B.; Lee, S.U.; Oh, H.; Kim, Y.-C. Asperlin from the marine-derived fungus *Aspergillus* sp. SF-5044 exerts anti-inflammatory effects through heme oxygenase-1 expression in murine macrophages. *J. Pharmacol. Sci.* **2011**, *116*, 283–295. [CrossRef]
116. Yoon, C.S.; Kim, D.C.; Lee, D.S.; Kim, K.S.; Ko, W.; Sohn, J.H.; Yim, J.H.; Kim, Y.C.; Oh, H. Anti-neuroinflammatory effect of aurantiamide acetate from the marine fungus *Aspergillus* sp. SF-5921: Inhibition of NF-kappaB and MAPK pathways in lipopolysaccharide-induced mouse BV2 microglial cells. *Int. Immunopharmacol.* **2014**, *23*, 568–574. [CrossRef]
117. Du, X.; Liu, D.; Huang, J.; Zhang, C.; Proksch, P.; Lin, W. Polyketide derivatives from the sponge associated fungus Aspergillus europaeus with antioxidant and NO inhibitory activities. *Fitoterapia* **2018**, *130*, 190–197. [CrossRef]
118. Wang, Y.; Qi, S.; Zhan, Y.; Zhang, N.; Wu, A.A.; Gui, F.; Guo, K.; Yang, Y.; Cao, S.; Hu, Z.; et al. Aspertetranones A-D, Putative Meroterpenoids from the Marine Algal-Associated Fungus *Aspergillus* sp. ZL0-1b14. *J. Nat. Prod.* **2015**, *78*, 2405–2410. [CrossRef] [PubMed]
119. Liu, S.; Wang, H.; Su, M.; Hwang, G.J.; Hong, J.; Jung, J.H. New metabolites from the sponge-derived fungus *Aspergillus sydowii* J05B-7F-4. *Nat. Prod. Res.* **2017**, *31*, 1682–1686. [CrossRef]
120. Fang, W.; Lin, X.; Wang, J.; Liu, Y.; Tao, H.; Zhou, X. Asperpyrone-Type Bis-Naphtho-gamma-Pyrones with COX-2-Inhibitory Activities from Marine-Derived Fungus *Aspergillus niger*. *Molecules* **2016**, *21*, 941. [CrossRef] [PubMed]
121. Gu, B.B.; Jiao, F.R.; Wu, W.; Jiao, W.H.; Li, L.; Sun, F.; Wang, S.P.; Yang, F.; Lin, H.W. Preussins with Inhibition of IL-6 Expression from *Aspergillus flocculosus* 16D-1, a Fungus Isolated from the Marine Sponge *Phakellia fusca*. *J. Nat. Prod.* **2018**, *81*, 2275–2281. [CrossRef] [PubMed]
122. Li, H.; Sun, W.; Deng, M.; Zhou, Q.; Wang, J.; Liu, J.; Chen, C.; Qi, C.; Luo, Z.; Xue, Y.; et al. Asperversiamides, Linearly Fused Prenylated Indole Alkaloids from the Marine-Derived Fungus *Aspergillus versicolor*. *J. Org. Chem.* **2018**, *83*, 8483–8492. [CrossRef]
123. Liu, M.; Sun, W.; Wang, J.; He, Y.; Zhang, J.; Li, F.; Qi, C.; Zhu, H.; Xue, Y.; Hu, Z.; et al. Bioactive secondary metabolites from the marine-associated fungus *Aspergillus terreus*. *Bioorg. Chem.* **2018**, *80*, 525–530. [CrossRef] [PubMed]
124. Wu, Z.; Li, D.; Zeng, F.; Tong, Q.; Zheng, Y.; Liu, J.; Zhou, Q.; Li, X.-N.; Chen, C.; Lai, Y.; et al. Brasilane sesquiterpenoids and dihydrobenzofuran derivatives from *Aspergillus terreus* [CFCC 81836]. *Phytochemistry* **2018**, *156*, 159–166. [CrossRef]
125. Wang, L.; Li, M.; Tang, J.; Li, X. Eremophilane Sesquiterpenes from a Deep Marine-Derived Fungus, *Aspergillus* sp. SCSIOW2, Cultivated in the Presence of Epigenetic Modifying Agents. *Molecules* **2016**, *21*, 473. [CrossRef]
126. Kim, K.S.; Cui, X.; Lee, D.S.; Sohn, J.H.; Yim, J.H.; Kim, Y.C.; Oh, H. Anti-inflammatory effect of neoechinulin a from the marine fungus *Eurotium* sp. SF-5989 through the suppression of NF-small ka, CyrillicB and p38 MAPK Pathways in lipopolysaccharide-stimulated RAW264.7 macrophages. *Molecules* **2013**, *18*, 13245–13259. [CrossRef] [PubMed]
127. Kim, K.S.; Cui, X.; Lee, D.-S.; Ko, W.; Sohn, J.H.; Yim, J.H.; An, R.-B.; Kim, Y.-C.; Oh, H. Inhibitory effects of benzaldehyde derivatives from the marine fungus *Eurotium* sp. SF-5989 on inflammatory mediators via the induction of heme oxygenase-1 in lipopolysaccharide-stimulated RAW264.7 macrophages. *Int. J. Mol. Sci.* **2014**, *15*, 23749–23765. [CrossRef]
128. Yang, X.; Kang, M.-C.; Li, Y.; Kim, E.-A.; Kang, S.-M.; Jeon, Y.-J. Asperflavin, an Anti-Inflammatory Compound Produced by a Marine-Derived Fungus, *Eurotium amstelodami*. *Molecules* **2017**, *22*, 1823. [CrossRef] [PubMed]
129. Yang, X.; Kang, M.-C.; Li, Y.; Kim, E.-A.; Kang, S.-M.; Jeon, Y.-J. Anti-inflammatory activity of questinol isolated from marine-derived fungus *Eurotium amstelodami* in lipopolysaccharide-stimulated RAW 264.7 macrophages. *J. Microbiol. Biotechnol.* **2014**, *24*, 1346–1353. [CrossRef]
130. Ha, T.M.; Ko, W.; Lee, S.J.; Kim, Y.C.; Son, J.Y.; Sohn, J.H.; Yim, J.H.; Oh, H. Anti-Inflammatory Effects of Curvularin-Type Metabolites from a Marine-Derived Fungal Strain *Penicillium* sp. SF-5859 in Lipopolysaccharide-Induced RAW264.7 Macrophages. *Mar. Drugs* **2017**, *15*, 282. [CrossRef] [PubMed]
131. Niu, S.; Xie, C.L.; Xia, J.M.; Luo, Z.H.; Shao, Z.; Yang, X.W. New anti-inflammatory guaianes from the Atlantic hydrotherm-derived fungus *Graphostroma* sp. MCCC 3A00421. *Sci. Rep.* **2018**, *8*, 530. [CrossRef]
132. Niu, S.; Xie, C.-L.; Zhong, T.; Xu, W.; Luo, Z.-H.; Shao, Z.; Yang, X.-W. Sesquiterpenes from a deep-sea-derived fungus *Graphostroma* sp. MCCC 3A00421. *Tetrahedron* **2017**, *73*, 7267–7273. [CrossRef]
133. Chen, S.; Wang, J.; Lin, X.; Zhao, B.; Wei, X.; Li, G.; Kaliaperumal, K.; Liao, S.; Yang, B.; Zhou, X.; et al. Chrysamides A-C, Three Dimeric Nitrophenyl trans-Epoxyamides Produced by the Deep-Sea-Derived Fungus *Penicillium chrysogenum* SCSIO41001. *Org. Lett.* **2016**, *18*, 3650–3653. [CrossRef]

134. Ko, W.; Sohn, J.H.; Kim, Y.C.; Oh, H. Viridicatol from Marine-derived Fungal Strain *Penicillium* sp. SF-5295 Exerts Anti-inflammatory Effects through Inhibiting NF-κB Signaling Pathway on Lipopolysaccharide-induced RAW264.7 and BV2 Cells. *Nat. Product. Sci.* **2015**, *21*, 240–247. [CrossRef]
135. Du, L.; Yang, X.; Zhu, T.; Wang, F.; Xiao, X.; Park, H.; Gu, Q. Diketopiperazine alkaloids from a deep ocean sediment derived fungus *Penicillium* sp. *Chem. Pharm. Bull.* **2009**, *57*, 873–876. [CrossRef]
136. Kim, D.C.; Lee, H.S.; Ko, W.; Lee, D.S.; Sohn, J.H.; Yim, J.H.; Kim, Y.C.; Oh, H. Anti-inflammatory effect of methylpenicinoline from a marine isolate of *Penicillium* sp. (SF-5995): Inhibition of NF-kappaB and MAPK pathways in lipopolysaccharide-induced RAW264.7 macrophages and BV2 microglia. *Molecules* **2014**, *19*, 18073–18089. [CrossRef]
137. Park, J.S.; Quang, T.H.; Yoon, C.-S.; Kim, H.J.; Sohn, J.H.; Oh, H. Furanoaustinol and 7-acetoxydehydroaustinol: New meroterpenoids from a marine-derived fungal strain *Penicillium* sp. SF-5497. *J. Antibiot.* **2018**, *71*, 557–563. [CrossRef] [PubMed]
138. Quang, T.H.; Ngan, N.T.T.; Ko, W.; Kim, D.-C.; Yoon, C.-S.; Sohn, J.H.; Yim, J.H.; Kim, Y.-C.; Oh, H. Tanzawaic acid derivatives from a marine isolate of *Penicillium* sp. (SF-6013) with anti-inflammatory and PTP1B inhibitory activities. *Bioorg. Med. Chem. Lett.* **2014**, *24*, 5787–5791. [CrossRef] [PubMed]
139. Ngan, N.T.; Quang, T.H.; Kim, K.-W.; Kim, H.J.; Sohn, J.H.; Kang, D.G.; Lee, H.S.; Kim, Y.-C.; Oh, H. Anti-inflammatory effects of secondary metabolites isolated from the marine-derived fungal strain *Penicillium* sp. SF-5629. *Arch. Pharm. Res.* **2017**, *40*, 328–337. [CrossRef]
140. Lee, D.S.; Ko, W.; Quang, T.H.; Kim, K.-S.; Sohn, J.H.; Jang, J.-H.; Ahn, J.S.; Kim, Y.-C.; Oh, H. Penicillinolide A: A new anti-inflammatory metabolite from the marine fungus *Penicillium* sp. SF-5292. *Mar. Drugs* **2013**, *11*, 4510–4526. [CrossRef]
141. Li, J.L.; Zhang, P.; Lee, Y.M.; Hong, J.; Yoo, E.S.; Bae, K.S.; Jung, J.H. Oxygenated hexylitaconates from a marine sponge-derived fungus *Penicillium* sp. *Chem. Pharm. Bull.* **2011**, *59*, 120–123. [CrossRef]
142. Ozkaya, F.C.; Ebrahim, W.; Klopotowski, M.; Liu, Z.; Janiak, C.; Proksch, P. Isolation and X-ray structure analysis of citreohybridonol from marine-derived *Penicillium atrovenetum*. *Nat. Prod. Res.* **2018**, *32*, 840–843. [CrossRef]
143. Shin, H.J.; Pil, G.B.; Heo, S.-J.; Lee, H.-S.; Lee, J.S.; Lee, Y.-J.; Lee, J.; Won, H.S. Anti-Inflammatory Activity of Tanzawaic Acid Derivatives from a Marine-Derived Fungus *Penicillium steckii* 108YD142. *Mar. Drugs* **2016**, *14*, 14. [CrossRef]
144. Toledo, T.R.; Dejani, N.N.; Monnazzi, L.G.S.; Kossuga, M.H.; Berlinck, R.G.; Sette, L.D.; Medeiros, A.I. Potent anti-inflammatory activity of pyrenocine A isolated from the marine-derived fungus *Penicillium paxilli* Ma(G)K. *Mediat. Inflamm.* **2014**, *2014*, 767061. [CrossRef] [PubMed]
145. Afiyatullov, S.S.; Leshchenko, E.V.; Sobolevskaya, M.P.; Antonov, A.S.; Denisenko, V.A.; Popov, R.S.; Khudyakova, Y.V.; Kirichuk, N.N.; Kuz'mich, A.S.; Pislyagin, E.A.; et al. New Thomimarine E from Marine Isolate of the Fungus *Penicillium thomii*. *Chem. Nat. Compd.* **2017**, *53*, 290–294. [CrossRef]
146. Li, L.; Zhang, Y.; Li, Z.; Yu, Z.; Sun, T. Stereochemical Investigation of a Novel Biological Active Substance from the Secondary Metabolites of Marine Fungus *Penicillium chrysogenum* SYP-F-2720. *J. Mex. Chem. Soc.* **2017**, *59*, 53–58.
147. Zhu, H.; Hua, X.-X.; Gong, T.; Pang, J.; Hou, Q.; Zhu, P. Hypocreaterpenes A and B, cadinane-type sesquiterpenes from a marine-derived fungus, *Hypocreales* sp. *Phytochem. Lett.* **2013**, *6*, 392–396. [CrossRef]
148. Renner, M.K.; Jensen, P.R.; Fenical, W. Mangicols: Structures and biosynthesis of A new class of sesterterpene polyols from a marine fungus of the genus *Fusarium*. *J. Org. Chem.* **2000**, *65*, 4843–4852. [CrossRef] [PubMed]
149. Hsiao, G.; Chi, W.C.; Pang, K.L.; Chen, J.J.; Kuo, Y.H.; Wang, Y.K.; Cha, H.J.; Chou, S.C.; Lee, T.H. Hirsutane-Type Sesquiterpenes with Inhibitory Activity of Microglial Nitric Oxide Production from the Red Alga-Derived Fungus *Chondrostereum* sp. NTOU4196. *J. Nat. Prod.* **2017**, *80*, 1615–1622. [CrossRef]
150. Chen, C.J.; Zhou, Y.Q.; Liu, X.X.; Zhang, W.J.; Hu, S.S.; Lin, L.P.; Huo, G.M.; Jiao, R.H.; Tan, R.X.; Ge, H.M. Antimicrobial and anti-inflammatory compounds from a marine fungus *Pleosporales* sp. *Tetrahedron Lett.* **2015**, *56*, 6183–6189. [CrossRef]
151. Lee, M.S.; Wang, S.W.; Wang, G.J.; Pang, K.L.; Lee, C.K.; Kuo, Y.H.; Cha, H.J.; Lin, R.K.; Lee, T.H. Angiogenesis Inhibitors and Anti-Inflammatory Agents from *Phoma* sp. NTOU4195. *J. Nat. Prod.* **2016**, *79*, 2983–2990. [CrossRef] [PubMed]
152. Zhang, P.; Li, Y.; Jia, C.; Lang, J.; Niaz, S.I.; Li, J.; Yuan, J.; Yu, J.; Chen, S.; Liu, L. Antiviral and anti-inflammatory meroterpenoids: Stachybonoids A–F from the crinoid-derived fungus *Stachybotrys chartarum* 952. *RSC Adv.* **2017**, *7*, 49910–49916. [CrossRef]
153. Zhang, P.; Jia, C.; Lang, J.; Li, J.; Luo, G.; Chen, S.; Yan, S.; Liu, L. Mono- and Dimeric Naphthalenones from the Marine-Derived Fungus *Leptosphaerulina chartarum* 3608. *Mar. Drugs* **2018**, *16*, 173. [CrossRef]
154. Wang, J.F.; Qin, X.; Xu, F.Q.; Zhang, T.; Liao, S.; Lin, X.; Yang, B.; Liu, J.; Wang, L.; Tu, Z.; et al. Tetramic acid derivatives and polyphenols from sponge-derived fungus and their biological evaluation. *Nat. Prod. Res.* **2015**, *29*, 1761–1765. [CrossRef]
155. Chen, Q.; Chen, T.; Li, W.; Zhang, W.; Zhu, J.; Li, Y.; Huang, Y.; Shen, Y.; Yu, C. Mycoepoxydiene inhibits lipopolysaccharide-induced inflammatory responses through the suppression of TRAF6 polyubiquitination [corrected]. *PLoS ONE* **2012**, *7*, e44890.
156. Liu, J.; Gu, B.; Yang, L.; Yang, F.; Lin, H. New Anti-inflammatory Cyclopeptides from a Sponge-Derived Fungus *Aspergillus violaceofuscus*. *Front. Chem.* **2018**, *6*, 226. [CrossRef]
157. Belofsky, G.N.; Anguera, M.; Jensen, P.R.; Fenical, W.; Köck, M. Oxepinamides A-C and fumiquinazolines H--I: Bioactive metabolites from a marine isolate of a fungus of the genus *Acremonium*. *Chem. Eur. J.* **2000**, *6*, 1355–1360. [CrossRef]
158. Ko, W.; Sohn, J.H.; Jang, J.H.; Ahn, J.S.; Kang, D.G.; Lee, H.S.; Kim, J.S.; Kim, Y.C.; Oh, H. Inhibitory effects of alternaramide on inflammatory mediator expression through TLR4-MyD88-mediated inhibition of NF-small ka, CyrillicB and MAPK pathway signaling in lipopolysaccharide-stimulated RAW264.7 and BV2 cells. *Chem. Biol. Interact.* **2016**, *244*, 16–26. [CrossRef] [PubMed]

159. Marra, R.; Nicoletti, R.; Pagano, E.; DellaGreca, M.; Salvatore, M.M.; Borrelli, F.; Lombardi, N.; Vinale, F.; Woo, S.L.; Andolfi, A. Inhibitory effect of trichodermanone C, a sorbicillinoid produced by *Trichoderma citrinoviride* associated to the green alga *Cladophora* sp., on nitrite production in LPS-stimulated macrophages. *Nat. Prod. Res.* **2019**, *33*, 3389–3397. [CrossRef]
160. Quang, T.H.; Kim, D.C.; Van Kiem, P.; Van Minh, C.; Nhiem, N.X.; Tai, B.H.; Yen, P.H.; Thi Thanh Ngan, N.; Kim, H.J.; Oh, H. Macrolide and phenolic metabolites from the marine-derived fungus *Paraconiothyrium* sp. VK-13 with anti-inflammatory activity. *J. Antibiot.* **2018**, *71*, 826–830. [CrossRef]
161. Lee, H.S.; Kang, J.S.; Choi, B.K.; Lee, H.S.; Lee, Y.J.; Lee, J.; Shin, H.J. Phenazine Derivatives with Anti-Inflammatory Activity from the Deep-Sea Sediment-Derived Yeast-Like Fungus *Cystobasidium laryngis* IV17-028. *Mar. Drugs* **2019**, *17*, 482. [CrossRef] [PubMed]
162. Lee, D.S.; Jang, J.H.; Ko, W.; Kim, K.S.; Sohn, J.H.; Kang, M.S.; Ahn, J.S.; Kim, Y.C.; Oh, H. PTP1B inhibitory and anti-inflammatory effects of secondary metabolites isolated from the marine-derived fungus *Penicillium* sp. JF-55. *Mar. Drugs* **2013**, *11*, 1409–1426. [CrossRef] [PubMed]
163. Hassan, H.M.; Boonlarppradab, C.; Fenical, W. Actinoquinolines A and B, anti-inflammatory quinoline alkaloids from a marine-derived *Streptomyces* sp., strain CNP975. *J. Antibiot.* **2016**, *69*, 511–514. [CrossRef]
164. Alvariño, R.; Alonso, E.; Lacret, R.; Oves-Costales, D.; Genilloud, O.; Reyes, F.; Alfonso, A.; Botana, L.M. Caniferolide A, a Macrolide from *Streptomyces caniferus*, Attenuates Neuroinflammation, Oxidative Stress, Amyloid-Beta, and Tau Pathology in Vitro. *Mol. Pharm.* **2019**, *16*, 1456–1466. [CrossRef] [PubMed]
165. Nam, S.-J.; Gaudêncio, S.P.; Kauffman, C.A.; Jensen, P.R.; Kondratyuk, T.P.; Marler, L.E.; Pezzuto, J.M.; Fenical, W. Fijiolides A and B, Inhibitors of TNF-α-Induced NFκB Activation, from a Marine-Derived Sediment Bacterium of the Genus Nocardiopsis. *J. Nat. Prod.* **2010**, *73*, 1080–1086. [CrossRef]
166. Alshawwa, S.Z.; Alshallash, K.S.; Ghareeb, A.; Elazzazy, A.M.; Sharaf, M.; Alharthi, A.; Abdelgawad, F.E.; El-Hossary, D.; Jaremko, M.; Emwas, A.H.; et al. Assessment of Pharmacological Potential of Novel Exopolysaccharide Isolated from Marine *Kocuria* sp. Strain AG5: Broad-Spectrum Biological Investigations. *Life* **2022**, *12*, 1387. [CrossRef] [PubMed]
167. Yan, X.; Zhou, Y.X.; Tang, X.X.; Liu, X.X.; Yi, Z.W.; Fang, M.J.; Wu, Z.; Jiang, F.Q.; Qiu, Y.K. Macrolactins from Marine-Derived *Bacillus subtilis* B5 Bacteria as Inhibitors of Inducible Nitric Oxide and Cytokines Expression. *Mar. Drugs* **2016**, *14*, 195. [CrossRef] [PubMed]
168. Rotter, A.; Barbier, M.; Bertoni, F.; Bones, A.M.; Cancela, M.L.; Carlsson, J.; Carvalho, M.F.; Cegłowska, M.; Chirivella-Martorell, J.; Conk Dalay, M.; et al. The Essentials of Marine Biotechnology. *Front. Mar. Sci.* **2021**, *8*, 629629. [CrossRef]
169. Bouchet, P.; Decock, W.; Lonneville, B.; Vanhoorne, B.; Vandepitte, L. Marine biodiversity discovery: The metrics of new species descriptions. *Front. Mar. Sci.* **2023**, *10*, 929989. [CrossRef]
170. Dias, D.A.; Urban, S.; Roessner, U. A historical overview of natural products in drug discovery. *Metabolites* **2012**, *2*, 303–336. [CrossRef]
171. Leal, M.C.; Puga, J.; Serodio, J.; Gomes, N.C.; Calado, R. Trends in the discovery of new marine natural products from invertebrates over the last two decades—Where and what are we bioprospecting? *PLoS ONE* **2012**, *7*, e30580. [CrossRef] [PubMed]
172. Qian, P.Y.; Cheng, A.; Wang, R.; Zhang, R. Marine biofilms: Diversity, interactions and biofouling. *Nat. Rev. Microbiol.* **2022**, *20*, 671–684. [CrossRef] [PubMed]
173. Dewapriya, P.; Kim, S.-K. Marine microorganisms: An emerging avenue in modern nutraceuticals and functional foods. *Food Res. Int.* **2014**, *56*, 115–125. [CrossRef]
174. Carroll, A.R.; Copp, B.R.; Davis, R.A.; Keyzers, R.A.; Prinsep, M.R. Marine natural products. *Nat. Prod. Rep.* **2020**, *37*, 175–223. [CrossRef] [PubMed]
175. Carroll, A.R.; Copp, B.R.; Davis, R.A.; Keyzers, R.A.; Prinsep, M.R. Marine natural products. *Nat. Prod. Rep.* **2023**, *40*, 275–325. [CrossRef] [PubMed]
176. Lindequist, U. Marine-Derived Pharmaceuticals-Challenges and Opportunities. *Biomol. Ther.* **2016**, *24*, 561–571. [CrossRef]
177. Sudek, S.; Lopanik, N.B.; Waggoner, L.E.; Hildebrand, M.; Anderson, C.; Liu, H.; Patel, A.; Sherman, D.H.; Haygood, M.G. Identification of the putative bryostatin polyketide synthase gene cluster from "Candidatus Endobugula sertula", the uncultivated microbial symbiont of the marine bryozoan *Bugula neritina*. *J. Nat. Prod.* **2007**, *70*, 67–74. [CrossRef]

Disclaimer/Publisher's Note: The statements, opinions and data contained in all publications are solely those of the individual author(s) and contributor(s) and not of MDPI and/or the editor(s). MDPI and/or the editor(s) disclaim responsibility for any injury to people or property resulting from any ideas, methods, instructions or products referred to in the content.

MDPI AG
Grosspeteranlage 5
4052 Basel
Switzerland
Tel.: +41 61 683 77 34

Marine Drugs Editorial Office
E-mail: marinedrugs@mdpi.com
www.mdpi.com/journal/marinedrugs

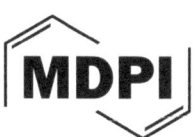

Disclaimer/Publisher's Note: The title and front matter of this reprint are at the discretion of the Guest Editor. The publisher is not responsible for their content or any associated concerns. The statements, opinions and data contained in all individual articles are solely those of the individual Editor and contributors and not of MDPI. MDPI disclaims responsibility for any injury to people or property resulting from any ideas, methods, instructions or products referred to in the content.

www.ingramcontent.com/pod-product-compliance
Lightning Source LLC
LaVergne TN
LVHW072334090526
838202LV00019B/2416